Therapeutic Recreation
in
Health Promotion
and
Rehabilitation

Therapeutic Recreation
in
Health Promotion
and
Rehabilitation

John Shank and Catherine Coyle
Temple University

Venture Publishing, Inc.
State College, PA

Production Manager: Richard Yocum
Manuscript Editing: Valerie Paukovits, Richard Yocum
Additional Editing: Michele L. Barbin
Cover Design by Echelon Design

Library of Congress Catalogue Card Number 2002104946
ISBN 1–892132–31–1

Acknowledgements

Writing a textbook is an enormous undertaking. It requires a firm belief in the value of the endeavor, and a commitment to persist despite distractions and, sometimes, doubt. Thus, no text of this magnitude could be written without important input and critique from others. This began with our students. Much of this text has been used in our teaching, so we have had chance to try it out and get reactions from students. We also deliberately solicited reactions from others. Most notably, we owe our deep gratitude to Susan "Boon" Murray for her thoughtful and helpful critique of each chapter. Boon challenged our thinking at times, and offered many useful suggestions. She is a generous colleague and friend. Throughout our writing we also received valuable feedback from practitioners and educators, including Susanne Lesnik-Emas, Chari Cohen, Jen Hilinski, Theresa Beck, Linda Buettner, Diane Groff, Patti Craig, Donna Gregory, Donna Long, Pat Theringer, and Linda Hutchison Troyer. We were privileged to benefit from their perspectives. We also want to acknowledge our Temple University colleagues, Rosangela Boyd and Terry Kinney, and their influence on our thinking about TR clinical practice. They have been partners on many projects, and we have benefited from their abilities and support. In particular, we want to acknowledge Terry's contribution to the psychosocial rehabilitation model presented in Chapter 6.

Finally, we want to acknowledge the unending support we received from our families. Their willingness to sacrifice family time and to endure our almost constant preoccupation was a significant factor in our finishing this text. We are very fortunate to have their love, support, and encouragement, and our thanks and appreciation is immeasurable.

Acknowledgements

Table of Contents

Part 1
Foundations of TR Practice

Part 2
Integrating Theory with TR Clinical Practice

Part 3
The TR Clinical Process

Part 4
Communicating Practice and Ensuring Competence

List of Tables, Figures, and Exhibits

Chapter 1

Chapter 2

Chapter 3

Chapter 4

Chapter 5

Chapter 6

Chapter 7

Chapter 8

Chapter 9

Chapter 10

Chapter 11

Introduction

During the last half of the 20th century, therapeutic recreation (TR) developed into a distinct professional discipline within health care and human services. During this time TR adjusted to various social, political, and economic forces that influenced health care and human services. These changes have caused the profession to continuously reaffirm its role and function. While TR is provided in a variety of settings to people who have illnesses, disabilities, and other constraints on health and life quality, the profession has one central and unifying purpose: *to promote and protect the importance of play, recreation, and leisure in achieving and maintaining health and life quality.*

As the 21st century unfolds, health care and human services are changing in ways that make TR's central purpose clearly relevant. For instance, health is being defined more holistically, and its impact on life quality is a primary concern for all health and human service systems. There is increasing attention to health promotion programs, and rehabilitation services are emphasizing the prevention of secondary health conditions. These changes and others represent opportunities for TR professionals to be valued and contributing members of health care and human service systems, and to be important advocates for people whose health and life quality are compromised or at risk. Yet, to do so depends on knowledgeable and skilled professionals who will practice with integrity, thoughtfulness, and discipline. Our hope for this text is that it can assist you, the reader, to develop and enhance your knowledge and skill to meet these challenges.

What This Textbook Is About

The purpose of this text is to describe TR practice, specifically TR *clinical practice.* TR clinical practice, as described in this text, is independent of any particular setting; it can occur in clients' homes, in community recreation centers and other human service agencies, or traditional medical facilities. An underlying assumption of clinical practice is that barriers or impediments to health and life quality exist, and that helping people avoid, manage, or overcome these barriers requires thoughtful and careful intervention. This involves a deliberate and purposeful use of activity-based interventions, supportive and accommodating environments, and therapeutic relationships with clients. Through these relationships clients learn about themselves, adapt to the challenges associated with illnesses and disabling conditions, and grow in ways that are meaningful and fulfilling. Ultimately, TR clinical practice is a process that facilitates a person's sense of personal control and competence in achieving and maintaining health and life quality through play, recreation, and leisure. It is a process in which clients learn, adapt, and grow as a result of our interventions.

While there are many ways to theoretically explain how clients learn, adapt, and grow, we orient practice around a *cognitive–behavioral* change process. We provide a theoretical framework based on a view of human behavior as being the end result of person–environment interactions. This *ecological perspective* recognizes the impact of the physical and social environment on a person's thoughts, feelings, and behavior related to one's quest for health and life quality. Thus, TR clinical practice addresses morale, motivation, and empowerment, as well as improvements in physical and social functioning. While interventions are focused largely on individual change, they must involve creating supportive and accommodating environments that are conducive to change and growth through play, recreation, and leisure. With a solid conceptual and theoretical framework as a foundation, the bulk of this text focuses on the essential aspects of clinical TR practice.

Overview of Content

This textbook is organized into four interrelated parts. **Part 1: Foundations of TR Practice** includes three chapters about the issues, concepts, and perspectives that provide a framework for understanding TR as a *health-related profession.* This framework accommodates the broad scope of TR practice reflected in the definitions advanced by the American Therapeutic Recreation Association (ATRA) and the National Therapeutic Recreation Society (NTRS).

Chapter 1: Contemporary Issues in Health and Human Services describes several forces shaping the organization and delivery of services and their impact on TR practice. These forces of change include demographics, economics, technology, and a stronger "voice" among consumers of services. These changes demand ethical as well as practical responses from all professions, including TR. While these changes can be viewed as either opportunities or threats to the TR profession, several conceptual shifts are also happening in health care and human services that are consistent with TR's core principles and practices.

Chapter 2: Changing Concepts within Health and Human Service Systems describes three significant conceptual shifts in health and human services, and give examples of how TR contributes positively to these shifts. The first conceptual shift is from a disease model of health care to a holistic model of disease prevention and health promotion. This broader health model presents opportunities for all aspects of TR practice that contribute to recovering and maintaining health. The shift toward more active involvement of clients as "partners" in their health care and health maintenance reflects an emphasis on self-determination, which is a core principle of TR. Also, an emerging emphasis on quality of life as the unifying focus for all health and human service systems presents opportunities for TR to be a real contributor to the entire service system.

Part 1 ends by explaining a "systems" approach to practice. *Chapter 3: Using a Client-System Perspective to Guide Practice* contains a model that represents a holistic perspective of a person. This includes the biological, psychological, social, and spiritual dimensions of the person, as well as the developmental, cultural, and environmental factors that influence a client's needs, wants, opportunities, and constraints. We also present psychosocial adaptation as a process that is common among clients who receive TR services as they cope with and adapt to chronic illnesses and disabilities.

Understanding, applying, and advancing TR clinical practice depends on a theoretical framework, which is addressed in **Part 2: Integrating Theory with TR Clinical Practice**. This portion of the text contains chapters that define TR clinical practice, both theoretically and practically. We begin Part 2 with *Chapter 4: Defining TR Clinical Practice*. Clinical practice is a purposeful use of activity-based interventions, supportive and accommodating environments, and therapeutic relationships with clients to facilitate learning, adaptation, and growth. It involves a systematic 5-phase process of assessing, planning, implementing, evaluating, and terminating services with clients. Whether delivered individually or through group work, TR clinical practice is aimed at supporting a client's personal control and sense of competence necessary for maintaining health and life quality through play, recreation, and leisure.

Chapter 5: Understanding Theories that Guide Practice begins with a discussion of social psychology as an appropriate and relevant theoretical framework for TR. We link this orientation to existing TR service models and contend that practice can be effective when it is based on an understanding of interaction between cognition and behavior and the role of the environment. Thus, we describe several theories that explain how beliefs about health and one's abilities to seek and maintain health through recreation and leisure help guide TR clinical practice. The chapter concludes with several common assumptions shared by these theories which can provide direction for theory-based clinical TR practice.

Finally, *Chapter 6: Applying Theories to Practice* offers readers an opportunity to understand how theory informs and guides TR practice. The chapter starts with an explanation of how change can happen with clients through TR interventions. This change process reflects assumptions about human behavior and behavior change presented in Chapter 5. To make the discussion of theory more practical, three case examples illustrating theory-based TR clinical practice are included. Additionally, several cognitive–behavioral strategies are described in this chapter, and each case example demonstrates how these strategies can be used in clinical TR practice.

Part 3: The TR Clinical Process contains six chapters. Each chapter takes the reader through the various phases found in the clinical TR process. *Chapter 7: Assessing Clients* discusses the purpose and procedures of TR assessments. The chapter provides a comprehensive and detailed overview of the types of information that can be gathered in each area of the client system. Enough information is presented to guide the assessment process no matter where or with whom you are working. Various assessment tools specific to TR practice as well as interdisciplinary methods such as the Inpatient Rehabilitation Facility–Patient Assessment Instrument and the Minimum Data Set are described. Issues related to reliability and validity are also discussed.

Chapter 8: Planning Interventions discusses how to use information from an assessment to design individualized intervention plans focused on rehabilitation and health promotion. The planning process is discussed generally without limiting this discussion to any particular setting or client population. The chapter reviews various team approaches to intervention planning, and TR's commitment to emphasizing client strengths and sharing responsibility with clients for determining needs and goals. It includes guidelines for writing goals and objectives, and factors to consider in selecting intervention strategies such as literacy, safety, motivation, and readiness to change.

Chapters 9 through 12 represent the principle elements of TR practice used during the implementation phase of clinical practice. *Chapter 9: Using Activity-Based Interventions* discusses the therapeutic potential found in activities that are commonly used in

TR practice, as well as guidelines for selecting activity-based interventions. Also included is an explanation of program protocols and an example of a community-based protocol, *Healthy Living through Leisure*. This chapter also contains an extensive description of activity-based interventions in the following categories: mind–body health, creative expression, physical activity and fitness, games, self-discovery, social skills, nature-based and education-based interventions.

Chapter 10: Incorporating the Environment addresses the importance of an ecological approach to practice. We describe ways in which the environment affects human behavior, and how TR practitioners can "humanize" care environments and structure them for therapeutic purposes. While the chapter contains specific commentary on pediatric and geriatric care environments, the concepts presented apply to all environments where clinical practice occurs. This includes group homes, adult day centers, social clubs, a client's home, and the community at large.

Chapter 11: Developing Therapeutic Relationships contains an overview of personal attributes and characteristic skills of effective helping professionals. We provide a detailed discussion of three essential competencies needed in therapeutic relationships: creating partnerships with clients, multicultural competencies, and communication competencies. The importance of carefully terminating relationships with clients is discussed, and several challenging issues that arise in client-therapist relationships are presented.

Part 3 concludes with *Chapter 12: Using Group Interventions*. While groups are used often in TR, we emphasize psychoeducational group interventions and present information about the structure and process of these groups. We include information drawn from the professional literature on therapeutic groups and relate it to TR practice, including information about types of groups, format, membership, and leadership issues. An extensive section on processing TR interventions and various techniques that can be used is also provided.

Part 4: Communicating Practice and Ensuring Competence concludes this text. It contains chapters that address procedures for monitoring and evaluating the clinical process. *Chapter 13: Documenting Practice* is about the oral and written procedures used to inform others about TR clinical practice. It includes a discussion about the various forms of charting and record keeping. Finally, *Chapter 14: Pursuing Competence: The Role of Reflection, Ethical Reasoning, and Clinical Supervision*, brings readers full circle. That is, this text begins with a claim that health care and human services are constantly changing and asserts that TR practitio-

ners must be prepared to think critically about their work because of this constant change. Thus, the willingness to be a "reflective practitioner" and to exercise judgment is paramount to effective clinical practice. Chapter 14 presents information that readers will find useful in their journey of reflection including information on ethics and clinical supervision.

Throughout this text, we have tried to provide a comprehensive framework that explains TR clinical practice, without limiting our discussion to any particular group of clients or service delivery setting. Readers will have to decide where, when, and with whom our guidelines for clinical practice can be applied. Ultimately, this is the truest test of a professional—the ability to make judgments about practice based on a solid foundation of knowledge and understanding. We hope that the contents of this text add to your preparedness and professionalism.

Features of This Book

This textbook contains an extensive amount of information relevant to practicing within health care and human services. We have purposefully included information drawn from other disciplines, which is often used in classes on TR principles and procedures but not found in other TR textbooks. For example, we include information on health promotion and disease prevention, such as *Healthy People 2000* and *Healthy People 2010*, the federal government's blueprints for a healthy America. We also include information on psychosocial adaptation, which can be a unifying focus for all TR practice. Given the comprehensive nature of this text, we believe it is a resource for several courses, especially courses on clinical aspects of practice and program planning and implementation. Much of the text can also be used by practitioners as a template for examining practice throughout each phase of the TR process.

Each chapter opens with a set of *Guided Reading Questions*. We encourage you to use these questions to orient yourself to the chapter's content and to reflect on what you learned after you have read the chapter. Throughout the text we use *Thinking Triggers* to provoke your thoughts and reactions to various issues raised in the chapter. These thinking triggers can be used to focus classroom discussion as well. A separate learner's guide and instructor manual contains chapter study questions and learning activities as well as PowerPoint presentations.

Throughout the text we refer to TR professionals as TR specialists, TR practitioners, and recreation therapists.

We use these titles interchangeably, similar to how they are used in practice. Regardless of title, TR clinical practice occurs in a variety of settings, and so we use many examples to illustrate practice. Several examples are quite detailed and so they are presented as free-standing *Exhibits*. Of course, we can never be all-inclusive. We encourage readers to develop other relevant examples of TR practice and practical applications of the concepts and theories contained in this text.

Part 1

Foundations of TR Practice

Chapter 1
Contemporary Issues in Health and Human Services

Guided Reading Questions

After reading this chapter, you should be able to answer the following:
- What forces are influencing change in health and human service systems?
- How is the role of consumers changing within health and human service systems?
- What ethical challenges result from the changes described in this chapter? What are the implications for all health care disciplines including therapeutic recreation?
- What are some of the essential competencies expected of health professionals in the 21st century?

Introduction

As the 20th century came to a close, a number of forces created significant changes within health and human services. These forces included economic constraints associated with the delivery of health care, advances in technology, and rapidly changing demographic patterns. There has also been noticeable downsizing of professional staff and the creation of new service delivery models. At times, ethical questions about priorities, procedures, and promises associated with care have been raised as health and human service systems respond to these pressures. Undoubtedly, these forces will continue to transform health and human services in the 21st century, and as they do every profession will be challenged to reaffirm its individual mission and scope of practice.

What is the future of therapeutic recreation (TR)? Do changes occurring in health and human services represent threat or opportunity for the profession? Some argue that innovative TR practice will be constrained by economic realities, and that our profession is ill-equipped and possibly unable to demonstrate its value within a system driven by outcome accountability (Mobily, 1996). Others believe that speculation about the future success of the profession is "contingent upon our abilities as a collective to be proactive in an ever-changing health care environment" (Skalko, 1999, p. 499). Will TR services be considered a worthy but unessential part of health and human services? We believe that TR can remain a viable part of health and human services within the 21st century. To contribute

worthwhile and effective services, however, TR professionals must have a sound understanding of these forces of change and their implications for practice.

In this chapter we explore some of the forces of change influencing the health and human service system and their impact on TR practice (see **Figure 1.1**). We include technological, demographic, and economic factors, as well as the increasing role of consumers in asserting their expectations for quality care. This chapter also includes some of the ethical implications resulting from rapid changes brought on by tension between consumers' needs and the system's priorities and ability to respond. Of course, these forces of change are confronting all health-related professions, including TR, and are pressing each profession with greater expectations for accountability. Thus, TR and

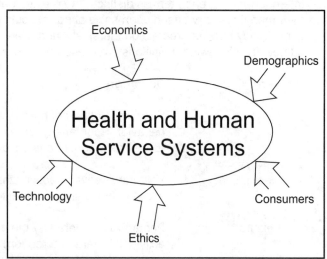

Figure 1.1: Forces influencing health and human service systems

all other health-related professions are challenged to "reinvent" themselves to accommodate these changes (O'Neil & the Pew Health Professions Commission, 1998).

While TR may be challenged to reinvent itself, we believe that the profession must remember its purpose within the community of health-related professionals: *Promoting and protecting the importance of play, recreation, and leisure in the lives of people with illnesses and disabling conditions.* As TR reinvents itself in the 21st century, it must accommodate the inevitable changes in the system without acquiescing to those forces that will challenge this core principle. Play, recreation, and leisure (see **Exhibit 1.1**) are important to achieving and maintaining health, functional independence, and quality of life for people who want to live well despite an illness or disabling condition. The profession must demonstrate the validity of this belief to remain a worthy and essential component within health and human services.

Forces of Change in Health and Human Service Systems

Health and human service systems constitute a complex mix of providers, consumers, payers, policy makers, and regulators. This mix is composed of both public and private, profit and nonprofit agencies. To survive

the challenges of the 21st century, TR professionals will need to communicate with this complex mix of parties and demonstrate how TR can contribute to the common goal shared by all health and human service providers: promoting health and life quality for all people and the communities in which they live. This is the overarching goal found in Healthy People 2000 and Healthy People 2010, both issued by the U. S. Department of Health and Human Services. These documents offer a common roadmap intended to unify the work of all health professionals. (For further information, see Chapter 2.)

Technological Forces

Unprecedented innovations in the delivery of health care services have occurred and will continue to occur as a result of technology. These changes will be observed in both indirect (administrative) and direct (client-focused) aspects of client care. Technology has influenced the creation of integrated information management and client care systems, which are redefining service delivery in health and human service agencies. Advances in telecommunication have resulted in the development of regional information networks and data banks that can be used to decrease paperwork/billing, identify cost-effective treatment, fight against false claims, streamline client care, and allow for innovation in the way health care information is utilized. Computerized medical records will become increasingly commonplace and their continued development

Exhibit 1.1: Definitions for play, recreation, and leisure (Adapted from Kelly, 1996)

The terms play, recreation, and leisure are used throughout this book. Even though they are often used interchangeably, each term is distinct. The precise definition of each term is difficult, however, because their meanings vary based upon societal norms, cultural traditions, and values. Consequently, the consistency between recreation therapists' and clients' understanding of the terms may not be assumed. The following definitions are presented to clarify the distinctions among these terms.

Term	Definition
Play	Fundamental part of human expression primarily associated with children's behavior. Spontaneity, creativity, and intrinsic meaning characterize play, as well as a nonserious suspension of reality.
Recreation	Voluntary nonwork activity that is organized for the attainment of personal and social benefits, including restoration and social cohesion.
Leisure	Primarily considered by the general public to be free or discretionary time or an activity (similar to recreation). Leisure researchers generally consider leisure to be the quality of an activity/experience characterized by perceived freedom, intrinsic motivation, and satisfaction.

and use within information networks will allow for further innovations as researchers are better able to track certain diseases as well as client responses to drugs and treatments. According to burlingame (1998), advances in technology have significant implications for the TR profession. In addition to becoming more familiar and comfortable with hardware and software, professionals will need to develop unified terminology and protocols in TR that can be used with regional and national data collection systems.

Technological advances have impacted client care, as well. New surgical procedures have dramatically shortened lengths of stay or have eliminated the need for hospitalization altogether. Innovations in assistive technology, such as functional electrical stimulation and robotics, will continue to allow individuals with disability-related limitations to enjoy greater independence in major life domains, including recreation. In fact, the National Center for Medical Rehabilitation and Research identified assistive technologies as a priority area for research (National Institutes of Health, 1993). Assistive technologies have infiltrated the domain of sport and recreation and have enabled people to incorporate physical activity as part of an overall healthier lifestyle. Likewise, augmentative communication devices have significantly changed the ability of people with communication disorders to interact and be more socially active. Because of these and other technological advances, accreditation guidelines issued by the Joint Commission on Accreditation of Healthcare Organizations (JCAHO) stipulate that all therapists, including recreation therapists, incorporate assistive technology into treatment and client education.

Furthermore, the use of the Internet will expand as a primary method for accessing health-related information for self-care. Use of the Internet, e-mail, and chat rooms will continue to grow as a method for social contact. For example, children who are hospitalized and want to communicate with children in similar situations are making use of the Internet to meet this need (Austin, 1999). The Internet has also proven very successful in promoting social contact and providing health-related information among youth with developmental disabilities (Johnson & Ashton-Shaeffer, 2001), older adults living in the community (Barol, 2000), and persons with head injuries (Zook & Luken, 2001). Other examples include the use of computerized games or video recordings as treatment modalities, and the creative use of virtual reality to simulate real world challenges (Broida-Kaufman & Germann, 1997; Yang & Poff, 2001). Undoubtedly, technology will continue to impact the delivery of health and human services and will have an important role in influencing clients' potential for achieving and maintaining health and well-being.

☆• • •Thinking Trigger

Is the Internet useful for accessing health information? How might the Internet influence TR practice? • • • ☆

Demographic Forces

The 2000 census revealed dramatic changes in the racial and ethnic composition of the United States (see **Table 1.1**). Projections had indicated that in 2000 one third of the North American population would be comprised of ethnic minorities and that this percentage would increase to 52% by 2010 (Aponte & Crouch, 1995). Comparisons with actual 2000 census findings indicate that the projections are quite close with the most notable rise occurring in the number of individuals who identify themselves as Hispanic or Asian and Pacific Islanders.

The changing demographic composition will put pressure on service delivery systems to recognize and

Table 1.1: Actual and projected demographic comparison for the years 2000 and 2050 (U. S. Census Bureau, http://www.census.gov)

Demographic Group	U.S. Census 2000 Data Year 2000	U.S. Census Projections Year 2000	Year 2050
Non-Hispanic White	69.1%	71.4%	52.8%
African American	12.1%	12.2%	13.2%
Hispanic	12.5%	11.8%	24.3%
Asian and Pacific Islander	3.7%	3.9%	8.9%
American Indian	0.7%	0.7%	0.8%

respond to cultural variations in the conceptualization, use, and need for health and human services. Health and human service systems will be challenged to overcome communication barriers and provide services that have relevance for increasingly diverse consumers who have different values, attitudes, and behaviors associated with health and health care. These differences are compounded by the disproportionate number of ethnic minorities with lower socioeconomic status, which is a powerful variable in health behavior patterns. Higher rates of risky health behavior, illiteracy, and a tendency not to use preventive health care services are associated with poverty (Ma & Henderson, 1999). The system must adjust to these demographic factors.

In addition to the sheer increase in the number of individuals from different demographic groups, health and human service systems will also need to be cognizant of the growing trend for individuals to have biracial or multiracial origins. Such individuals may not identify with the racial group that they appear most similar to, they may choose to reject the heritage of one of their parents, or they may identify with different racial groups than their siblings (Sheldon & Dattilo, 1997). Health and human service providers will need to ascertain which heritage such individuals choose to honor and be aware of the influence this choice may have on health-related beliefs, values, and behaviors.

Likewise, health and human services will also need to respond to the increasing number of individuals who are living longer, and the associated health concerns and social service issues they present. Adults aged 65 years or older numbered 33.9 million in 1996. They represented 12.8% of the U.S. population (U.S. Department of Health and Human Services, 2000). The fastest growing segment of this aging population is women and men aged 85 and older (Dychtwald, 1999). According to the Health Insurance Association of America (1997), an estimated 62.5% of those who are 85 years of age or older have such significant disabling conditions that they are unable to manage basic activities of daily living without much assistance. These later years of life present the most challenge as the incidence of diseases associated with the aging brain (e.g., Alzheimer's disease) increases the strain on an already taxed service delivery system. This older adult population requires access to a range of health and human services including home health care, adult day care, assisted living, nursing home care, and hospice care. These services will be needed despite the growing trend to try and maintain elderly individuals within their families and community. This trend has resulted

in an enormous burden on family caregivers, which increases their risk for declines in health (Bedini & Phoenix, 1999).

Health and human service agencies are recognizing this demographic reality and are responding by reforming long-term care services. According to the U.S. Department of Health and Human Services (2000):

Long-term care crosses the boundaries of different types of care, from health to social and intensity of services, from periodic home health and homemaker visits to round-the-clock subacute care. Access to the full range of long-term care services continues to be a problem because of financial barriers and the limited availability of specific services. (section 1, p. 15)

For this reason, increasing the availability of a wide variety of long-term care services to the aging population has been identified as a target goal of *Healthy People 2010*. This goal and other related needs of this population group will continue to influence the services provided by health and human service systems in the 21st century.

Another demographic change to which the system must respond is the increase in the number of individuals living with disabilities or chronic illnesses. According to McNeil (1997), an estimated 54 million Americans, or nearly 20% of the population, currently live with a disability that impairs one or more of their daily activities. Estimates made in 1993 indicated that 35 to 45 million Americans had a disabling condition, 13 million of whom required assistance with activities of daily living. Another 9.7 million were unable to carry on major life activities compared to peers without disabilities (NIH, 1993). According to the National Institute on Disability and Rehabilitation Research (1997) the increase in persons with chronic illness or disability is seen at every age group (see **Figure 1.2**). For instance, disability rates increased from 1990 to 1994. There was a 33% increase in activity limitations among girls; a 40% increase in activity limitations among boys; and a 16% increase in activity limitations among adults 18 to 44 (U.S. Department of Health and Human Services, 2000).

Advances in medical emergency care, pharmacology, and surgical techniques will continue to contribute to a growing increase in the number of people living with disabling conditions. The needs and unique challenges of providing cost-effective health and human services to this segment of the population will shape health and human services in the 21st century. Needs of these people will certainly extend well beyond primary medical care since many of their conditions will be chronic. There will be an increased concern with susceptibility to secondary health problems and an increased need for health promotion services that will enable these individuals to live, learn, work, and play in communities of their choosing.

Economic Forces

The cost of health care in the United States has continued to escalate at an extraordinary rate. In the 1940s the United States spent $4 billion on health care. By 1992 the amount had increased to three quarters of a trillion dollars. This sum was expected to triple in 1999 (van Servellen, 1997). The direct medical and indirect annual costs associated with disability alone are more than $300 billion, or 4% of the gross domestic product (Institute of Medicine, 1997). This estimate of disability-related costs includes $160 billion in medical care expenditures (1994 dollars) and $155 billion in lost productivity costs.

Despite exorbitant expenditures for health care, access to services is and will remain a significant problem for many. "Economists describing the problem of accessibility estimate that up to 38 million people may be uninsured despite the fact that the United States spends more of the Gross National Product (GNP) on health care than any other country in the world" (van Servellen, 1997, p. xvii). Recent estimates indicate that approximately 44.3 million persons lacked health insurance in 1998. Unemployment is typically seen as the problem; however, this is not always the case as many individuals who are uninsured or underinsured are employed in low paying jobs that do not provide health care benefits to employees.

Issues associated with affordability and access to health care have and will continue to redefine the structure and delivery of health and human services. Retrospective payment systems, which were once commonplace, are now obsolete. Managed care systems, including health maintenance organizations (HMOs), prospective payment systems (PPS), and fee-for-service plans emerged as a means to deal with runaway health care costs. However, containing escalating health care costs remains a vexing issue, and these coverage systems have created an additional set of problems related to accessing health care. First, some managed care systems are reluctant to enroll *high cost* individuals (i.e., individuals with chronic illnesses or disabilities). The need for services directed at preventing the occurrence of secondary health problems, such as skin ulcers in individuals with spinal cord injury, are

rarely considered *medically necessary*. Many managed care systems have shifted the decision-making authority from providers of care to the payers of that care. Consequently, insurance intermediaries rather than the direct care provider are making decisions about the course of care (e.g., types of services, length of time, location of services). Managed care scrutinizes reimbursement for all but the most medically necessary services. Recreation therapists, in particular, are challenged with articulating the importance of their services to be considered for reimbursement. The reluctance to reimburse is not just a matter of unfamiliarity with the potential benefits of TR. It is also largely a question of the medical relevance of these services and whether there is evidence to support the outcomes that are claimed to occur as a result of TR interventions.

Evidence-Based Practice

A consequence of these economic pressures has been the development of an almost exclusive focus on value-added services. Such services are considered to be medically necessary to the treatment or rehabilitation of the individual and are instrumental in achieving outcomes that are efficient and effective (Skalko, 1999). They meet the definition of *active treatment*, which means that the services are delivered through an individualized intervention plan, monitored by a physician, and are expected to result in improvement in the client's condition, as well as reduce the need for continued medical care. Since the mid-1980s there has been an increasing call for evidence-based recreation therapy in many sectors of practice. The TR profession's quest to be viewed as a value-added

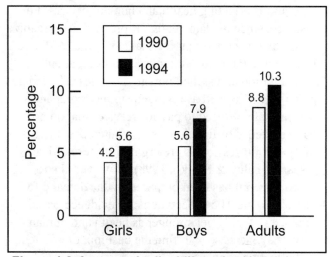

Figure 1.2: Increase in disability-related activity limitations (National Institute on Disability and Rehabilitation Research, 1997)

service and an equal player among allied health professions has been met with a demand for evidence. Such services must demonstrate that valued outcomes result from TR interventions. At times, TR has been able to make a persuasive case for inclusion. For instance, when the Agency for Health Care Policy and Research (AHCPR) established a protocol to guide post-stroke rehabilitation services, it included TR services. The AHCPR is the lead agency for the federal government's Department of Health and Human Services and is charged with supporting research that improves quality health care. The AHCPR, now called the Agency for Healthcare Research and Quality (AHRQ), believed that recreation therapy was instrumental in assisting persons who survived a stroke with adapting to functional impairments and resuming a socially active lifestyle.

The profession's involvement with accrediting bodies, such as the Joint Commission on Accreditation of Healthcare Organizations (JCAHO), the Commission on Accreditation of Rehabilitation Facilities (CARF), and the Centers for Medicare and Medicaid Services (CMS) (formerly the Health Care Financing Administration), has helped to clarify the contributions TR can make. Yet the amount of efficacy research and other outcome data to support TR as an active treatment is very limited. *Efficacy research* involves studies that demonstrate client outcomes that result from TR interventions. The need for evidence of efficacy (or effectiveness) is apparent each time recreation therapists advocate for services with case managers. They need to describe TR services in terms of interventions that will result in valued outcomes for individual clients. Such data is also needed when TR professional organizations meet with legislators and other government officials to advocate for changes in legislation and regulations effecting health and human services. For instance, since the late 1990s TR professional organizations have been pressing for changes in the Medicare Prospective Payment System used for outpatient rehabilitation and skilled nursing facilities. The federal government, as well as private insurance companies, has basically refused to pay for services that do not have evidence of functional client outcomes. Increasingly, TR professionals are urging for more efficacy research (Riley & Skalko, 1998). However, the response overall has been outpaced by the demand for outcome data. The expectations for evidence-based practice will only get stronger as health and human service agencies seek to find the best mix of efficient and effective services.

⚡• • •Thinking Trigger

Have you been (or will you be) prepared to contribute to the development of efficacy research in TR? Who has the most responsibility to conduct such research—university faculty or TR practitioners?   • • •⚡

Structural Changes in Health and Human Service Systems

Major changes in the structure of the U.S. health care system have occurred during the 1990s and will continue into the 21st century as a function of the increasing influence of market forces, welfare reform, and the rapid growth of managed care. These influences have resulted in new venues for service delivery. For instance, to streamline costs and maintain their client base, hospitals have created integrated systems of care where clients can receive services from a variety of providers that are part of an interrelated network. Increasingly service delivery has shifted from inpatient hospital stays to day surgeries, outpatient services, clinics, and in-home health care. Rehabilitation services have also undergone structural changes in response to market forces and payment and delivery systems. Traditional inpatient rehabilitation programs have experienced a decrease in the amount of time available for inpatient therapy. This shortened length of stay has resulted in innovative service delivery options including the expansion of outpatient and day treatment programs for persons needing rehabilitation. This same pattern has been seen in psychiatric care/behavioral health programs. Inpatient stays of 3–5 days that focus on symptom management and crisis intervention are very common. Consequently, there has been a greater reliance on community mental health services. Mental health services are also being delivered through intensive community case management and psychiatric home care programs (Haber, 1997).

Because of the rising costs associated with inpatient hospital stays and the growing focus on prevention in both physical medicine and behavioral health care, the next decade will undoubtedly see an increase not only in therapy-based community programs but also in health promotion programs provided in community-based settings. This new integrated system of services will be characterized by its emphasis on community-based primary care and prevention, and will be a *seamless* system of continuous care. Therapeutic recreation practice will have to adjust to these changing service delivery venues and create services that are relevant to the mission of complex systems.

The Consumer's Voice

Lack of accountability in health care outcomes, exorbitant costs, and unreasonable restrictions in health insurance plans regarding covered services have resulted in a backlash from consumers—the neglected party in health care. Increasingly, consumers are making their voices heard. Legislators and consumers are joining together to legislate changes and restore consumer confidence. For example, under the Clinton administration, a bipartisan commitment to support client rights was initiated. The Consumer Bill of Rights and Responsibilities was introduced in an effort to strengthen consumer confidence while holding participants in the system (e.g., medical personnel and organizations) accountable for improving the quality of care (President's Advisory Commission on Consumer Protection and Quality in the Health Care Industry, 1998). This initiative materialized into bills introduced in both the House and Senate in 1999. Although different in scope, these bills were designed to increase consumers' access to accurate, easily understood information related to choice of a health plan, availability of specialty care, confidentiality of medical records, and a guaranteed appeal process when insurance companies deny medical care. While a Consumer's Bill of Rights and Responsibilities has not yet been passed into law, the public sentiment for reaffirming the role of the consumer, and fighting the insurance industry's control of health care is quite clear.

Similarly, consumers of mental health services are asserting themselves. "Consumer and family organizations, which formed out of concern over frequent fragmentation of mental health services and lack of accessibility to such services, have assumed a substantial role in supporting development of mental health services" (U.S. Department of Health and Human Services, 2000, section 18, p. 6). The 1999 Surgeon General's Report on Mental Health identified the emergence of powerful consumer and family movements as one of four defining trends in the mental health field (U.S. Department of Health and Human Services, 1999). The goals of this consumer movement include overcoming stigma and discrimination in health care policies, encouraging self-help, and focusing on recovery that is sensitive to special needs associated with age, gender, race, and culture. As a result of consumer pressure, the Mental Health Parity Act (P. L. 104-204), which was passed in 1998, closed the gap in disparities between coverage for mental health and other health services. While there still continues to be far less coverage for mental health, the consumer's voice is evident in changing the system.

Consumer groups are also asserting their views on what ought to constitute health services. This is evident in recent actions by the *Consortium for Citizens with Disabilities* (CCD), one of the strongest lobbying groups in Washington, DC. The CCD represents more than 30 consumer and provider organizations that share a commitment to advocacy action through public education and legislative lobbying. The CCD has placed health promotion and disease prevention high on its agenda for 2000 and beyond. It is committed to lobbying for changes in health and human services in response to known facts indicating that the majority of health conditions and impairments leading to disability and secondary conditions can be reduced through healthy behavior and active lifestyles. The CCD has created a Prevention Task Force to formulate strategies to promote legislation aimed at disease prevention and health promotion for persons with disabilities. The Task Force will spearhead collaborative efforts among such groups as Easter Seals, the Arthritis Foundation, the National Alliance for the Mentally Ill, the National Therapeutic Recreation Society, and the American Therapeutic Recreation Association.

> ✫• • •Thinking Trigger
>
> What has been your experience with advocating for your own health care? Was this easy or difficult to do? • • •✫

These examples reflect advocacy work done by consumers to affect national public policy issues. But, hearing the consumer's voice is important on an individual level as well. The Picker Commonwealth Group from Boston conducted an important study that captured the personal views of clients as they experienced health care. The resulting book, entitled *Through the Patient's Eyes* (Gerteis, Edgman-Levitan, Daley & Delbanco, 1993), offers a guide to providing care that is truly client centered.

Ethical Challenges

Contemporary issues related to technology, increasing demands for varied and complex services, and especially economic constraints have created many ethical questions related to *good* care, *fair* care, and *honest* care. Difficult decisions about client rights and competing interests and values have always been a part of health care; yet, the issue of ethics and ethical conduct has been receiving even greater attention now that the limits to health care resources are apparent. Increasingly the general public is made aware of many of these issues through newspaper and magazine reports that highlight ethical struggles around such issues as terminal care and decision making on behalf of incapacitated clients. Occasionally the media details stories about researchers who falsified outcomes to gain an advantage in the highly competitive search for research dollars, or about clients who were discharged from facilities due to insurance constraints despite clear evidence of their continuing need for medical care.

Changes that have been brought about by managed care have also created moral and ethical conflicts for service providers. Difficult decisions regarding the distribution of health care resources inevitably result in services for some at the expense (exclusion) of others. Restrictive regulatory standards or minimal health care coverage plans have also led to an unprecedented level of false insurance claims. A recent study reported in the American Medical Association's *Archives of Internal Medicine* found that 58% of physicians surveyed considered it ethical to lie to an insurance company to secure coverage for treatment if clients could not get treatment any other way (Freeman, Rathore, Weinfurt, Schulman & Sulmusy, 1999).

Finally, changes in health care regulations and practices go to the heart of certain fundamental issues, such as the meaning of autonomy and control in the process of health care, and the ultimate intent of medicine and rehabilitation (Collopy, 1996). For instance, while medical technology can prolong life and enable people to live with chronic illnesses, questions are raised about the system's responsibility for the quality of these lives. Other moral and ethical questions are provoked by the commercialization of the health and human service system (Lahey, 1998). Competition for limited health care dollars has practically transformed health care into an industry operating within a business model. The profit motive has diverted the system from its original goals. "Unfortunately, the trend in health care seems to be away from caring as

more and more energy is put into the business side of the health care industry" (Lahey, 1998, p. 492). Consequently, all health-related professionals need to examine the influence of economic pressures on their fundamental values and beliefs.

> Marketplace pressures and priorities exist within every profession, and it is the task of each profession to deal with economic realities in terms of its basic philosophical and moral commitment. When a profession faces dramatic widening or narrowing of economic opportunities, it becomes critically important for it to identify and critique the relationship between its marketplace and other priorities, the relationship between its own goals and the goals of its clients. (Lahey, 1996, p. 23)

Lahey (1998) warns the TR profession that the economic pressures described above can lead to a survival mode whereby the profession becomes preoccupied with competing for its share of dwindling resources. Consequently, the profession's self-interest causes it to lose sight of larger moral issues and its professional values and goals.

Sylvester (1996) articulated this concern as well because of the health care system's apparent preoccupation with efficiency and economics. This orientation, according to Sylvester, has brought pressure upon the TR profession to emphasize its contribution to client care in ways valued by the health care system rather than in ways valued by clients. In other words, an exclusive focus on measurable functional outcomes valued by the system may result in an unfortunate disregard for those things that give meaning, purpose, and worth to clients' lives. Thus, TR has a moral and ethical obligation to have a balanced focus on functional outcomes that are "instrumental" for living, and "existential" outcomes that represent meaning in the client's life (Richter & Kaschalk, 1996; Murray & Burton, 1997).

Perhaps a brief example can help clarify the difference between these two types of outcomes and how they can be addressed simultaneously. Consider Harold, a 78-year-old widower who had a stroke and is now in a rehabilitation facility receiving physical therapy to regain strength and mobility. His investment in rehabilitation, however, is minimal. Rosalina, the recreation therapist, arranges to bring Harold's dog Lucky into the hospital three times a week so that Harold is reminded of why he might want to get stronger and recover. Rosalina recognizes that Harold's relationship with his dog is his primary form of recreation and leisure and a source of significant meaning and purpose in his life. She incorporates this awareness into her sessions with Harold, arranging for him to work on strength and mobility while attending to his dog. Thus, Harold's rehabilitation involves both instrumental and existential outcomes. Harold not only regains his abilities to walk—he has a *reason* to walk.

Practitioners of the 21st Century

The rapid changes that have occurred in the health and human service system in the last decade have also raised questions about the qualities and characteristics needed by health-related professionals in the twenty-first century. In response to these changes, the Pew Health Professions Commission (O'Neil & the PHPC, 1998) issued its fourth and final report outlining recommendations for health professionals to "reinvent" themselves to most effectively address the challenges of the new century. The report concluded, "Health professionals must continually reconsider, in fundamental ways, how they best add value to the delivery of health services" (p. i). The Pew Health Professions Commission identified twenty-one competencies needed by health care providers in the twenty-first century (see **Exhibit 1.2,** p. 12). Aimed at all health professional groups, these recommendations provide an excellent reference point for therapeutic recreation students, educators, and practitioners alike. They can guide us as we endeavor individually and collectively to become the most competent and responsive professionals possible. Many of these competencies are reflected, directly or indirectly, throughout this text.

Summary

The TR profession faces several significant forces of change related to technology, changing demographics, complex structuring of health systems, and economics. Ethical questions are also being raised in addition to and as a consequence of these changes. Change is inevitable; you cannot expect otherwise. It is widely believed that health and human service systems known today are not the same systems that existed five years ago, nor will today's systems be the same five years from now. The perspective taken on change, however, has much to do with the responses made in the face of change. As suggested at the beginning of this chapter, change can be seen as a threat or an opportunity. Therefore, the TR profession must seize opportunities to contribute to the positive impact change can have on health and human services. Rather than simply reacting to change, TR practitioners have opportunities to assert themselves and help transform the system in ways that reflect the values of the profession and the desires of consumers. These characteristics will influence the response of health and human service systems to the challenges reviewed in this chapter. To TR's advantage, the systems are donning characteristics congruent with fundamental values of the TR profession. The next chapter will explore conceptual shifts being created by these particular characteristics, and the opportunities they provide for TR to assert a legitimate and important role in emerging systems of care.

Exhibit 1.2: Twenty-one competencies for the twenty-first century (O'Neil & PHPC, 1998)

1. *Embrace a personal ethic of social responsibility and service.* Emphasize the value of altruism in professional training and practice.

2. *Exhibit ethical behavior in all professional activities.* Honor professional codes of conduct, including our duties to clients, colleagues, and society.

3. *Provide evidence-based, clinically competent care.* Incorporate the latest knowledge from research and best practice guidelines.

4. *Incorporate the multiple determinants of health in clinical care.* In addition to the physiological determinants of health, consider the importance of emotional, psychosocial, cultural, economic, environmental, geographic, and political influences on the health of individuals and communities.

5. *Apply knowledge of the new sciences.* Strive to understand and evaluate new knowledge (e.g., genetics, psychoneuroimmunology) and its economic, social, and ethical implications.

6. *Demonstrate critical thinking, reflection, and problem-solving skills.* Develop the capacity to recognize and reflect on problems that fall outside the current scope of knowledge and practice, thereby developing a response readiness when new situations arise and dilemmas are encountered.

7. *Understand the role of primary care.*

8. *Rigorously practice preventive health care.* Use educational approaches to help people learn self-management skills, and serve as role models and resources for ways to adopt health-promoting behaviors.

9. *Integrate population-based care and services into practice.*

10. *Improve access to health care for those with unmet health needs.* Help improve access to basic health care services by helping to distribute resources widely and efficiently and acting as advocates for people with unmet health needs.

11. *Practice relationship-centered care with individuals and families.* Develop skills necessary for open, empathetic communication and the abilities to convey compassion for the contextual meaning of health to each individual served.

12. *Provide culturally sensitive care to a diverse society.* Learn about the culturally learned values, customs, and beliefs that affect people's health behavior.

13. *Partner with communities in health care decisions.* Support the right to self-determination and choice by individuals, families, and communities.

14. *Use communication and information technology effectively and appropriately.* Work cooperatively with information systems officials to build and effectively use information technologies to benefit clients and service delivery systems.

15. *Work with interdisciplinary teams.* Develop and maintain attitudes and skills that foster communication and cooperation, mutual respect, trust, and support. Learn to work interdependently.

16. *Ensure care that balances individual, professional, system, and societal needs.* Join with all other participants in the health care environment—practitioners, payers, and consumers of care—to balance value and quality with costs.

17. *Practice leadership.* Learn to "work effectively across complex integrated organizational and institutional boundaries. This will require health professionals that can think and act from the perspective of a system" (O'Neil & PHPC, 1998, p. 40).

18. *Take responsibility for quality of care and health outcomes at all levels.* Accept accountability for individual competence and ensure that one's performance adheres to professional standards of practice.

19. *Contribute to continuous improvement of the healthcare system.*

20. *Advocate for public policy that promotes and protects the health of the public.*

21. *Continue to learn and help others learn.* Embrace career-long commitment to continuous learning.

References

Aponte, F. A. and Crouch, T. R. (1995). The changing ethnic profile of the United States. In J. F. Aponte, R. Y. Rivers, and J. Wohl. *Psychological interventions and cultural diversity* (pp. 1–20). Boston, MA: Allyn & Bacon.

Austin, D. (1999). *Therapeutic recreation: Processes and techniques*. Champaign, IL: Sagamore Publishing.

Barol, J. (2000, May). *Using the Internet to improve our service to clients*. Paper presented at the 24th Annual Meeting of the Mideastern Symposium on Therapeutic Recreation, Philadelphia, PA.

Bedini, L. and Phoenix, T. (1999). Addressing leisure barriers for caregivers of older adults: A model leisure wellness program. *Therapeutic Recreation Journal, 33*(3), 222–240.

Broida-Kaufman, J. and Germann, C. (1997). Enhancing accessibility through virtual environments. *Parks & Recreation, 34*(5), 94–97.

burlingame, j. (1998). The role of information technologies. In Brasile, F., Skalko, T., burlingame, j. (Ed.), *Perspectives in recreational therapy: Issues of a dynamic profession* (pp. 463–486). Ravensdale, WA: Idyll Arbor.

Collopy, B. (1996). Bioethics and therapeutic recreation: Expanding the dialogue. In C. Sylvester (Ed.), *Philosophy of therapeutic recreation: Ideas and issues, Volume I* (pp. 10–19). Ashburn, VA: National Recreation and Park Association.

Dychtwald, K. (1999). *Healthy aging: Challenges and solutions,* Gaithersburg, MD: Aspen.

Freeman, V., Rathore, S., Weinfurt, K., Schulman, K., and Sulmusy, D. (1999, October 25). Lying for patients: Physician deception of third-party payers. *Archives of Internal Medicine, 159*(19), 2263–2270.

Gerteis, M., Edgman-Levitan, S., Daley, J., and Delbanco, T. (Eds.). (1993). *Through the patient's eyes: Understanding and promoting patient-centered care.* San Francisco, CA: Jossey-Bass.

Haber, J. (1997). Delivery of mental health services. In J. Haber, B. Krainovich-Miller, A. Leach McMahon, and P. Price-Hospkins (Eds.), *Comprehensive psychiatric nursing* (5th ed., pp. 2–15). St. Louis, MI: Mosby Year Book, Inc.

Health Insurance Association of America (1997). Guide to long-term care insurance. In Institute of Medicine, *Enabling America: Assessing the role of rehabilitation science and engineering.* Washington, DC: National Academy Press.

Institute of Medicine. (1997). *Enabling America: Accessing the role of rehabilitation science and engineering.* Washington, DC: National Academy Press.

Johnson, D. and Aston-Shaeffer, C. (2001). Using the Internet to facilitate social connections. Paper presented at the meeting of the American Therapeutic Recreation Association's National Conference, New Orleans, LA.

Kelly, J. (1996). *Leisure* (3rd ed.). Boston, MA: Allyn & Bacon.

Lahey, M. (1996). The commercial model and the future of therapeutic recreation. In Sylvester, C. (Ed.), *Philosophy of therapeutic recreation: Ideas and issues, Volume II* (pp. 20–29). Ashburn, VA: National Recreation and Park Association.

Lahey, M. (1998). Impact of global trends. In F. Brasile, T. Skalko, and j. burlingame. (Eds.), *Perspectives in recreational therapy: Issues of a dynamic profession* (pp. 489–498). Ravensdale, WA: Idyll Arbor.

Ma, G. and Henderson, G. (1999). *Rethinking ethnicity and health care.* Springfield, IL: Charles C. Thomas.

McNeil, J. M. (1997). Americans with disabilities 1994-95. *Current Populations Report*, P7061:3–6.

Mobily, K. (1996). Therapeutic recreation philosophy revisited: A question of what leisure is good for. In C. Sylvester (Ed.), *Philosophy of therapeutic recreation: Ideas and issues, Volume II* (pp. 57–70). Ashburn, VA: National Recreation and Park Association.

Murray, S. and Burton, A. (1997, September). More than fun and games: Recreational therapists are value-adding team members. *Team Rehab Report, 8*(9), 31–35.

National Institutes of Health (1993). *Research Plan for the National Center for Medical Rehabilitation Research.* U. S. Department of Health and Human Services, NIH Publication No. 93-3509.

National Institute on Disability and Rehabilitation Research (1997). *Trends in disability prevalence and their causes: Proceedings of the fourth national disability statistics and policy forum.* Washington, DC: U.S. Department of Education.

O'Neil, E. H. and the Pew Health Professions Commission (1998, December). *Recreating health professional practice for a new century: The 4th report of the Pew Health Professions Commission.* San Francisco, CA: Pew Health Professions Commission.

President's Advisory Commission on Consumer Protection and Quality in the Health Care Industry. (1998). *Quality first: Better health care for all Americans: Final report to the President of the United States.* Washington, DC: U.S. Government Printing Office.

Richter, K. and Kaschalk, S. (1996). The future of therapeutic recreation: An existential outcome. In C. Sylvester (Ed.), *Philosophy of therapeutic recreation: Ideas and issues, Volume II* (pp. 86–91). Ashburn, VA: National Recreation and Park Association.

Riley, B. and Skalko, T. (1998). The evolution of therapeutic recreation. *Parks & Recreation, 33*(5), 64–71.

Sheldon K. and Dattilo, J. (1997). Multiculturalism in therapeutic recreation: Terminology clarification and practical suggestions. *Therapeutic Recreation Journal, 31*(3), 148–158.

Skalko, T. K. (1999). The future of the profession. In F. Brasile, T. K. Skalko, and j. burlingame. *Perspective in recreational therapy: Issues of a dynamic profession,* (pp. 499–515). Ravensdale, WA: Idyll Arbor.

Sylvester, C. (1996). Instrumental rationality and therapeutic recreation: Revisiting the issue of means and ends. In C. Sylvester (Ed.), *Philosophy of therapeutic recreation: Ideas and issues, Volume II* (pp. 92–103). Ashburn, VA: National Recreation and Park Association.

U.S. Census Bureau. (2000). Retrieved from http://www.census.gov

U.S. Department of Health and Human Services (1999). *Mental health: A report of the surgeon general: Executive summary.* Rockville, MD: Author.

U.S. Department of Health and Human Services (2000). *Healthy People 2010 (Conference Edition, in Two Volumes).* Washington, DC: U. S. Government Printing Office.

van Servellen, G. (1997). *Communication skills for the health care professional: Concepts and techniques.* Gaithersburg, MD: Aspen.

Yang, H. and Poff, R. (2001). Virtual reality therapy: Expanding boundaries of therapeutic recreation. *Parks & Recreation, 36*(5), 52–57.

Zook, B. and Luken, K. (2001). Building technology bridges for brain injury support groups. *Parks & Recreation, 36*(5), 82–88.

Chapter 2
Changing Concepts within Health and Human Service Systems

Guided Reading Questions

After reading this chapter, you should be able to answer the following:

- What is the holistic model of health?
- How does the holistic model differ from the medical model?
- What impact will a holistic model have on the delivery of health care?
- What are health promotion and disease prevention?
- What is meant by quality of life?
- What roles do health promotion and disease prevention have in maintaining health and quality of life?
- How can TR services address health maintenance, health promotion, and disease prevention?
- Why is quality of life an important outcome in rehabilitation?
- How can TR services promote and maintain life quality?

Introduction

Chapter 1 highlighted several contemporary factors that are changing the nature of health and human services, including new demographic patterns, cost containment, technology, and consumerism. These factors not only create changes in the structure of service delivery systems but also challenge the medical and physical science paradigms that have traditionally driven the conceptualization of health and subsequent service orientations. In this chapter, we will explore three particular conceptual shifts that are gaining prominence in health care and human services and the implications they have for TR (see **Figure 2.1**). We will illustrate how each of these shifts is consistent with fundamental principles of TR practice.

The first conceptual shift is the move away from a *disease model* of health toward a *holistic model* of health, which includes health promotion and wellness. This newer model presents health as more than the absence of disease; rather, it is a dynamic process aimed at achieving a sense of balance and integration between body, mind, and spirit. A holistic conceptualization of health (often referred to as *wellness*) places particular emphasis on the physical, psychological, social, and environmental determinants of health and the capacity of the individual, in concert with his or her community and culture, to define, determine, and manage personal health and well-being. Thus *self-*

determination is the second conceptual shift emerging in health and human services. This shift results in a recognition of clients as partners in maintaining health. The third shift seen in contemporary health and human services is the increasing emphasis on *life quality* as the ultimate outcome of services.

Within this text *rehabilitation* is broadly defined to include both habilation services and rehabilitation services. *Habilitation services* traditionally involve helping clients acquire abilities and skills associated with normal development. In contrast *rehabilitation services* traditionally involve helping clients restore or regain functioning that may have been lost or altered due to illness or disability. Rehabilitation has also begun to concentrate on facilitating the individual's

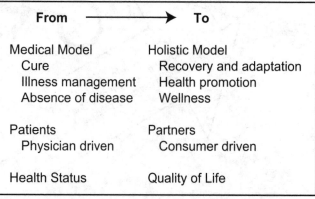

From ⟶	To
Medical Model	Holistic Model
Cure	Recovery and adaptation
Illness management	Health promotion
Absence of disease	Wellness
Patients	Partners
Physician driven	Consumer driven
Health Status	Quality of Life

Figure 2.1: Conceptual shifts in health and human service systems

adjustment to disability as well as social and community integration (Renwick & Friefeld, 1996). Both habilitation and rehabilitation involve many disciplines concerned with the individual's physical, emotional, cognitive, and social functioning in major life areas, including recreation. In this text, we merge these two types of services under the rubric of rehabilitation.

Shift toward Holistic Health

Western medicine and health care have been oriented around a medical model that focused on pathology and causes and subsequent cure for disease and illnesses. The portion of the body (e.g., circulatory system, respiratory system) that was the source of symptoms was the focus of study, not the person experiencing the conditions. Symptoms needed to be eliminated, illnesses needed to be cured, and clients needed to be returned to an illness/disease-free state. Within the medical model, little emphasis was placed on understanding the

ways in which the illness/disease influenced the client's life, or on the effects of the environment on an individual's health.

In contrast, a holistic approach to health suggests that health is not a state to be achieved but rather an ever-changing dimension of one's life that is influenced by physical, mental, social, emotional, spiritual, and environmental factors. "Health is a quality of life, involving social, emotional, mental, spiritual, and biological fitness on the part of the individual, which results from adaptation to the environment" (Dubos, 1968, p. 15). While this holistic perspective toward health has existed since the 1940s when the World Health Organization's (WHO) introduced a broader conceptualization of health as a state of complete physical, mental, and social well-being, it has in recent years gained increasing prominence. The term "health" has become synonymous with the term "wellness." *Wellness* is seen as a dynamic process in which individuals recognize the interrelatedness that exists among each of the dimensions of health (see **Figure**

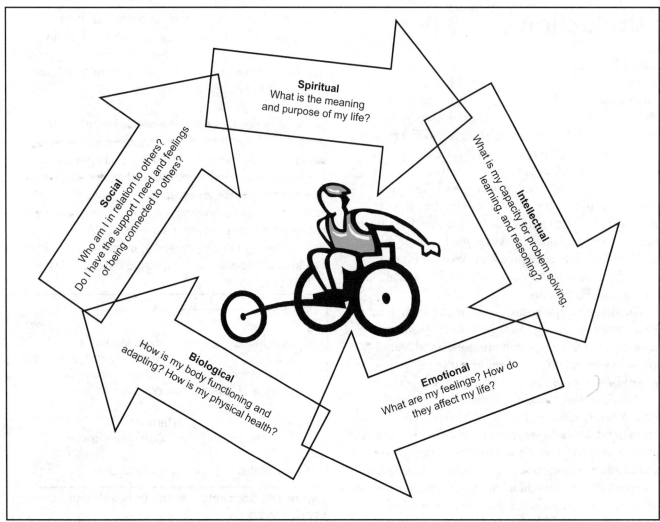

Figure 2.2: Dimensions of health

2.2). Wellness also involves accepting responsibility for becoming aware of and making choices to create a healthier lifestyle and striving to achieve a sense of balance between body, mind, and spirit.

The growing acceptance of a holistic view of health has resulted in a reorientation of health and human service systems away from treatment exclusively and toward a greater reliance on health promotion and disease prevention. The health promotion/disease prevention orientation stems from consumers' desire for information that helps with healthy living. In addition, growing awareness of public health issues also contributes to this new orientation. As a result, health and human service agencies are beginning to include disease prevention and health promotion programs that focus on societal problems such as domestic violence, alcohol and drug abuse, teen pregnancy, and at-risk behaviors of youth.

Likewise, health promotion strategies for persons with disabilities are emerging in response to a growing awareness that the existence of a disability does not preclude wellness. In other words, people can learn to live well with a disabling condition. Increased acceptance of a holistic health orientation within health and human service systems and the resulting orientation toward health promotion and disease prevention are clear opportunities for the TR discipline to assert itself as an important contributor to responsive health and human services in the 21st century.

Health Promotion and Disease Prevention

The traditional disease-oriented, biomedical model of health care is slowly giving way to a more complex, holistic model of health and well-being. For instance, self-healing and complementary and alternative medicine such as herbal therapies, acupuncture, and homeopathy are increasingly blended with conventional Western medicine. According to a report in the *New England Journal of Medicine* (Eisenberg, Kessler, Foster, Norlock, Calkins & Delbanco, 1993), approximately 34% of Americans were using at least one type of alternative therapy. Clients visited alternative practitioners 425 million times in 1990. This represents approximately 40 million more visits to alternative therapy providers than to primary care physicians. The widespread use of these approaches by consumers in their quest for health and wellness has forced traditional medicine to take notice. These topics and other aspects of mind–body health and healing have gained

such prominence that they have been incorporated into traditional medical school curricula.

☼• • •Thinking Trigger

Do you or any family member currently use a form of alternative or complementary medicine? What motivated this use?

• • •☼

There has also been a significant increase in scientific investigations of the mind–body connection. This research, which examines how the brain affects the body's immune system, is known as psychoneuroimmunology or behavioral medicine (Hafen, Karren, Frandsen & Smith, 1996). The National Institutes of Health (NIH) recognize this growing trend. In 1998 the National Center for Complementary and Alternative Medicine (NCCAM) was established by congressional mandate as a part of NIH. NCCAM (2002) is charged with evaluating the effectiveness of alternative medical treatment modalities, supporting research in this area, and disseminating credible information. Fiscal support for NCCAM rose from $2 million in 1993 to $68.7 million in 2000. NCCAM has classified approaches to complementary and alternative medicine into seven major categories. **Exhibit 2.1** (p. 18) presents two categories of complementary and alternative medicine that have relevance to current TR practice.

In addition to the increasing use of alternative medicine to maintain health, the growing prominence of health promotion and disease prevention also results from financial pressures within the health and human service system. An overriding concern in the system is cost containment. According to van Servellen (1997) the economic viability of the United States will be significantly threatened in the 21st century if some type of reform to reduce the costs of health care does not occur. One way to minimize costs associated with health and human services is to include health promotion and disease prevention programs as part of comprehensive health care. This translates into an approach to services focused on keeping people out of (or shortening the amount of time spent in) expensive inpatient care facilities. The American health care system is changing from an acute care hospital model to a community-based model of care. Community-based systems "will stress health promotion and active participation on the part of clients who are no longer the passive recipients of health care" (van Servellen, 1997, p. xx).

Health promotion activities combine educational, organizational, financial, and environmental supports to help people eliminate negative health behaviors and promote positive change (Donatelle & Davis, 1999). According to Donatelle and Davis (1999), such programs provide information that educates individuals about the benefits they can derive from making lifestyle changes (e.g., the benefits derived from being physically active during leisure time). They also provide programs and/or services that encourage an individual's efforts at making change (e.g., discounts for attending an exercise class). Health promotion programs might also provide procedures to guide an individual's efforts at making change (e.g., developing individualized exercise programs or personalized nutrition plans). Health promotion programs may also encourage a client to develop supports that facilitate lifestyle change (e.g., obtaining an exercise buddy or personal trainer). Finally, most health promotion programs would encourage clients to identify an incentive or reward system to help them maintain their motivation toward making health promoting lifestyle changes. Health promotion programs enhance the likelihood that once a person decides to change an unhealthy lifestyle behavior, the education, supports, and incentives are available to promote success.

Exhibit 2.1: Categories of the National Center for Complementary and Alternative Medicine Classification System relevant to TR practice (Weaver, 1999)

Mind–Body Medicine involves behavioral, psychological, social, and spiritual approaches to health. There are 4 subcategories of mind–body medicine.

1. *Mind–Body Systems* involve whole systems of mind–body practice used largely as primary interventions for disease. These are usually delivered in combination with lifestyle interventions.

2. *Mind–Body Methods* involve individual modalities used in mind–body approaches. When these approaches are applied to a medical condition for which they are not usually used they are considered complementary and alternative medicine (CAM). This category is further divided into three approaches. Modalities that are not commonly used, accepted, or available in conventional medicine are designated as CAM. Approaches that fall mainly within the domains of conventional medicine are designated as behavioral medicine. Practices that can fit either category are considered overlapping.

>   CAM: yoga, internal qigong, tai chi
>   Behavioral Medicine: psychotherapy, meditation, imagery, support groups, hypnosis, biofeedback
>   Overlapping: art therapy, music therapy, dance therapy, journaling, humor

3. *Religion and Spirituality* deals with nonbehavioral aspects of spirituality and religion and their relationship to biological functioning or clinical conditions. Examples include confession, nontemporality, spiritual healing, and soul retrieval.

4. *Social and Contextual* refers to social, cultural, symbolic, and contextual interventions that are not covered in other areas. Examples include holistic nursing, pastoral care, placebos, community-based approaches to healing such as Alcoholics Anonymous, Native American "sweat rituals," and support groups.

Lifestyle and Disease Prevention involves theories and practices designed to prevent the development of illness, identify and treat risk factors, or support the healing and recovery process. This category is concerned with integrated approaches for the prevention and management of chronic disease in general or the common determinants of chronic disease. There are 3 subcategories of lifestyle and disease prevention.

1. *Clinical Preventive Practices* refer to unconventional approaches used to screen for and prevent health-related imbalances, dysfunction, and disease (e.g., functional cellular enzyme measures).

2. *Lifestyle Therapies* refer to complete systems of lifestyle management that include behavioral changes, dietary changes, exercise, stress management, and addiction control. The changes in lifestyle must be based on a nonorthodox system of medicine or be applied in unconventional ways.

3. *Health Promotion* involves laboratory and epidemiological research on healing, the healing process, health promoting factors, and autoregulatory mechanisms.

Primary, Secondary, and Tertiary Prevention

Generally all health promotion programs include disease prevention activities. Prevention activities focus on averting an illness or disabling condition by getting individuals to take action that will hinder the occurrence of the health problem. Prevention activities are classified as primary, secondary, or tertiary (see **Table 2.1**).

Primary prevention activities are directed at precluding the development of a health problem. Vaccination and inoculation programs, cancer screening programs, and/or nutrition education programs are examples of primary prevention interventions used by nurses and physicians. Support groups, friendship clubs, or community-based fitness and recreation programs are examples of primary prevention interventions that can be implemented by recreation therapists to assist individuals with averting health problems associated with sedentary, isolated lifestyles.

More recently, some recreation therapists have become involved in presenting primary prevention programs to specific high-risk population groups. For instance, **Exhibit 2.2** (p. 20) illustrates two primary prevention programs implemented by the Jefferson Health System in Philadelphia, Pennsylvania, that often use TR practitioners to provide educational information to youth to prevent the occurrence of spinal cord and head injuries.

Secondary prevention activities are directed at reducing the nature, severity, or duration of the illness or disability by restoring health through health promo- These programs also aim to prevent

secondary complications that often accompany the primary disability, such as deconditioning, social isolation, or weight gain. Programs designed to minimize the occurrence of pressure ulcers in individuals with mobility impairments are an example of a secondary prevention focus for TR practice.

Tertiary prevention activities are focused on reducing the nature, extent, and severity of limitations that result from a long-term disability or chronic illness. Medication, surgery, counseling, client education, family education, and rehabilitation services (including physical, occupational, and/or recreation therapy) are examples of tertiary prevention services. Because the client has experienced a chronic illness or disability, the individual may or may not return fully to his or her pre-illness level of health or functioning. Tertiary prevention efforts are directed at assisting the individual to obtain the highest level of health and wellness possible.

Wellness

The growing orientation toward health promotion and disease prevention has also been influenced in large part by consumers' willingness to assume greater responsibility for their own health and well-being. This increased attention to self-care is a fundamental tenet of wellness and is helping to shape a paradigm shift in health and human services. "Wellness is an active process of becoming aware of and making choices to create a healthier lifestyle, in all of life's dimensions" (Donatelle, Snow-Harter & Wilcox, 1995, p. 7). It is characterized by a personal sense of responsibility to seek out information and necessary social supports to create and maintain conditions that allow an optimal level of health within one's limits and potential. Additional characteristics of wellness include a holistic approach to health and a belief in the importance of balance among the five dimensions of self—physical, psychological, intellectual, social, and spiritual (see **Figure 2.3**, p. 21). It is also reflected in the motivation that one has to achieve health and wellness. Health promotion programs, therefore, play a key role in assisting people to achieve an optimum level of health through wellness.

The National Health Agenda

Beyond cost containment and consumer choices, additional impetus for a greater emphasis on disease prevention and health promotion programs, especially for persons with disabilities, can be found in governmental

	ention approaches
	Focus of Intervention
	Intervention designed to stop problems before they start.
on	Intervention instituted early in the development of a health problem to eliminate the cause of the problem before more serious health conditions develop.
Tertiary Prevention	Intervention designed to treat and/or rehabilitate a long-term health problem.

and accrediting agencies' policies and recommendations. One of the first publications for advancing health promotion and disease prevention for people with disabilities was the Institute of Medicine's publication, *Disability in America: Toward a National Agenda for Prevention* (Pope & Tarlov, 1991). The recommendations made in this publication include:

- Expand research on preventive and therapeutic interventions for persons with disabilities

- Develop new health service delivery strategies for persons with disabilities

- Develop new health promotion models for persons with disabilities

- Examine the longitudinal effects of these programs on the health and wellness behaviors of individuals with disabilities

In addition, in 1979 the U.S. Department of Health and Human Services began to identify national health objectives for all American citizens and a timeline for achieving them. Three reports that identify health promotion and disease prevention goals have been issued:

- *Healthy People: The Surgeon General's Report on Health Promotion and Disease Prevention* (1979)

- *Healthy People 2000* (1990)

- *Healthy People 2010* (2000)

The first report significantly enhanced the status of public health and preventive medicine and was the predecessor to more recent documents. The national health objectives proposed in *Healthy People 2000* broaden the national prevention and health promotion agenda to include individuals with disabilities. However, a 1997 review found that none of the targets listed in *Healthy People 2000* for people with disabilities had been met (U.S. Department of Health and Human Services, 1995). Because health promotion and disease prevention have been underemphasized for people with disabilities, there have been increased occurrences of secondary health problems in this population. These include medical, social, emotional, family, or community problems secondary to the primary disabling condition. For example, individuals with chronic mental illness often experience significant social isolation, and individuals with chronic illnesses like multiple sclerosis or arthritis often experience economic and role constraints that create high levels of

Exhibit 2.2: Sample primary prevention programs

Think First

Think First, a national primary prevention program founded in 1986 by the American Association of Neurological Surgeons and the American College of Neurological Surgeons, is directed at preventing head and spinal cord injuries through education and community awareness. At Magee Rehabilitation Hospital, the Think First program has been presented to more than 27,000 students annually in Philadelphia, South Jersey, and Northern Delaware. Presented at school assembly programs, Think First features the award winning film, *Harms Way,* that depicts the how and why of head and spinal cord injuries. A Magee health professional, often a recreation therapist, presents educational material about how injuries occur to the brain and spinal cord while a paramedic provides information about appropriate bystander behavior. The program closes with personal stories from survivors of head and spinal cord injuries. The Think First program is designed to show adolescents that life altering injuries can easily occur and that they should recognize the dangers associated with weapons, drinking and driving, riding in a car without a seatbelt, biking without a helmet, and other risky behaviors. Prevention by "thinking first" is stressed in the program.

Cruisin' not Boozin'

Regional prevention programs are also developed when local agencies recognize a need. Such was the case with Bryn Mawr Rehabilitation Hospital's Cruisin' not Boozin' program. Developed in 1989, the Cruisin' not Boozin' program focuses on the prevention of death and injuries associated with drug and alcohol use among adolescents. The Cruisin' not Boozin' program includes individuals who sustained traumatic brain injuries during a drunk driving accident telling adolescents the perils of driving under the influence of drugs and alcohol. These individuals vividly describe their own personal stories and the daily struggles they encountered within the rehabilitation process to regain each tiny bit of functioning. Having won several awards, the Cruisin' not Boozin' program has been widely disseminated and is recognized for its success in the educating adolescents about the dangers of drunk driving.

stress in their lives. Therefore, *Healthy People 2010* devoted an entire chapter to identifying ways to promote the health of people with disabilities, prevent secondary conditions, and eliminate disparities between those with and without disabilities.

> The health promotion and disease prevention needs of people with disabilities are not nullified because they are born with an impairing condition or have experienced a disease or injury that has long-term consequence. Having a long-term condition increases the need for health promotion that can be medical, physical, social, emotional, or societal. (U.S. Department of Health and Human Services, 2000, section 6, p. 5).

A historical view of efforts directed at advancing the health promotion concerns of people with disabilities within the national health agenda is discussed thoroughly in *Issues in Disability and Health* (Simeonsson & McDevitt, 1999). **Exhibit 2.3** (p. 22) identifies the national health promotion and disease prevention goals for persons with disabilities identified in *Healthy People 2010*.

TR's role in Health Promotion/ Disease Prevention

Health care providers, insurers, and educators are joining forces with TR professionals to provide health promotion programs to individuals with disabilities. The ProMotion Fitness Center, located at Shepherd Center in Atlanta, Georgia, is a community wellness center for people of all abilities. Staffed by recreation therapists, the center strives to assist individuals to maintain their health through exercise. The Steadward Centre for Personal & Physical Achievement, located at the University of Alberta, Edmonton, is an example of a health promotion center designed specifically for adults with physical disabilities. Other examples of TR in health promotion include wheelchair sport programs sponsored by many rehabilitation centers, such as the HealthSports Program at Harmerville Rehabilitation Hospital in Pittsburgh, Pennsylvania. One of the most recent TR-based health promotion programs is Project PATH (see **Exhibit 2.4**, p. 23). This health promotion program in New Hampshire is designed for individuals with physical disabilities. Project PATH provides individualized, community-based health promotion and recreation information, instruction, and consultation to individuals in their homes and communities. It is quite likely that approaches such as these will continue to expand in TR.

According to Kraus (2000) leisure services providers are also challenged to strengthen their identity as a health-related field by designing programs aimed at health and wellness outcomes and systematically documenting and communicating these findings to the general public. Kraus reported on a survey of recreation and leisure educators regarding trends, issues, and challenges facing the field at the beginning of the 21st century. The seventh most important trend (out of 18) was "the increased recognition of leisure as a health-related field." This was based on numerous studies that demonstrated the value of physically active forms of leisure, especially those pursued in a social context, to total health and wellness.

Innovative health promotion/disease prevention programs such as *Active Options* (see **Exhibit 2.5**, p. 25) are already emerging. It can be inferred from this trend that general recreation and leisure service providers may be open to increased collaboration with TR professionals on health promotion programs designed for persons with disabilities. Whereas in the past the primary focus for collaboration was on social integration and inclusion of people with disabilities, there may be increased opportunities to also collaborate on health promotion and wellness services. Leisure service providers and TR specialists may now recognize a shared commitment to health and wellness.

Shared collaboration between community and therapeutic recreation practitioners makes good sense. Recreation and leisure involvement can play an important part in health promotion and disease prevention.

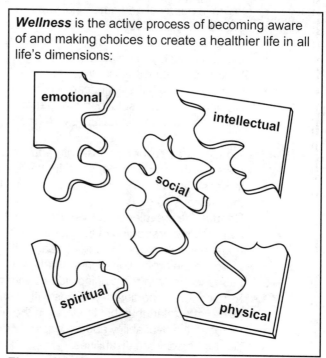

Wellness is the active process of becoming aware of and making choices to create a healthier life in all life's dimensions:

emotional

intellectual

social

spiritual

physical

Figure 2.3: Wellness

According to Coleman and Iso-Ahola (1993) leisure behavior can be a moderator of health status. Increased participation in physically and socially active leisure buffers the stress associated with life crises and other challenges in daily life.

✷• • •Thinking Trigger

Suppose a family member or friend was sick or dealing with a chronic illness. How would you talk with this person about the possible role of recreation as a stress reducer?   • • •✷

A variety of research studies have demonstrated the role of leisure in enhancing health and decreasing the incidence and severity of secondary conditions among persons with disabilities (Brock, 1988; Coyle & Santiago, 1995; Coyle, Shank, Kinney & Hutchins, 1993; Green, 1989; Mahon & Bullock, 1992; McGuire, Boyd & James, 1992; Rancourt, 1991; Santiago, Coyle & Kinney, 1993). An emerging line of research

suggests that quality leisure and recreation experiences have the potential to promote *hardiness*, a personality disposition that allows individuals to be more resilient when facing stress (see **Exhibit 2.6**, p. 26). The issue of resilience and the need for enhanced coping skills among individuals who are at risk for psychological distress have also been identified by the recent *Healthy People 2010* report as key areas for preventive interventions and research. Recreation involvement, therefore, is a critical ingredient in health promotion programs targeting stress reduction.

Documents such as *Disability in America: Toward a National Agenda for Prevention*, *Healthy People 2000* and *Healthy People 2010* provide direction for health and human services agencies to develop programs that go beyond traditional treatment and rehabilitation. TR should be a natural service provider in this emerging arena, but TR practitioners must assert themselves and demonstrate leadership by incorporating a health promotion focus into their practice.

Exhibit 2.3: Healthy People 2010 goals and targets for persons with disabilities

Promote the health of people with disabilities

Prevent secondary conditions
- Diminish depression
- Diminish anxiety
- Increase the number of healthy days for persons with activity limitations
- Improve personal and emotional support
- Increase life satisfaction
- Expand print size on medicines, and patient instructions material
- Increase employment rates
- Include children with disabilities in regular education programs
- Comply fully with the Americans with Disabilities Act
- Eliminate environmental barriers, generally physical or "built" barriers
- Enhance disability surveillance and health promotion programs

Eliminate disparities between people with and without disabilities in the U.S. population
- Increase the proportion of individuals with disabilities reporting good or excellent health
- Increase proportion of individuals with disabilities reporting at least 26 days of good health within the previous 30 days
- Reduce the prevalence of overweight adults, adolescents, and children
- Increase the proportion of individuals with disabilities above 6 years of age who regularly engage in light to moderate physical activity for an extended number of minutes
- Increase the proportion of individuals with mobility impairments who use assistive devices
- Increase the proportion of individuals with disabilities who receive case coordination services
- Reduce the proportion of persons with disabilities above 18 years of age who report adverse health effects attributable to stress in the previous 12 months
- Increase the availability and accessibility of physical activity and fitness centers within communities for person with disabilities

From Patient to Care Partner

One of the forces of change influencing a shift in health and human services is a stronger consumer voice. Consumer activism on the part of individuals with disabilities represents a demand for self-determination. People with disabilities desire to be viewed as *partners*

with care providers. The disability rights movement begun in the 1970s (see **Exhibit 2.7**, pp. 28–29) will continue to challenge health and human service systems to no longer view disability as something that needs to be "fixed." Some care recipients have become militant due to harm they incurred while a client. Reading about their personal stories and their activism in magazines like *MOUTH* and *Disability Rag* can help sensitize you to consumers' concerns and encourage you to incorporate

Exhibit 2.4: Project PATH—A TR-based health promotion/disease prevention program

Project PATH: Promoting Access, Transition, and Health is a health promoting intervention designed by Certified Therapeutic Recreation Specialists (CTRS) for people with spinal cord injuries (SCI). Not only does Project PATH reflect the emerging role of therapeutic recreation within the health promotion/disease prevention paradigm, it also reflects current trends within health care toward multiagency collaboration and community-based services. Project PATH is a multiagency collaboration of the following:

- University of New Hampshire's Recreation Management and Policy Department
- Northeast Passage: Affiliate of Disabled Sports USA
- HealthSouth Rehabilitation Hospitals (Woburn, MA; Portland, ME; and Concord, NH)
- Northeast Rehabilitation Health Network (Salem, NH)
- Spaulding Rehabilitation Hospital (Boston, MA)

Pilot funding for the program was obtained through New Hampshire's Department of Health and Human Services Healthcare Transition Fund and the UNUM Foundation, a leading provider of long-term disability insurance in the United States. The 3-year research study was funded by the National Institute on Disability and Rehabilitation Research (NIDRR) through their field-initiated projects. The program was designed to be responsive to the needs of both consumers and the healthcare industry.

Designed for individuals who have recently acquired a SCI, the program aimed to empower individuals to take responsibility for their own health via the development of a lifestyle that includes positive health behaviors and less dependency on the health care system. The services provided by Project PATH include barrier awareness and management, wellness education, personalized fitness instruction and monitoring, and leisure education (including leisure skill instruction). The program developed out of the recognition that with the shorter length of stay in rehabilitation settings, individuals with a SCI were often discharged having only been exposed to new skills required for life in the community. Project PATH "solves issues that arise once home that threaten independence, and helps establish positive behaviors that will prevent the onset of many of the most costly secondary conditions" (Sable & Gravink, 1999, p. 37).

The standard 12-month involvement with Project PATH begins while consumers are still receiving rehabilitation services. The CTRS assigned to Project PATH works to assure a smooth transition from the hospital setting by meeting with clients prior to discharge from the hospital to acquaint them with the project, obtain leisure lifestyle information, and discuss key issues and concerns. In addition, the CTRS meets with the inpatient treatment team for clarification of issues or concerns. One-to-one interventions begin in the consumer's home 1 to 3 months postdischarge. The interventions include a wellness education series, individualized fitness program, individual/family recreation skill development, practical functional skill development, community reintegration, resource file and network development, and peer mentoring. Individuals have many opportunities to practice leisure activities, explore community resources, learn to use adaptive equipment, explore personal modifications that can enhance their recreation involvement, and initiate and maintain a personalized fitness program in their home or community.

Project PATH recognizes the influence of social support on successful outcomes, and accordingly utilizes peer mentors, family members, and significant others in the treatment process. The overall intention of the program is that as consumers learn ways to engage more fully in community life, they will experience greater life quality, pursue more health promoting activities, and decrease their healthcare utilization (e.g., fewer and less severe secondary conditions).

Explanation of the program can be found in the *Annual in Therapeutic Recreation* (Sable & Gravink, 1999, pp. 33–34) and the *Therapeutic Recreation Journal* (Sable, Craig & Lee, 2000, pp. 348–361).

the concept of a care partner in your daily practice. These stories are especially compelling in mental health where activists like Jeanine Grobe (1995) relate stories about humiliating experiences and callous labeling that sometimes occurs. Consumer activism will challenge health and human service providers not only to examine the environmental and structural barriers to independence for persons with disabilities, but also to recognize individuals with disabilities as active partners in shaping health and human services to best meet their needs. This demand for self-determination is clearly represented in the disability community's slogan: *Nothing about me without me.*

Care providers and health and human service systems are responding slowly with a growing awareness that clients must have a voice in decisions. Care providers increasingly recognize clients as key decision makers. This is most clearly evident in service systems for people with developmental disabilities that practice *person-centered* planning. This process looks to the client to identify and express needs and interests, to set goals, and to select and use preferred strategies for meeting these goals. This conceptual shift also occurs within agencies that serve persons with head injuries. According to Cathy Terrill, vice president for the Brain Injury Association:

> Self-determination is being in charge of your life, having control and being an equal partner. The principles of self-determination include freedom, authority, responsibility, respect, choice, support and opportunity. People with disabilities want to be active partners in the determination of their life goals. (2000, p. 9)

Newer approaches to mental health services also emphasize an involvement of clients as partners in the care process (Carling, 1995). This is influenced by a shift in the perceived role and function of clients and providers. For instance, providers now assume roles of supporters, while clients are viewed as persons rather than disabled clients. Clients are increasingly being seen as citizens who exercise self-determination through circles of support, which include the formal mental health system, natural relationships, and community resources. "The goal of both formal and informal support systems is to maximize the extent to which people take charge over their own lives and are able to make substantive decisions about life goals, directions, and choices" (Carling, 1995, p. 58).

Self-care and shared medical decision making will also be at the center of medical practice in the 21st century.

By tapping the wisdom, experience and expertise of countless willing and able medical care consumers, we can reinvent the patient's role in health care, and, by doing so, we can improve quality and reduce cost. This vision reframes the traditional divide between patient and provider. Rather than being a passive recipient of medical services, the new health care consumer is recognized as a capable, essential member of the health care team. In partnership with physicians [*and other health care providers*] these new medical consumers provide appropriate home care, share in medical decisions and assume partial responsibility of outcomes. (Mettler, 1999, p. 317; emphasis added)

Empowering medicine, which provides individuals with opportunities to share the responsibility for their own health, will increasingly be used to help clients optimize their health by accessing and using information and knowledge to develop and maintain healthy lifestyles.

TR's Contribution to Partnerships

Supporting self-determination has been a cornerstone of therapeutic recreation philosophy and practice. In a review of TR practice models that guide service delivery, Bullock and Mahon (1997) identified self-determination as a core foundation apparent in every practice model proposed by the TR discipline. TR practice has repeatedly emphasized a commitment to ultimately enabling clients to determine the role and meaning of leisure in their lives. In addition, self-determination is a core characteristic of leisure experiences and a basis for leisure's contribution to health (Coleman & Iso-Ahola, 1993). Beyond that, sharing with clients the responsibility for change and growth is a fundamental tenet of effective helping relationships. With greater demand by consumers to be partners in the care process, TR practitioners may now have an increased opportunity to lead by example and to demonstrate how play, recreation, and leisure can be the basis for clients to take greater control of their physical, psychological, social, and spiritual health. TR practice must emphasize a *shared responsibility* to build *individual capacities* (competence, knowledge, beliefs, and abilities) that can be exercised in *environmental contexts* that promote health and well-being, or quality of life.

Quality of Life

These conceptual shifts, which begin to define contemporary health and human services, also contribute to an increased focus on quality of life as the ultimate outcome of services. When health and human service systems maintain a holistic view of the individual interacting with a supportive and health-promoting environment that emphasizes self-determination, the conditions necessary for life quality are set. The assumed outcome of care has always been that clients would experience better life quality resulting from cured illnesses and improved functioning. An expanded view of life quality maintains that holistic health does not necessitate the complete absence of disease, and that cure is not the ultimate intention of care. This is illustrated in mental health services where there has been a shift in its underlying philosophy from *curing* to *caring* and *comfort* (McCormick, 1999). According to McCormick, mental health services, especially those concerning individuals with persistent mental illness, are now considering indicators of

Exhibit 2.5: Active options—Health promotion in community recreation and park settings

Within a comprehensive rehabilitation framework, the transition from supervised outpatient rehabilitation to community health promotion programs and services is critical to the completion of the rehabilitative process. Successful transition ensures the likelihood of long-term compliance with the changes needed in one's lifestyle to regain and to maintain health. According to Payne, Orsega-Smith, Spangler, and Godbey (1999), the ideal recovery process, following a major health event (e.g., a heart attack), would be comprised of these stages:

1. Medical treatment for the health event (e.g., bypass surgery)
2. Clinical rehabilitation (e.g., outpatient physical therapy, occupational therapy, speech therapy)
3. Community based health promotion/disease prevention program (e.g., physical activity and social program sponsored by a local recreation and park department)
4. Recreation and park participation (e.g., participation in public recreation and park services)

Within this model, community recreation and park programs are well-positioned to provide a valuable and needed service to the larger health care system.

The nature of community agencies makes them an ideal setting for this step (i.e., *health promotion*) in the health care continuum. Besides being affordable, accessible, and attractive, local park and recreation agencies offer a wide variety of programs and facilities. [italics added] (Payne, Orsega-Smith, Spangler & Godbey, 1999, p. 74)

In addition to programs that promote physical activity (e.g., exercise, swimming, yoga, tai chi), many community recreation and park programs offer opportunities in other interest areas such as the arts, hobbies, trips, social clubs, and social events. Involvement in these broader activities may promote some physical activity but more likely they promote psychological outcomes, such as improved mood, that may lead to improved health.

For this reason, the National Recreation and Park Association (NRPA) is working with the Centers for Disease Control and Prevention and NIH's Heart, Lung and Blood Institute to illustrate to the medical and allied health professions how recreation and park agencies can be used for health promotion programs. Collaborating with researchers from Pennsylvania State University and staff from the Foothills, Colorado, Park and Recreation District, NRPA is involved in the evaluation of a senior wellness program called Active Options. Active Options staff have worked collaboratively with Kaiser Permanente and other health organizations to promote the program to their clients. Active Options includes fitness testing, adapted exercise classes, and individualized leisure counseling/advising as part of its affordable and accessible recreation program for senior citizens. Evaluation strategies target uncovering the program's value at promoting health and well-being among its participants. In-depth interviews, questionnaires, and physical testing reveal a variety of positive outcomes. Participants showed improvements in cardiovascular fitness, muscle strength, and flexibility. Their self-perceptions about health and their abilities to stay healthy improved. Participants also liked the convenience, low cost, and fun setting in which to interact with their peers (Orsega-Smith, Payne, Katzenmeyer & Godbey, 2000). Given its success, Active Options is being replicated in many recreation and park agencies across the country. This model can be extended to other groups that experience health risks. Such expansion creates opportunities for a collaborative health promotion work among TR and other recreation professionals.

improved life quality as treatment outcomes. For instance, the ability to use coping skills and community-based social supports are now acceptable as relevant quality of life outcomes for people with chronic mental illness.

The growing focus on quality of life within health and human service agencies is not at the neglect of health concerns. Rather, this increases an awareness of the complex relationship between quality of life and health. Health is often viewed as a determinant of quality of life, yet the quality of one's life (e.g., financial resources, access to care, self-enrichment opportunities, social support) also influences one's health. The interactive relationship between these two constructs requires that health and human service agencies focus on both health and quality of life as reciprocating outcomes of their services.

> Let us be honest with ourselves. We are not only interested in how well people can feed themselves or how independent they can be,

but also in how they feel about themselves and the world and how they will face themselves and that world. (Morris, 1994, p. 7)

Quality of life is also a matter of the individual in interaction with his or her environment. Thus life quality will be shaped by the opportunities and supports that exist in the physical and social environment, which enable clients to achieve and maintain physical health, a sense of belonging, and various personal aspirations that give meaning and purpose to life. **Exhibit 2.8** (p. 30) details a conceptual model developed by multidisciplinary researchers from the Quality of Life Research Unit at the Centre for Health Promotion (CHP), University of Toronto (Renwick & Brown, 1996). The CHP model attempts to describe the personal and environmental elements that contribute to life quality for all individuals. Three fundamental areas of life that are critical aspects of being human form the framework for the model: *being, belonging,* and *becoming.* This model offers TR practitioners and

Exhibit 2.6: Hardiness

The personality disposition *hardiness* was developed through the stress research conducted by psychologist Susanne Kobasa (1979) and her colleague Salvatore Maddi (Maddi & Kobasa, 1984). Hardiness is a psychological construct used to explain why some individuals thrive under conditions in which other individuals experience extreme stress and dysfunction.

Hardiness is comprised of three Cs: challenge, commitment, and control. Challenge refers to an outlook in which change is viewed as a challenge for new growth rather than a threat. Hardy individuals have a positive attitude toward change. Commitment refers to the investment of energy and effort in life, which results in feelings of engagement. It is an attitude of involvement in life, whether through work, family, or other forms of self-expression (e.g., leisure and recreation). Hardy people have a sense of commitment to solve problems. Control refers to the belief that individuals can utilize resources to handle problems as they arise and they can influence life outcomes. Hardy individuals tend to take charge of situations. Together, these three traits produce a "disease-resistant" personality that can ultimately influence whether an individual engages in health-promoting behaviors.

According to Maddi, hardiness can be developed through exercises that change one's perception of control. Rather than fretting about situations and events one cannot control, Maddi recommends selecting an area in one's life that can be controlled and that can be a source of personal growth. Often this is a leisure pursuit. The individual is guided in a process of focusing energies on new challenges, things they have never tried or never had time for. Involvement in these new activities challenges the individual and evokes feelings of commitment, confidence, and control thereby promoting hardiness. People who learn to incorporate the three Cs into their lifestyle reportedly experienced less anxiety, felt calmer, and had more energy. Scheduling time for things they never were able to do before makes life busier and the individual hardier (Kindy, 1998).

Witman (1999) also discussed the concept of hardiness and its relevance to TR practice. Witman suggested that TR programs could be developed to promote the three Cs and provide clients with opportunities to practice getting along with others, to encourage trust and cooperation, to facilitate the development of support networks, and to create a sense of commitment. Control can be incorporated into programming by offering clients choices and allowing them (when appropriate) opportunities to design, lead, and evaluate programs. Control can also be incorporated by providing opportunities for clients to identify, use, and develop their strengths. Challenge means that TR programming should include opportunities for novel experiences, tasks that involve risk and adventure, and a balance between clients' competence levels and the activity requirements.

researchers an integrative framework from which to explore leisure and recreation's contribution to quality of life for persons with and without disabilities. It is also a concrete way of conceptualizing relevant outcome areas for TR practice.

TR's Contribution to Quality of Life

The focus on quality of life issues within health and human service settings serves the TR discipline well. Quality of life has been a systematic theme addressed in TR practice (Wenzel, 1997). Numerous research studies have focused on the role of leisure in enhancing life satisfaction among individuals with disabilities (Bullock & Howe, 1991; Coyle, Lesnik-Emas & Kinney, 1994; Coyle, Shank, Kinney & Hutchins, 1993; Haight, 1992; Hawkins, 1993; Kinney & Coyle, 1992; Lee, 1990; Ross, 1993). Evidence exists throughout these studies that attitudes, perceptions, and beliefs about one's leisure, and the particular activities in which one engages influence quality of life. For instance, our research with Kinney and Hutchins highlighted the relationship between leisure involvement and life satisfaction in adults with secondary complications related to spinal cord injury. Those individuals who had acquired a disability and who reported the same or increased involvement in personal, family, and social leisure were more satisfied with their life than peers reporting declines in their leisure involvement since injury. Bullock and Howe (1991) reported similar findings in their research on the effect of transitional community-based leisure education and counseling. Participants showed "improved behavioral functioning, adjustment to disability, autonomy, and enhanced quality of life" as a result of the leisure education program (p. 16). Lee (1990) and Hawkins (1993) focused their research on the relationship between leisure involvement and life satisfaction among adults with developmental disabilities. Findings from these research studies supported an association between *leisure involvement* and life satisfaction. Other researchers have focused on the relationship between *leisure satisfaction* and life satisfaction (Allison, 1991; Haavio-Mannila, 1971; Kinney & Coyle, 1992; London, Crandall & Seals, 1977; Ragheb, 1993; Ragheb & Griffith, 1982; Trafton & Tinsley, 1980). In general, these studies found that leisure satisfaction was a strong predictor of life satisfaction.

The service and research focus on quality of life provides a foundation on which the discipline of TR

can build. As Pope and Tarlov (1991) suggest, "quality of life" is a unifying theme that can guide and organize disability-related research and facilitate cooperative relationships and service provision within and among medical and nonmedical disciplines.

*** • • •Thinking Trigger**

What do you think can be included as a quality of life outcome?   • • • ⚙

A System Perspective

It should be evident in the three conceptual shifts presented in Figure 2.1 (p. 15) that TR has tremendous opportunity to make important contributions to responsive and effective health and human services in the 21st century. However, in order to assume a viable role within health and human service agencies, it will be necessary for TR practitioners to adopt a system perspective. The Pew Commission (O'Neil & PHPC, 1998) stated that a system perspective was essential for competent practice in the 21st century. A *system* is a complex whole comprised of many interrelated parts that function together to give definition and meaning to the entity. A *system perspective* is being able to see how the overall functioning of the system is a result of the interaction between and among many distinct yet interconnected parts. This perspective is integrating rather than fragmenting. This view applies to our perspective of health and human services, and to the clients we serve.

For instance, throughout much of this chapter we have referred to the health and human service system, an entity comprised of multiple agencies, providers, consumers, payers, and policy makers. Therapeutic recreation, as a professional discipline and as a distinct set of services, is simply one part of the overall system. For TR to respond to changes, it will need to understand itself *in relation to* each of the other parts of the system. Likewise, consumers of health services need to be viewed as more than their biological selves. They too must be viewed holistically. Accordingly, TR can make helpful contributions to systems of care and the consumers of that care if the following points pertaining to a system perspective are understood.

- *Health care and human services are a complex whole comprised of health promotion and disease prevention as well as disease-oriented medical interventions.* The mix of services includes education-oriented services that can be empowering to clients in their quest to be responsible for their health and wellness. The extent to which intervention, health promotion, and disease prevention complement each other determines the overall quality of the system.

- *A complex mix of health and human service professionals, each having a distinct identity and purpose yet sharing a common mission, comprise the health and human service system. In addition, clients are now expecting to be included as members of the "team."* The extent to which these team members communicate, collaborate, and cooperate around their shared commitment to mutually desired goals will determine the overall effective functioning of the system.

- *Consumers of care must be viewed individually as a bio/psycho/social/spiritual system, whose health is a function of the interrelatedness of these multiple dimensions and the environment.* Failure to recognize the interrelatedness of these aspects of an individual results in fragmented and sometimes less successful and more costly care.

- *Human behavior and the relative quality of one's life must be viewed holistically. Holism represents a view of the person as a system interacting with his or her physical and social environment.* Accordingly, health and human services are aimed at creating conditions (e.g., opportunities and supports) that allow the person to achieve and maintain health and well-being.

Exhibit 2.7: Ed Roberts and the Independent Living Movement

In 1962 Ed Roberts quietly began a civil rights movement that would reshape the world for people with disabilities. Roberts, who was paralyzed as a result of polio, was beginning his studies at the University of California–Berkeley. Having convinced school and rehabilitation authorities to allow him to attend college, Roberts utilized paid attendants to assist him with activities of daily living, push his wheelchair, and assist him as he navigated the many architectural and environmental barriers on the Berkeley campus. By 1967 Roberts was joined in his studies at Berkeley by 11 other students with severe disabilities. Housed together on the third floor of the university's Cowell Hospital—the only university building with floors strong enough to support the weight of the 800-pound iron lung that Roberts used to help him breathe most hours of the day— the students called themselves the Rolling Quads.

In late night bull sessions on the hospital floor, Roberts and his friends, in wheelchairs and iron lungs, would strategize constantly about breaking down the common barriers they faced—from classrooms they could not get into to their lack of transportation around town—and dissect the protests for self-determination of minority students. (Shapiro, 1993, p. 48)

From the experiences and responses of this group, the Independent Living Movement was born. Shaprio (1993) details three important events occurring between 1968 and 1970 that dramatically influenced the formation of the Independent Living Movement. First, in 1968 California's Department of Rehabilitation began to run the dormitory on the third floor of Cowell Hospital as a formal program. A rehabilitation counselor tried to evict two students from the dormitory due to low grades. Roberts lead the Rolling Quads in a rebellion targeting university administrators and liberal Berkley students.

It was unfair, he argued, for the freewheeling campus to apply stricter rules of behavior to a pocket of disabled students. Thinking back to his own fight to get into Berkeley—and then the protest movements he had seen on campus—Roberts put in telephone calls to local newspapers, radio, and television stations. Within a few weeks, the counselor was reassigned. (Shapiro, 1993, p. 48)

Second, in 1969 the Rolling Quads battled with the city of Berkeley. As curb cuts were not yet a standard part of street design, Berkeley was renovating the main shopping street south of campus without including curb cuts in the design. Eight students with disabilities showed up in their wheelchairs at a city council meeting and won a commitment of $50,000 a year to ramp city streets so that they and others could move about freely.

Third, in 1970 the Physically Disabled Students Program (PDSP), a support group for students with disabilities, was established. Funded primarily by a grant from the Department of Health, Education, and

Summary

This chapter provided an overview of several shifts occurring in the conceptualization of health and their impact on service delivery within the health and human service system. This has included a shift from a disease-oriented biomedical approach to holistic and prevention-oriented approaches. Furthermore, there is a shift from viewing the client as only a passive recipient of care to someone who can share decision making and responsibility in the care process. Increasingly the ultimate outcome focus for the health and human service system is greater quality of life for its consumers. As these conceptual shifts unfold, contemporary health and human services become increasingly complex and require that professionals develop a system perspective in their work. As illustrated throughout the chapter, there is evidence that TR is compatible with these changing conceptualizations. Consequently, we contend that opportunities exist for TR to claim its rightful place in the fabric of health and human services—not as followers, but as leaders.

> By proactively embracing change, assuming advocacy roles, cooperating and coordinating, and promoting the benefits of therapeutic recreation in the health care puzzle, therapeutic recreation is virtually guaranteed to remain a vital component of consumers' well-being in the new millennium. (Carter, 1999, p. 25)

To ensure that we respond effectively to change and that we move practice forward in ways that shape change, we need a framework for guiding practice. That framework is a system perspective of individual clients and the process of psychosocial adaptation, the focus of the next chapter.

Exhibit 2.7: Ed Roberts and the Independent Living Movement (continued)

Welfare, PDSP was designed to assist students with disabilities to live independently. Designed by Roberts and his friends, the program primarily utilized people with disabilities as employees and provided students with disabilities assistance in finding accessible apartments, personal attendants, wheelchair maintenance and adaptive equipment design, student advocacy, and referral services.

The overwhelming success of the PDSP resulted in similar requests for assistance from individuals with disabilities who were not Berkeley students. In 1972 the Center for Independent Living (CIL) was incorporated. CIL was designed to work on the same principles as PDSP.

It would be run by disabled people; approach their problems as social issues; work with a broad range of disabilities; and make integration into the community its chief goal. Independence was measured by an individual's ability to make his own decisions and the availability of the assistance necessary—from attendants to accessible housing—to have such control. (Shapiro, 1993, p. 54)

The CIL started in Berkeley in 1972 has the distinction of being the first independent living center and remains one of the most active and thriving centers. The movement spread across the United States and in 1978 Congress allowed states to receive federal monetary support to operate independent living centers through Title VII of the Rehabilitation Act. The independent living movement represents the efforts of individuals with disabilities to organize, to become political, and to take greater control over their lives. Typically, independent living centers are guided by the following principles:

- Those who know best the needs of persons with disabilities and how to meet those needs are the individuals with disabilities themselves.

- The needs of the persons with disabilities can be met most effectively through comprehensive programs, which provide a variety of services.

- People with disabilities should be integrated as fully as possible into their community.

Four core services are provided to individuals with disabilities and their communities through independent living centers: information and referral, advocacy services, peer support, and independent living training (including financial management, safety, and attendant care). Today many independent living centers exist throughout the United States. These centers focus on consumer empowerment, independence, and inclusion. The centers and the individuals with disabilities that utilize them are a consumer force that health and human service agencies must recognize. They endorse a view of health and health care that emphasizes looking at the whole person in his or her environment (Shapiro, 1993).

Exhibit 2.8: The Centre for Health Promotion (CHP) Quality of Life Model

In the CHP model, quality of life is "the degree to which the person enjoys the important possibilities of his or her life" (Rootman et al., 1992, p. 23). The term "enjoyment" refers to the attainment of meaningful things (e.g., life goals, achievements, accomplishments) and the pleasure or satisfaction such attainment provides to the individual. The term "possibilities" refers to the opportunities and constraints that operate in a person's life as well as the balance between them. Possibilities may occur by chance (e.g., gender, genetics, parents' socioeconomic status) or by choice (e.g., decisions about how to spend time, money, join groups, eat, exercise). In the CHP model, "opportunities and constraints occurring by chance and by choice interact to produce the things that are possible in a person's life" (Renwick & Brown, 1996, p. 81). The CHP quality of life model focuses on the person's possibilities in three fundamental areas of life: being, belonging, and becoming.

Being is comprised of the most fundamental aspects of the person. *Physical being* is concerned with a person's health, nutrition, fitness, physical mobility, and hygiene. This category includes any aspect of a person's physical self. *Psychological being* refers to a person's emotional state. It is concerned with a person's feelings, cognitions, self-confidence, self-control, and ability to initiate positive behaviors. *Spiritual being* refers not to religion (although it does include religious beliefs) but to the personal values and standards by which a person lives.

Belonging reflects a person's social nature. *Physical belonging* pertains to the connectedness and acceptance that a person has in his or her physical environments (e.g., home, work, community). Aspects of this category include the amount of privacy and safety a person experiences in these environments as well as the freedom a person has to display their personal possessions in these environments. *Social belonging* focuses on meaningful relationships. It is concerned primarily with one's satisfaction with their relationships including familial and intimate relationships as well as friends, colleagues, coworkers, neighbors, and members of the community. *Community belonging* relates to an individual's connectedness to resources that are typically available in a community such as employment, housing, health care, social services, recreation, education, and other community programs or events.

Becoming is concerned with the attainment of personal goals, hopes, and dreams. *Practical becoming* refers to purposeful activities or routines that are done regularly. It includes housework, chores, employment, volunteer work, participation in school or other structured educational programs, and activity in which the individual searches for needed services such as health care or social services. *Leisure becoming* refers to the individual's involvement in leisure or recreation activities for pleasure. It includes activities that are brief, like involvement in a game or socializing with friends, or activities that span a longer time frame, like a vacation. While leisure is only explicit in the becoming dimension, we believe play, recreation and leisure activities are equally relevant as an opportunity for being and belonging. *Growth becoming* involves activities that promote the development of new skills, knowledge or capabilities in the individual, or allow the individual to adapt to changes in his or her life.

References

Allison, M. (1991). Leisure, sport and quality of life: Those on the fringes. In P. Oja and R. Telama (Eds.), *Sport for all* (pp. 45–55). New York, NY: Elsvier Science Publishers.

Brock, B. (1988). Effects of therapeutic horseback riding on physically disabled adults. *Therapeutic Recreation Journal, 22*(3), 34–43.

Bullock, C. C. and Howe, C. Z. (1991). A model therapeutic recreation program for the reintegration of persons with disabilities into the community. *Therapeutic Recreation Journal, 25*(1), 7–17.

Bullock, C. and Mahon, M. (1997). *Introduction to recreation services for people with disabilities. A person-centered approach.* Champaign, IL: Sagamore Publishing.

Carling, P. J. (1995). *Return to community building support systems for people with psychiatric disabilities.* Guilford Press: New York, NY.

Carter, M., 1999. Serving a brave new world. The millennium vision: Exploring the future of parks and recreation. *Parks & Recreation*, 20–25.

Coleman, D. and Iso-Ahola, S. (1993). Leisure and health: The role of social support and self-determination. *Journal of Leisure Research, 25*(2), 111–128.

Coyle, C., Lesnik-Emas, S., and Kinney, W. (1994). Predicting life satisfaction among adults with spinal cord injuries. *Rehabilitation Psychology, 39*(2), 95–112.

Coyle, C. and Santiago, M. (1995). Exercise and depression in adults with physical disabilities. *Archives of Physical Medicine and Rehabilitation, 76*, 647–652.

Coyle, C., Shank, J., Kinney, W., and Hutchins, D. (1993). Psychosocial functioning and changes in leisure lifestyle among individuals with chronic secondary health problems related to spinal cord injury. *Therapeutic Recreation Journal, 27*(4), 239–252.

Donatelle, R. and Davis, L. (1999). *Health: The basics* (3rd ed). Needham Heights, MA: Allyn & Bacon.

Donatelle, R., Snow-Harter, C., and Wilcox, A. (1995). *Wellness: Choices for health and fitness.* Reading, MA: Benjamin/Cummings Publishing.

Dubos, R. (1968). *So human the animal.* New York, NY: Scribners.

Eisenberg, D. M., Kessler, R. C., Foster, C., Norlock, F., Calkins, D., and Delbanco, T. (1993). Unconventional medicine in the United States. Prevalence, costs, and patterns of use. *New England Journal of Medicine, 328*, 246–252.

Green, J. (1989). Effects of a water aerobic program on the blood pressure, percentage of body fat, weight, and resting pulse rate of senior citizens. *Journal of Applied Gerontology, 8*(1), 132–138.

Grobe, J. (1995). *Beyond bedlam: Contemporary women psychiatric survivors speak out.* Chicago, IL: Third Side Press.

Haavio-Mannila, E. (1971). Satisfaction with family, work, leisure, and life among men and women. *Human Relations, 24,* 585–601.

Hafen, B., Karren, K., Frandsen, K., and Smith, L. (1996). *Mind, body, health.* Needham Heights, MA: Allyn & Bacon.

Haight, B. (1992). Long-term effects of a structure life review process. *Journal of Gerontology, 47,* 312–315.

Hawkins, B. (1993). An exploratory analysis of leisure and life satisfaction of aging adults with mental retardation. *Therapeutic Recreation Journal, 27*(2), 98–109.

Kindy, K. (1998, February 27). He professes to teach the weak to be strong: Some are "hardy" professor says. Others can learn. *The Philadelphia Inquirer,* p. E16.

Kinney, W. and Coyle, C. (1992). Predicting life satisfaction among adults with physical disabilities. *Archives of Physical Medicine and Rehabilitation, 73*(9), 863–869.

Kobasa, S. (1979). Stressful life events, personality, and health: An inquiry into hardiness. *Journal of Personality and Social Psychology, 37*, 1–11.

Kraus, R. (2000). *Leisure in a changing America: Trends and issues for the 21st century* (2nd ed.). New York, NY: Allyn & Bacon.

Lee, L. (1990). *Leisure involvement and the subjective well-being of young adults with mental retardation.* Unpublished doctoral dissertation, University of Illinois at Urbana-Champaign, Champaign.

London, M., Crandall, R., and Seals, G. W. (1977). The contribution of job and leisure satisfaction to quality of life. *Journal of Applied Psychology, 61*, 328–334.

Maddi, S. and Kobasa, S. (1984). *The hardy executive: Health under stress.* Chicago, IL: Dow Jones-Irwin Dorsey.

Mahon, M. and Bullock, C. (1992). Teaching adolescents with mild mental retardation to make decisions in leisure through the use of self-control techniques. *Therapeutic Recreation Journal, 27*(1), 9–25.

McCormick, B. (1999). Contributions of social support and recreation companionship to the life satisfaction of people with persistent mental illness. *Therapeutic Recreation Journal, 33*(4), 304–319.

McGuire, F., Boyd, R., and James, A. (1992). Therapeutic humor with the elderly. *Activities, adaptation and aging.* 17(1), 1–96.

Mettler, M. (1999). Past, present, and future of self-care. In K. Dychtwald (Ed.), *Healthy aging: Challenges and solutions,* (pp. 317–331). Gaithersburg, MD: Aspen.

Morris, J. (1994). Some cautions when using functional assessment scales. *Topics in Geriatric Rehabilitation, 9*(3), 2–7.

National Center for Complementary and Alternative Medicine. (2002). About NCCAM. Available online: http://www.NCCAM.nih.gov

O'Neil, E. H. and the Pew Health Professions Commission (December, 1998). *Recreating health professional practice for a new century: The 4th report of the Pew Health Professions Commission.* San Francisco, CA: Pew Health Professions Commission.

Orsega-Smith, B., Payne, L., Katzenmeyer, C., and Godbey, G. (2000). Community recreation and parks: The benefits of a healthy agenda. *Parks & Recreation, 35*(10), 69–74.

Payne, L., Orsega-Smith, E., Spanger, K., and Godbey, G. (1999, October). Local parks and recreation: For the health of it. *Parks & Recreation,* 34(10), 72–77.

Pope, A. and Tarlov, A. (1991). *Disability in America: Toward a national agenda for prevention.* Washington, DC: National Academy Press.

Ragheb, M. G. (1993). Leisure and perceived wellness: A field investigation. *Leisure Sciences, 15,* 13–24.

Ragheb, M. G. and Griffith, C. A. (1982). The contribution of leisure participation and leisure satisfaction to life satisfaction of older persons. *Journal of Leisure Research, 14,* 295–306.

Rancourt, A. (1991). An exploration of the relationships among substance abuse, recreation, and leisure for women who abuse substances. *Therapeutic Recreation Journal, 25*(3), 9–18.

Renwick, R. and Brown, I. (1996). The Centre for Health Promotion's conceptual approach to quality of life: Being, belonging, becoming. In R. Renwick, I. Brown, and M. Nagler (Eds.), *Quality*

of life in health promotion and rehabilitation: Conceptual approaches, issues, and applications (pp. 75–88). Thousand Oaks, CA: Sage Publications, Inc.

Renwick, R. and Friefeld, S. (1996). Quality of life and rehabilitation. In R. Renwick, I. Brown, and M. Nagler (Eds.), *Quality of life in health promotion and rehabilitation: Conceptual approaches, issues, and applications* (pp. 26–38). Thousand Oaks, CA: Sage Publications, Inc.

Rootman, I., Raphael, D., Shewchuk, D., Renwick, R., Friefeld, S., Garber, M., Talbot, Y., and Woodill, D. (1992). *Development of an approach and instrument package to measure quality of life of persons with developmental disabilities.* Toronto, ON: University of Toronto, Centre for Health Promotion.

Ross, J. (1993). *Young adults with recent spinal cord injuries: Transition from rehabilitation hospital to community living.* Unpublished doctoral dissertation, University of Illinois at Urbana-Champaign, Champaign.

Sable, J. R. and Gravink, J. (1999). Project PATH (Promoting Access Transition and Health): A health promoting intervention for people with spinal cord injuries. *ATRA Annual, 8,* 33–41.

Sable, J., Craig, P., and Lee, D. (2000). Promoting health and wellness: A research-based report. *Therapeutic Recreation Journal, 34*(4), 348–361.

Santiago, M., Coyle, C., and Kinney, W. (1993). Aerobic exercise effect on individuals with physical disabilities. *Archives of Physical Medicine and Rehabilitation, 74,* 1192–1198.

Shapiro, J. P. (1993). *No pity.* New York, NY: Times Books.

Simeonsson, R. and McDevitt, L. (1999). *Issues in disability and health: The role of secondary conditions and quality of life.* Chapel Hill, NC: University of North Carolina, FPG Child Development Center.

Terrill, C. (2000). A look ahead at the 21st century and how it may affect the brain injury community. *Brain Injury Source, 4*(1), 8–9.

Trafton, R. and Tinsley, H. (1980). An investigation of the construct validity of measures of job, leisure, dyadic and general life satisfaction. *Journal of Leisure Research, 12,* 34–44.

U.S. Department of Health and Human Services. (1979). *Healthy people: The Surgeon General's report on health promotion and disease prevention* (DHEW

Publication number 79-55071). Washington, DC: U. S. Department of Health, Education and Welfare.

U.S. Department of Health and Human Services. (1990). *Healthy people 2000: National health promotion and disease precaution objectives*. Washington, DC: U.S. Government Printing Office.

U.S. Department of Health and Human Services (1995). *Healthy people midcourse review and 1995 revisions.* Washington, DC: Author.

U.S. Department of Health and Human Services. (2000). *Healthy People 2010 (Conference Edition in Two Volumes)*. Washington, DC: U.S. Government Printing Office.

van Servellen, G. (1997). *Communication skills for the health care professional: Concepts and techniques*. Gaithersburg, MD: Aspen.

Weaver, S. (Ed.). (1999). *Holistic health promotion and complementary therapies: A resource for integrated practice*. Gaithersburg, MD: Aspen.

Wenzel, K. (1997). *Therapeutic recreation specialists: The quality of life professionals*. Ashburn, VA: National Recreation and Park Association.

Witman, J. (1999). Letters to the guest editors of the practice models series. *Therapeutic Recreation Journal*, 33(4), 342–343.

Chapter 3
Using a Client–System Perspective
to Guide Practice

Guided Reading Questions

After reading this chapter, you should be able to answer the following:

- What is the client–system perspective? Why is it important to the clinical practice of TR?
- What is psychosocial adaptation?
- What factors influence psychosocial adaptation?
- How do lifestyle, culture, and developmental stage influence psychosocial adaptation?
- What is an ecological perspective of disability? How does it influence psychosocial adaptation?
- What are some targets for TR interventions that can assist clients with the psychosocial adaptation process?

Introduction

The perspective TR professionals have toward their work and the clients they serve will influence their responses to various changes occurring in health care and human services. In the last chapter we suggested that a system perspective would help TR professionals understand their work in relation to all other parts of the service delivery system, thus increasing the chances for effective communication and collaboration with other service providers. Beyond that, a system perspective also applies to understanding clients, their health, and the relevance of TR interventions to the disability experience.

Along with a paradigm shift away from a purely medical model of health and health care, a newer model of human functioning and disablement has emerged. A revision to the *International Classification of Impairment, Disabilities, and Handicaps* (ICIDH–2) now reflects changes in health and human services and a new social understanding of disability (World Health Organization, 2001). This new classification, entitled the *International Classification of Functioning, Disability and Health* (ICF), is a biopsychosocial model of human functioning and disablement that offers a common framework for planning, managing, and evaluating services, and an international language for policy development and research.

This model (see **Figure 3.1**, p. 36) views human functioning and disablement as outcomes resulting from interactions between a person's health conditions and his or her physical and social environment. The full range of human functioning is conceptualized at three levels: the body or body part, the whole person, and the whole person in a social context. Disablement refers to dysfunctioning that may result from losses of bodily function, activity limitations, and restrictions to participation. Interventions, therefore, are needed at each of these levels. This includes rehabilitation services to improve and maintain functioning and preventive services that reduce participation restrictions by making environmental changes that accommodate activity limitations and equalize opportunities. (For more information on ICF, see http://www3.who.int/icf/icftemplate.cfm).

This chapter presents a system perspective of clients and the process of psychosocial adaptation, explaining much of the overall intent of the ICF model. First, we provide a holistic view of the client as a system. This includes the biological, psychological, social, and spiritual dimensions as interrelated parts comprising a whole person. We include developmental stage, culture, and lifestyle because they affect these dimensions of the person. Additionally, a client–system perspective incorporates the individual's environment as a significant determinant of health and life quality and thus a relevant target for interventions. Health and life quality of many clients are threatened by a combination of factors that include conditions within the client (e.g., activity limitations) and conditions external to the client (e.g., lack of social support). Addressing both individual and environmental factors is the essence of a system approach to health and rehabilitation services, and is consistent with the WHO's ICF model. Finally, we close the chapter with a discussion of psychosocial adaptation, which we consider to be a focal point for the work of all TR practitioners. *Psychosocial adaptation* is a process by which clients adjust to illnesses or disabling conditions and find an optimal fit between their needs and aspirations and the resources and opportunities within their environment.

Understanding the Client–System Perspective

The client–system perspective requires that you view a person holistically (see **Figure 3.2**). This perspective maintains that every individual is composed of numerous dimensions including the biological, psychological (including emotional and mental functioning), social, and spiritual dimensions. While each dimension is distinct, a client–system perspective maintains that no single dimension can be completely understood in isolation from the others. This holistic perspective appreciates the interrelationship and interdependence among all four dimensions of the person; yet, the essence and true meaning of an individual's health is more than simply the sum of these parts. Health, when

understood holistically, is best defined by the individual. Consequently, no matter what one's functional limitations may be, a personal sense of health and well-being can be quite high.

The client–system perspective also takes into consideration the influence of culture, development, and lifestyle on functioning and personal identity. Additionally, the client–system perspective involves appreciating the physical and social environment's impact on the individual's functioning, identity, expectations, and aspirations. The individual is understood as functioning within a larger social system comprised of family and friends, and other social, economic, political, religious, and health and human service institutions. As such, understanding the individual is incomplete without understanding the interaction the individual has with the social system. Together, these dimensions or subsystems have unlimited potential to interact with one another and to affect health and life quality.

Despite emerging paradigms of health discussed in Chapter 2, there is a tendency, particularly in medical healthcare, to view the dimensions of a client singularly rather than holistically. Often one dimension of the individual is emphasized over others. The educational preparation of the service provider and/or the orientation of the health and human service agency influence the area emphasized. For instance, in physi-

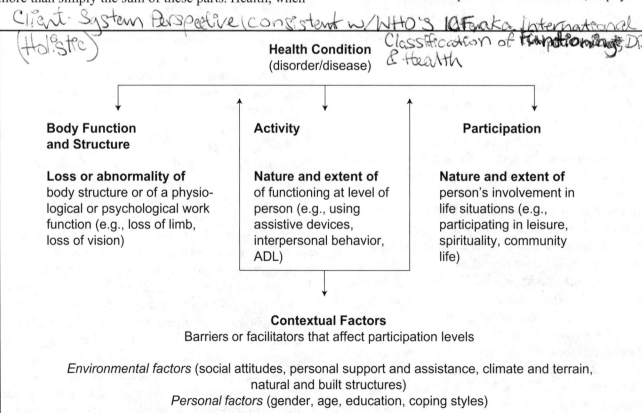

Figure 3.1: ICF model (Adapted from WHO, 2001)

cal rehabilitation facilities, there is a tendency to primarily focus on the disease process and the physical aspects of client care due to the long-standing influence of the medical model. This piecemeal approach to client care fragments the client and does not fully address the client's needs. Rarely does a physical problem fail to affect other aspects of the person's life. For this reason, a holistic or client–system approach to care is recommended.

Understanding the Bio/Psycho/Social/Spiritual Aspects of the Client–System Perspective

An individual's health and life quality is influenced by the interplay between biological, psychological, social, and spiritual factors. Biological factors can be thought of as those things that influence one's physical health. These might include things such as the body's size and shape, the relative health of the major body systems, body functioning, physical fitness levels, sensory acuity, and susceptibility to diseases and disorders. Psychological factors are those things that influence one's mental and emotional health. Mental health refers to the person's cognitive abilities and would include the person's ability to learn and to utilize intellectual capabilities. Emotional health deals with feelings related to self-esteem, trust, and love and would include the person's ability to express emotions appropriately. Social factors refer to the person's ability to have satisfying relationships with others, the ability to adapt to different social settings, and to develop and maintain a support system. Spiritual factors guide individuals in making sense of things that happen in their lives and finding meaning and value in life. Spirituality has been associated with a person's will to live, capacity to adjust to losses, or to deal with life's uncertainty. Spiritual beliefs may also include feelings of unity with nature or the universe or a person's beliefs about and relationships with supreme beings or organized religion. The spiritual beliefs of an individual become enfolded into that person's being and incorporate a person's values, meaning, and purpose in life (Dossey, 1997).

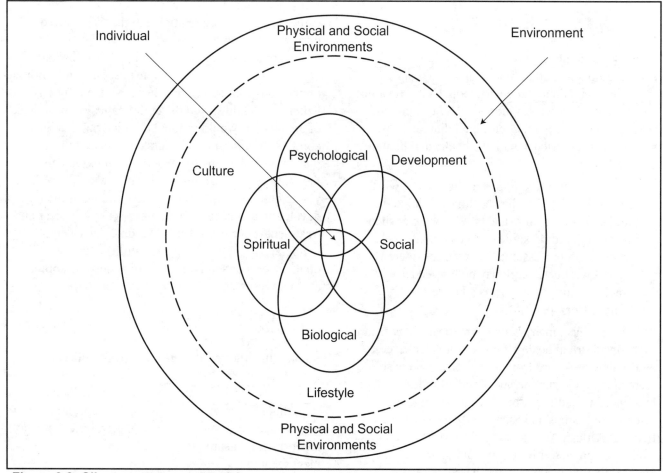

Figure 3.2: Client–system perspective

These four dimensions of a person are interdependent and interrelated. Because of the reciprocal interactions that occur among these dimensions, no two individuals will be alike. In terms of health and quality of life, each person's unique combination of biological, psychological, social, and spiritual dimensions will influence their perceptions of health, their experience of illness and recovery, and the meaning of disability, healing, leisure, and even death.

Understanding the Cultural, Developmental, and Lifestyle Aspects of the Client–System Perspective

The biological, psychological, social, and spiritual dimensions are not static. They are shaped by and expressed through one's culture, stage of development, and lifestyle behaviors (Figure 3.2). Consequently, health-related professionals must also be cognizant of these factors when assisting an individual to attain or maintain a state of wellness.

Culture

The cultural dimension refers to the values, beliefs, and behaviors that an individual has as a result of identification with a particular group. Cultural values and beliefs will affect an individual's behavior and reaction to different situations, including one's perspective and experience with the health and human service system.

> Culture determines, in part, beliefs about what constitutes illness, when health care should be sought and by whom, and how to behave when sick or injured. In some cultures, seeking help from health professionals may be considered a sign of weakness, or it may be viewed as a practice to be taken only as a last resort. (Falvo, 1999, p. 87)

For instance, many Native Americans may tend to first consult tribal healers for health-related issues before they seek care from a physician. Likewise, recreation and leisure behavior and attitudes are also influenced by culture. Consider the findings from the research of Stamps and Stamps (1985), which identified that African Americans tend to participate in similar leisure activities throughout their adult life and are heavily involved in church-based recreation. In

contrast, Caucasians tend to participate in a larger number of novel recreation activities. Questions have also been raised about the suitability of recreation as a purposeful rehabilitation intervention for diverse cultures. McIntosh (1986) found distinctions among African American, American Indian, and Latino/Mexican American inmates in terms of their attitude toward a rehabilitative recreation program. Only African American inmates expressed acceptance of the recreation interventions being facilitated. American Indian and Latino/Mexican inmates expressed nonacceptance of the activities because the recreation interventions did not match their lifestyle and values (Peregoy & Dieser, 1997).

Development

The developmental dimension refers to the point at which a client is in his or her lifecycle. Development will influence a person's experience of health and illness, as well as recovery and healing. This occurs in two ways. First, a health crisis or acquired disability can disrupt the individual's attainment of developmental tasks. For instance, a health problem may interfere with developmental tasks associated with friendship formation among children, or the aspirations for a career or an intimate relationship that is expected during young adulthood.

Second, the stage of the lifecycle will also influence the biological, psychological, social, and spiritual dimensions themselves. For instance, the religious beliefs of a child would differ dramatically from those of an adult, as would rational thinking and intellectual abilities. A child might understand illness to be a punishment, perhaps from God, for thinking bad thoughts or other wrongdoing. Thus, working with young children requires an understanding of their developmental capacities to make sense of illness and treatment procedures. Likewise, an elderly person may deliberately emphasize spiritual fulfillment over all other aspects of self and this choice must be appreciated and respected.

Lifestyle

Finally, the lifestyle dimension refers to the constellation of day-to-day behaviors of the individual that can promote or impede health and wellness. It includes such things as eating and sleeping patterns, amount of physical activity, substance use (e.g., tobacco, alcohol, other drugs), leisure involvement, and stress management techniques.

Lifestyle can have an enormous impact on the prognosis for adopting health behaviors. One's lifestyle is typically an engrained pattern of living that is not easily changed. Consider, for instance, a 60-year-old man being treated for a cardiovascular accident (CVA). His premorbid lifestyle was characterized by minimal socialization outside of his work setting, no physical exercise, and weekend leisure-time devoted primarily to television viewing. Thus, a recreation therapist would want to recognize that making recommendations to be more physically active would be insufficient to effect behavioral changes given his premorbid lifestyle.

Further Comments on Development and Culture

Development and culture are critical elements in the client–system perspective because they influence a client's lifestyle as well as psychosocial adaptation. Unfortunately, their influence on individuals' lifestyle behaviors and attitudes toward health, recreation, and recovery is often overlooked. Therefore, a more extensive discussion of these elements in the client–system perspective is warranted.

Developmental Theory and Life Stage Perspective

Models of human development illustrate the typical issues, problems, and potential challenges that people face throughout their life span. Each developmental period or stage preoccupies the individual with needs and expectations that are typically linked to social expectations and responsibilities. Such knowledge is fundamental to effective TR practice. Understanding developmental theory helps to anticipate potential intervention needs of individuals at different life stages. It serves not only as a guideline for assessing an individual's functional abilities, but also as a guideline for determining potential environmental stressors, whether they be intrapersonal, interpersonal, or extrapersonal in nature (e.g., onset of a disabling condition or chronic illness, moving to a new living environment such as a nursing home). With this knowledge, TR practitioners are better able to use intervention strategies that are based on the client's stage of development, and to design suitable interventions that can minimize the effect of developmental stressors and assist clients in maintaining a sense of health and wellness.

For example, adolescents will struggle with separation and individuation. They seek more independence. Therefore, being confined to a hospital bed or having limited capacity to take care of themselves will create some internal conflict. Similarly, acquiring a disability during adulthood may threaten a person's ability to continue with parenting responsibilities or earning a living through work. TR practitioners must realize these important developmental issues and present recreation and leisure to clients in ways that make it relevant to their developmental concerns and the adaptation process. Thus, providing adolescents with a place to have "space" from parents and other figures that represent control, or teaching a parent who has acquired a disability how to recreate with their children despite their physical limitations are examples of developmentally sensitive TR practice.

It should be noted, however, that many developmental theories portray "typical" patterns of development. Classical theories of human development (e.g., Piaget, Erikson) represent stage theories (see **Table 3.1,** p. 40 and **Table 3.2,** p. 41). These stages are presumed to be normative and found across the human species. These explanations of development reflect a biological or ontogenetic view. They assume a set of consistent, predictable changes across the life span.

There are, however, other influences on human development. Mannell and Kleiber (1997), citing the work of Baltes, Cornelius, and Nesselroade (1980), describe how significant historical events within one's life course can shape development and subsequent leisure behavior. For instance, they point to evidence that people who grew up during the Depression place less value on leisure, and tend to justify any right they have to it by using their leisure productively. Mannell and Kleiber also refer to the influence of unexpected life events on human development. For instance, the loss of a parent or spouse early in the life course or acquiring a disability can have a significant effect on attitudes and behavior. The capacity to respond to social expectations may be altered dramatically by significant life events and challenge the notion of a "normative" course of development. Consider the heroic reception received by World War II veterans compared to the social rejection that many Vietnam veterans experienced and how it may have influenced Vietnam veterans' thoughts about assuming civic and social responsibilities immediately after the war.

Finally, Mannell and Kleiber point out that the array of lifestyles that exist today reflects diverse developmental paths. These may reflect differences in gender, sexual identity, and cultural backgrounds.

Popular developmental models (e.g., Erikson, Levinson) have been criticized as being androcentric and ethnocentric—they apply to the experience of boys and men only and have not been established as valid theories for different cultures. Therefore, it is also important to remember that one's gender and culture can have a bearing on the significance of certain developmental milestones. For example, the meaning ascribed to physical changes associated with puberty, or the expectations for children to serve as surrogate parents to their siblings may be an acceptable and expected event in only certain cultures and communities.

Having a developmental perspective is necessary if operating from a client–system and psychosocial perspective. This is why the certification standards from the National Council on Therapeutic Recreation Certification (NCTRC) require coursework in human development as an educational prerequisite for all Certified Therapeutic Recreation Specialists (CTRS). A developmental perspective requires that, in addition to traditional and well-referenced theories of development, TR practitioners should leave open the possibil-

 • • •Thinking Trigger

What significant life events of your generation have influenced the course of your development and subsequent views about health and leisure behaviors? What impact might exposure to violence, sexual promiscuity, and AIDS have on the leisure and recreation attitudes and behaviors of youth?

• • •

ity that clients may have a unique developmental path. While clients share common developmental issues shaped by changing physical, cognitive, social, and emotional capacities, each has a unique developmental path shaped by historical events, unexpected life circumstances, and cultural heritage. The individual's course of development will influence identity, attitudes, beliefs, needs, and expectations.

Table 3.1: Erikson's (1963) Psychosocial Theory of Development

---

Trust vs. Mistrust (infancy: 0–1 yrs.)
- Child is challenged to develop a basic sense of trust in the world and assurance that needs will be met

Autonomy vs. Shame/Doubt (early childhood: 1–3 yrs)
- Child is challenged to develop a sense of being able to meet demands placed upon him or her while asserting his or her own will in exploring the world

Initiative vs. Guilt (preschool: 3–5 yrs)
- Child is challenged to develop a sense of his or her own ability to initiate action and learn self-restraint

Industry vs. Inferiority (elementary school: 6–11 yrs.)
- Child is challenged to learn cultural values such as loyalty, industriousness, responsibility, and to develop sense of personal competence

Identity vs. Role Confusion (adolescence: 12–19 yrs.)
- Adolescent is challenged to make choices and commitments in developing a future path in a complex world

Intimacy vs. Isolation (young adulthood: 20+ yrs.)
- Adult is challenged to reconcile sense of identity and independence with need to develop intimate, sharing relationships with others

Generativity vs. Stagnation (middle adulthood)
- Adult is challenged to guide and protect the future of humankind, to become community-minded and less self-focused

Ego Integrity vs. Despair (late adulthood)
- Adult is challenged to face limits and losses associated with aging and mortality and to reflect on the shape of his or her life in attempt to reconcile feeling regarding mortality

Culture

Berger (1995) defines culture as a pattern of beliefs, values, and behaviors that are socially transmitted from one generation to the next through spoken and written word and through the use of certain objects, customs and traditions. Culture influences all aspects of one's life (e.g., political, social, educational, financial). Each person, therefore, has a cultural identity and in many instances multiple cultural memberships. Race, nationality, ethnicity, or religion are usually identified as the basis of cultural groups. However, one should not forget that other individual characteristics such as gender, sexual orientation, social class, geographic location, or physical ability may influence cultural identity (Sheldon & Dattilo, 1997).

The relevance of multiculturalism to TR practice is not only noted in those aspects of culture that would affect how a client may respond to services, but also in the unique way that culture influences each client's leisure/recreation interests and participation patterns. Peregoy and Dieser's (1997) discussion of multicultural issues suggests that recreation therapists must understand differences in their client's behavior, values, and attitudes that arise as a result of cultural influences. For instance, some cultures have experienced a history of oppression and discrimination in which policies and procedures were used as a control mechanism. Individuals from such cultures may have difficulty trusting the motives and recommendations made by individuals of other cultures and may, therefore, question whether the health care provider's recommendations are truly in their best interest (Falvo, 1999).

Table 3.2: Piaget's (1952) Cognitive Theory of Development

Sensorimotor (0–2 yrs.)
- Intentional exploration of the world through sensory experiences and motor actions
- Progression from reflexive instinctual action to beginning of symbolic thought (i.e., being able to look at object and imagine manipulating it before doing so)
- Emerging ability to understand that objects still exist even when not in view (object permanence)
- Self-centered (egocentric) focus with clear display of likes and dislikes

Preoperational (2–7 yrs.)
- Thought process is largely prelogical (intuitive) and egocentric (i.e., inability to distinguish own thoughts and perspective from someone else's)
- Ability to think symbolically is evident in pretend play and representational acts like drawing and language (e.g., a stick is a sword; child is mommy and the doll is baby)
- Solitary play slowly advances toward greater awareness and inclusion of others
- Reasoning or judging right and wrong is based on consequences of action, not intentions

Concrete Operations (7–11 yrs.)
- Rules are observed but little agreement exists on what are the rules
- Mental actions about real concrete objects are reversible, and the properties of objects can be classified (e.g., relatives comprise a "family tree") and are understood in relation to each other (e.g., a mom can be a woman, mother, and parent)
- Logical reasoning replaces intuitive thought but cannot be applied to hypothetical or abstract problems
- Able to infer intentionality and wonder about the motives of others

Formal Operations (after 11–12 yrs.)
- Able to apply logic to all stages of problems including concrete, hypothetical, and future-oriented scenarios
- Advanced language skills are reflected in use of metaphors (i.e., an implied comparison between two ideas conveyed by an abstract meaning—a piece of glass is like love because both can be shattered)
- Tendency to reduce all reasoning to what is logical thereby creating conflicts between ideals and reality
- Codification of rules, agreement as to what rules are, willingness to change rules by consensus
- Moral reasoning considers both intentions and circumstances

Adult Cognitive Development
- Piaget's Theory of Cognitive Development does not extend past 15 years of age. Piaget thought that knowledge continued to be acquired during adult years, but not intelligence, which is according to him, the ability to solve new problems.

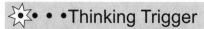

• • •Thinking Trigger

Has your cultural background influenced
your views on health or recreation? **• • •**

Additionally, Peregoy and Dieser also suggest that TR practitioners must examine their own cultural biases as well as those that exist in the conceptual foundations of TR practice. They argue that TR is a profession that operates predominately from a Western worldview that values individualism. Focusing their argument on the construct of independence in TR research and functional independence in TR practice, these authors suggest that TR's emphasis on independence may create conflict when working with clients from different cultural groups that do not value independence and individualism. Defined as "collectivist cultures," such cultures emphasize the goals of one's group (often the family) over the goals of the individual (Myers, 1993). According to Peregoy and Dieser, TR practitioners should be cognizant of this differing value orientation when working with clients from minority groups that traditionally orient towards collectivism, including American Indians, Mexican Americans and Latinos, Asian Americans, and African Americans. While there is a legitimate basis for Peregoy and Dieser's challenge to the TR discipline, having a client–system perspective will help practitioners to appreciate the influence of culture and practice in a culturally

sensitive manner. (Cultural competence is addressed further in Chapter 10.)

Understanding the Environmental Aspects of the Client–System Perspective

An understanding of the client–system perspective is incomplete without consideration of the physical and social environment. The client–system approach maintains that the client is an "open" system. This implies that environmental forces, which can be either physical or social or both, can influence the client's state of wellness. In **Figure 3.2** (p. 37), the broken circle surrounding the bio/psycho/social/spiritual dimensions depicts this open aspect of the client–system. The environment may support or weaken the client's capacity to achieve and maintain health or wellness. An environment that has inadequate resources is obviously detrimental and stressful, whereas an environment with consistent and reliable resources serves a major role in supporting and maintaining health. Because the client is viewed as an open system, the client both influences and is influenced by the environment.

To view individuals from the client–system perspective and to aid them in the process of psychosocial adaptation requires that TR practitioners examine

Exhibit 3.1: Environmental supports: Focus on community

Craig Rehabilitation Hospital in Denver developed the ***Therapeutic Recreation Community Liaison Program*** (TRCL) for clients with traumatic brain injury. The recreation therapist in charge of the TRCL program is responsible for a multidimensional facilitation approach focused on transition and community involvement (Baker-Roth, McLaughlin, Weitzenkemp & Womeldorff, 1995). TRCL works with local community agencies to assist with the greater inclusion of clients with brain injuries into community recreation programs. Service providers receive consultation and education from TRCL regarding the cognitive limitations and necessary supportive techniques that providers can use when clients with brain injuries seek to be involved in programs at the agency. They also help clients identify, locate and use recreation opportunities at these agencies. This liaison process is instrumental in minimizing barriers that are deterrents to health-promoting behaviors.

Reintegration through Recreation (RTR) was developed by the Center for Recreation and Disabilities Studies in the Curriculum for Leisure Studies and Recreation Administration at the University of North Carolina at Chapel Hill for individuals with severe and persistent mental illness. The program offered individualized therapeutic recreation services using the individual's community. RTR staff worked with clients preparing to leave the hospital and with clients already residing in their community. Clients in the RTR program worked with a CTRS to establish individualized goals. The CTRS then met individually with clients on a weekly basis to facilitate learning while doing. Often sessions focused on discussing client's independent follow-through (or lack there of) on self-selected recreation activities, supporting the client during actual community activity participation, developing life skills of relevance to the client, and evaluating these new experiences. The ultimate outcome of these services was to increase community integration and life quality.

environmental issues that may be unique to the individual. Assistance must be offered to the person to deal with barriers that impede his or her functioning in a variety of environmental contexts, including the home and the community at large. According to Renwick, Brown, and Nagler (1996), health and rehabilitation professionals "need to accord more attention than they currently do to such environmental issues as social support, access to vocational and leisure programs and services, and attitudes toward disability" (p. 29) since such issues are as important, and perhaps even more important than personal characteristics in the adjustment process.

An Ecological Perspective

Understanding the client in relation to his or her environment is also known as having an ecological perspective. According to Howe-Murphy and Charboneau (1987), the ecological perspective is a generic model, or way of thinking about the nature and scope of professional practice. An ecological perspective maintains that people are in constant transaction with their physical and social environment in an effort to adjust, adapt, and to have a sense of balance. The end result of successful transactions would be identity, autonomy, competence, and relatedness. All of these outcomes are hallmark indicators of health and wellness. While a traditional medical model approach to health and rehabilitation assumes the locus of change to be within the client, an ecological approach recognizes the impact of environmental factors in a client's capacity to achieve and maintain health and life quality. **Exhibit 3.1** describes two TR interventions, the Therapeutic Community Liaison program and the Reintegration through Recreation program. Both are directed at facilitating adjustment via the provision of community-based environmental supports.

Therapeutic recreation practice has traditionally understood the importance of the physical and social environment to the health and well-being of people. Howe-Murphy and Charboneau (1987) defined therapeutic recreation as "a planned process of intervention directed toward specific environmental or individual change" (pp. 9–10). While these authors specifically mentioned environmental intervention in their definition of TR, Bullock and Mahon (1997) maintained that virtually all definitions of TR imply the importance of the environment in understanding clients and in assisting them to achieve and maintain health and life quality. They refer to this as a *contextualized* approach to practice. "The contextualized process is one that

takes into consideration who a person is, where she has come from, where she is returning, and what her support systems are" (Bullock & Mahon, 1997, p. 382). TR practitioners can impact a person's health and life quality by focusing on the environment. For instance, the level of social contact and support that comes from family and friends directly affects a client's health and life quality. Awareness of the detrimental effect of dysfunctional, overstressed, or overburdened support systems on the health and life quality of individuals with disabilities has led to programs designed specifically for caregivers. **Exhibit 3.2** describes a role for TR practitioners within such programs.

TR practitioners also need to be especially attentive to the assets and limitations associated with clients' homes and communities. This is particularly important in terms of opportunities for play, recreation, and leisure. Such is the case when TR practitioners work

Exhibit 3.2: Environmental supports: Focus on family

An emerging focus of TR research and model demonstration projects is caring for the caregiver. Due to the ever-increasing cost of health care and the restrictive nature of health care coverage, the number of family members who function as primary caregivers for chronically ill relatives is growing rapidly. The burden on caregivers is more than economic; the health and well-being of the caregiver is compromised. Bedini and Guinan (1996) provide a compelling argument for the leisure needs of family caregivers, and the opportunities for TR to respond. Caregivers have reported numerous losses resulting from the expectations and demands of caregiving, including loss of time for oneself, loss of opportunities for socializing with friends, and a general loss of interest in all activities. Of particular interest to these researchers is the dramatic decline in caregiver leisure. Based on the recommendations of professional focus groups, Bedini and Phoenix (1999) proposed a leisure wellness program for caregivers consisting of four interrelated units: resource identification and utilization, leisure education, stress management, and mental and physical wellness (e.g., time management, social support, coping, problem solving). This program encourages caregivers to care for themselves and pursue their own recreation involvement to decrease their stress. In turn, greater support for caregivers can have secondary benefits for their loved ones.

with pediatric clients. **Exhibit 3.3** describes the national toy-lending program, LEKOTEK, which can be used by recreation therapists to create productive home environments for their pediatric clients.

Another reason TR practitioners need to be attentive to environmental issues in the home is the increasing prevalence of excess disability. Excess disability is used to describe the condition of a client whose impairment is greater than expected for the specific disease process (Katsinas, 1998). Excess disability "encompasses a decline of functional abilities, alertness, cognitive status, orientation, communication, physical status and socialization attributed to the environment and not specifically the disease process" (p. 311). This phenomenon has gained significant attention and seems to be more prevalent among individuals who live with chronic illnesses and disabilities. Interventions directed at reducing excess disability aim to modify the physical environment and to reeducate significant others within the individual's social environment so that an individual's functioning is consistent with or better than what would be expected for a particular disease process. At Home with the A.R.T.S, a home-based recreation program for clients with Alzheimer's disease is described in **Exhibit 3.4**. *At Home with the A.R.T.S.* strives to reduce excess disability by infusing the home environment with recreation activities (Daly, 2002).

The Client–System Perspective Summarized

The client–system perspective is a multidimensional model that allows practitioners to understand and describe the complex nature of an individual's identity, health, and well-being. Clients are viewed holistically, comprised of biological, psychological, social, and spiritual dimensions. They are also understood to be an open system in constant transaction with the physical and social environment. These transactions shape behavior as do culture, development, and daily lifestyles. This reciprocal exchange not only affects behavior but it also influences attitudes and beliefs about health, recover, disability, and leisure. Thus, TR practitioners have the mission of ensuring that play, recreation, and leisure contributes to each dimension of the individual in their quest for health and life quality. This perspective can be used as a guide for designing and delivering interventions when a client's health is threatened and there is a need for assistance in coping with and adapting to illness and disabling conditions. These interventions would target the entire client–system, including the environment.

Promoting Psychosocial Adaptation

Therapeutic recreation interventions aim to help people restore and maintain an optimal level of health to have the capacity to experience quality of life. Restoring and

Exhibit 3.3: Creating productive environments

When an ecological assessment suggests that appropriate play opportunities in the home are lacking, pediatric recreation therapists can refer parents to LEKOTEK, a national toy-lending program for families of children with disabilities. LEKOTEK offers parents and children a chance to try out various developmentally appropriate toys. Many battery-operated toys are modified by LEKOTEK staff using adaptive switches that allow for independent play. Attentiveness to such environmental constraints and appropriate interventions and referrals often results in an increase in the actual play and recreation experiences within households, and reportedly, a reduction in stress for all family members.

Exhibit 3.4: Building environmental supports

At Home with the A.R.T.S. (Alzheimer's Recreation Therapy Services) is a home-based recreation intervention program designed for people with Alzheimer's disease or related disorders and who cannot attend adult day care. Clients and their caregivers participate in weekly recreation activities in their home conducted by a CTRS. Clients' interests, abilities, and resources are determined by an in-home assessment and the CTRS designs activities that are consistent with the assessment findings. Particular attention is paid to the physical and social environment. The CTRS also provides educational sessions for clients' caregivers. These sessions teach caregivers about music, movement, and recreation activities that can be utilized with their significant other. Caregivers are also given assistance to purchase materials suited to the abilities of their loved one. The intent of the program is to minimize the occurrence of excess disability by providing physical (e.g., equipment) and social support (e.g., information and guidance) for caregivers.

maintaining one's health and life quality involves engaging clients in the process of psychosocial adaptation. Often recreation therapists encounter clients who are in the midst of a health crisis, either brought about by an acute illness or the challenges of rehabilitation. At other times, while the immediate health crisis may be past, clients are at risk for diminished health and well-being due to internal and external stressors related to coping and adapting to chronic illness or disabling conditions. For some clients this means improving physical or cognitive functioning (e.g., recovering from a stroke) while for others it means adapting to the constraints imposed by the environment (e.g., relocating to a nursing home). No matter what the precipitating circumstances are to providing interventions, having a client–system perspective is essential to facilitating the process of psychosocial adaptation.

Defining Psychosocial Adaptation

Psychosocial adaptation is defined within disability literature as an evolving process whereby individuals find a suitable and comfortable fit between personal needs and aspirations and the resources and opportunities available in their environment. According to Livneh and Antonak (1997) psychosocial adaptation is

an evolving, dynamic, general process through which the individual gradually approaches an optimal state of person-environment congruence manifested by (1) active participation in social, vocational, and avocational pursuits; (2) successful negotiation of the physical environment; (3) awareness of remaining strengths and assets as well as existing functional limitations. (p. 8)

It does not imply that individuals are "cured" necessarily, or that illnesses or impairments no longer exist. Rather, the process of psychosocial adaptation means that, even for those who continue to need on-going medical or other specialty care, things valued and important to the individual (which were lost or perceived as lost) are recovered. This idea of *recovery* has been used most recently in relation to individuals with chronic mental illness, but it has relevance to others who are coping and adapting to physical disabilities and other functional limitations. According to Ragins (2000), losses that people experience as a result of a health crisis or disability can be grouped into three broad categories of recovery:

- *Functions may be recovered*—as in the ability to read, to sleep restfully, to walk, to work, to have coherent conversations, to make love, to raise children, to drive a car, to go fishing
- *External things may be recovered*—as in an apartment, a job, friends, playing in a band, a spouse, a car, family relationships, a stereo, a TV, educational programs
- *Internal states can be recovered*—as in feeling good about oneself, peace, self-identity other than disability, responsibility for oneself, optimism, hopefulness

For some individuals these possessions, competencies, or internal states may not have existed before. Yet they may represent reasonable expectations for a meaningful life that ought to be aspired to despite the existence of functional limitations. Psychosocial adaptation is a *process of recovery* in which individuals find a *balance between their needs and aspirations* and the *resources and opportunities* provided in their environment. For example, young people who acquire spinal cord injuries as a result of skiing accidents often feel that they will never again participate in their former high-risk active sports. They are often amazed when a recreation therapist shows them exciting possibilities for participating in wheelchair sports or activities like adapted skiing or scuba diving.

Based on a review of several models of psychosocial adaptation, Livneh and Antonak (1997) categorized common conceptual features associated with psychosocial adaptation into four areas, displayed in **Figure 3.3** (p. 46) Elements in Class 1, Class 2, and Class 3 represent the *psychological dimension* of the adaptation process. Elements in Class 4 represent the *social dimension* involved in adaptation. (Hence, the term *psychosocial adaptation*.) Variables in Class 1 (disability-related), Class 2 (sociocultural and demographic-related) or Class 3 (personality and behavioral attributes) interact with elements from the variables in Class 4 (physical and social environment) to affect the speed, course, and degree of psychosocial adaptation seen in individuals. Consequently, the interaction of these four classes of variables results in wide variations in psychosocial adaptation among individuals who are recovering from a health crisis or adapting to a disability.

Livneh and Antonak's (1997) classification scheme can be used to help you understand the complex process of psychosocial adaptation. This scheme can also be used as a guide to aid in developing appropriate interventions and research studies on psychosocial adaptation. You can see how the classification scheme incorporates all of the variables presented in the section on the client–system perspective. Bio/psycho/social/spiritual aspects are considered in Livneh and Antonak's classification scheme, as are cultural, developmental, lifestyle, and environmental influences. Thus understanding and facilitating psychosocial adaptation via this model is consistent with the client–system approach to TR practice.

Variable Interactions in the Psychosocial Adaptation Process

While Livneh and Antonak (1997) divide the factors influencing the psychosocial adaptation process into discreet categories, they also recognize that these variables influence one another and the subsequent adjustment process. They provide the following example to explain the interaction effect they are proposing in their model.

Two individuals with similar physical disabilities (e.g., little variation among Class 1 variables) could conceivably show widely differing patterns of psychosocial adaptation to their condition

because of differing interactions among the variables in Class 2 (e.g., upper vs. lower socioeconomic status), Class 3 (e.g., use of active vs. use of passive coping modes) or Class 4 (e.g., social isolation vs. close family network). (Livneh & Antonak, 1997, p. 432)

Livneh and Antonak also identify how two different individuals, who may have different disabling conditions (e.g., Parkinson's disease, spinal cord injury), may experience a very similar psychosocial adaptation process due to similarities in Class 2, 3, and 4 variables (e.g., age of onset, personal values, socioeconomic status, family support, accessible home environments).

A similar pattern of interaction among these variables can be used to explain the widely varying psychosocial adaptation results seen within behavioral healthcare. For instance, two individuals with the same diagnosis of schizophrenia may display very different adaptation patterns as a result of differences in Class 2 (e.g., young adulthood vs. middle age), Class 3 (e.g., active vs. passive coping style) and Class 4 (e.g., employed vs. unemployed, family support vs. no support) variables.

Similar examples of the interactions among these categories and their subsequent effect on the psychoso-

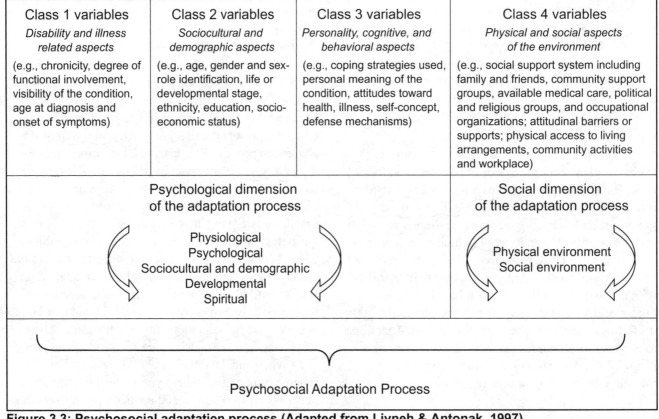

Figure 3.3: Psychosocial adaptation process (Adapted from Livneh & Antonak, 1997)

cial adjustment process could be developed for clients in any TR service setting. Regardless of diagnosis or service setting, the degree and speed of psychosocial adaptation that a client attains is linked to interactions among the variables in each category. Furthermore, clients' attitudes, beliefs, and behavior in relation to play, recreation, and leisure will be shaped by these myriad variables as well. Understanding the psychosocial adaptation process necessitates a client–system approach to practice whereby TR interventions are personalized and contextualized rather than simply selected based on the client's diagnostic label.

Facilitating Psychosocial Adaptation through TR Interventions

To assist clients with the psychosocial adaptation process, TR practitioners can develop primary, secondary, and tertiary interventions aimed at both the person and their environment. These interventions are relevant to all TR practitioners regardless of service setting. In addition to helping clients improve specific physical, cognitive, social, or affective skills, interventions would also help clients cope and adapt to changes brought about by functional limitations. Interventions could include teaching clients appropriate coping skills needed to buffer stress and to function in the community. Interventions could also focus on knowledge acquisition. Such interventions would target clients' perceptions about their disability and its impact on their lifestyle. Examples include client education groups focused on providing accurate information about health conditions, explaining the role of physically and socially active recreation in preventing secondary health conditions or the recurrence of symptoms, and exploring the use of assistive devices and self-management skills for recreation involvement. Interventions could also target modification in the physical and social environment such as family education about recreation and leisure strategies. For example, a program called "Sober Olympics" teaches recreation skills to people in recovery and their families as part of a weekend recreation program.

Summary Comments on Psychosocial Adaptation

The process of psychosocial adaptation is a framework around which all TR practice can converge, whether one works in acute care, hospice care, assisted-living centers, behavioral healthcare, physical medicine, community recreation agencies, independent living centers, group homes, or nursing homes. It has relevance to TR practice that is primarily aimed at restoring functional capacities as much as it does to TR practice that is aimed at maintaining healthy lifestyles through physically and socially active leisure involvement. All TR practice is directed at helping clients recover actual or perceived losses (including lost opportunities such as inclusive community living experiences). Ultimately all TR practice is directed at psychosocial adaptation and its outcome—life quality.

By maintaining a client–system perspective and remaining cognizant of the process of psychosocial adaptation, you will continually recognize that each person has a unique way of adapting shaped by one's culture and developmental level. Physical and social resources of the environment, including economic, political, religious, and health care institutions will also shape adaptation. Thus, when you provide services directed at assisting clients with adapting and improving life quality, you must understand and recognize the interplay between the client–system and psychosocial adaptation.

Summary

Along with a paradigm shift toward holistic health, there has been an expanded view of disability. Persons with disabilities are now viewed as more than their medical diagnosis alone, and their health conditions are being understood as outcomes of an interaction between the person and their physical and social environment. Just as a system perspective is valuable for understanding health and human services as a complex whole, a client–system perspective is most appropriate for identifying client needs and planning interventions. In this chapter we have described a client–system perspective to guide TR practice. The client system is comprised of four interrelated dimensions of personhood (bio/psycho/social/spiritual) shaped by developmental level, culture, and lifestyle. Disablement, which refers to an individual's capabilities and limitations are further affected by the person-environment transaction.

Using a client–system perspective helps with understanding the complex process of psychosocial adaptation in response to chronic illness and disability. Psychosocial adaptation involves a process of adjustment and recovery, motivated by a person's desire to feel competent in finding a suitable and comfortable fit between their needs and desires and the resources and opportunities in the environment. Thus TR practice involves developmentally appropriate and culturally sensitive interventions aimed at enhancing clients' sense of competence, holistic health, and life quality. Interventions are also aimed at modifying environments so that resources and opportunities support clients' sense of competence.

The client–system perspective and a focus on psychosocial adaptation form a common framework for all aspects of TR services. These perspectives also have relevance to the overall health and human service system, despite the nagging persistence of the medical model. They are consistent with the conceptual shifts challenging health and human service systems. By embracing these perspectives, you not only have a framework for competent practice, but also a common language and frame of reference that will become increasingly germane across a variety of disciplines and service delivery settings.

References

Baker-Roth, S., McLaughlin, E., Weitzenkamp, D., and Womeldorff, L. (1995). The impact of a therapeutic recreation community liaison on successful reintegration of individuals with traumatic brain injury. *Therapeutic Recreation Journal, 29*(4), 316–323.

Baltes, P., Cornelius, S., and Nesselroade, J. (1980). Cohort effects in developmental psychology. In J. R. Nessleroade and P. B. Baltes (Eds.), *Longitudinal research in the study of behavior and development* (pp. 61–87). New York, NY: Academic Press.

Bedini, L. and Guinan, D. (1996). The leisure of caregivers of older adults: Implications for CTRS in nontraditional settings. *Therapeutic Recreation Journal, 30*(4), 274–288.

Bedini, L. and Phoenix, T. (1999). Addressing leisure barriers for caregivers of older adults: A model leisure wellness program. *Therapeutic Recreation Journal, 33*(3), 222–240.

Berger, A. A. (1995). *Cultural criticism: A primer of key concepts.* Thousand Oaks, CA: Sage.

Bullock, C. and Mahon, M. (1997). *Introduction to recreation services for people with disabilities. A person-centered approach.* Champaign, IL: Sagamore Publishing.

Daly, F. (2002). *A study of the relationship between a home-based TR program and the reduction of excess disability in persons with early to mid-stage Alzheimer's disease.* Unpublished dissertation, Temple University. Philadelphia, PA.

Dossey, B. (1997). Holistic Nursing Practice. In Dossey, B. (Ed.), *Core curriculum for holistic nursing.* Gaithersburg, MD: Aspen.

Erikson, E. H. (1963). *Childhood and society.* New York, NY: W. W. Norton & Company.

Falvo, D. (1999). *Effective patient education: A guide to increased compliance.* Gaithersburg, MD: Aspen.

Howe-Murphy, R., and Charboneau, B. (1987). *Therapeutic recreation intervention: An ecological perspective.* Englewood Cliffs, NJ: Prentice-Hall.

Katsinas, R. (1998). Excess disability. In F. Brasile, T. Skalko, and j. burlingame, (Eds.), *Perspectives in recreational therapy: Issues of a dynamic profession,* (pp. 311–322). Ravensdale, WA: Idyll Arbor, Inc.

Livneh, H. and Antonak, R. (1997). *Psychosocial adaptation to chronic illness and disability.* Gaithersburg, MD: Aspen.

Mannell, R. and Kleiber, D. (1997). *A social psychology of leisure.* State College, PA: Venture Publishing, Inc.

McIntosh, M. (1986). The attitudes of minority inmates toward recreation programs as a rehabilitative tool. *Journal of Offender Counseling, Services and Rehabilitation, 104*(4), 79–86.

Myers, D. G. (1993). *Social psychology* (4th ed.). New York, NY: McGraw-Hill Inc.

Peregoy, J. and Dieser, R. (1997). Multicultural awareness in therapeutic recreation: Hamlet Living. *Therapeutic Recreation Journal, 31*(3), 173–187.

Piaget, J. (1952). *The origins of intelligence in children.* New York, NY: International Universities Press.

Ragins, M. (2000). Recovery: Changing from a medical model to a psychosocial rehabilitation mode. *The Journal, 5*(3) Available online: http://www.mhsource.com/hy/j53.html

Renwick, R., Brown, I., and Nagler, M. (1996). *Quality of life in health promotion and rehabilitation: Conceptual approaches, issues, and applications.* Thousand Oaks, CA: Sage Publications.

Sheldon K. and Dattilo, J. (1997). Multiculturalism in therapeutic recreation: Terminology clarification and practical suggestions. *Therapeutic Recreation Journal, 31*(3), 148–158.

Stamps, S. and Stamps, M. (1985). Race, class and leisure activities of urban residents. *Journal of Leisure Resarch, 17*(1), 40–55.

World Health Organization (2001). *International classification of functioning, disability, and health.* Geneva, Switzerland: Author.

Part 2

Integrating Theory with TR Clinical Practice

Chapter 4
Defining Clinical Practice in TR

Guided Reading Questions

After reading this chapter, you should be able to answer the following:
- What is meant by clinical practice?
- How is the clinical practice of TR different from providing general recreation services to people with disabilities?
- What are the key characteristics of TR clinical practice?
- What five phases occur in TR clinical practice?
- What is meant by competence?
- How does competence relate to TR clinical practice?

Introduction

The issues, concepts, and perspectives presented in Part 1 provide a framework for understanding TR as a health-related discipline. This framework accommodates the broad scope of TR practice reflected in the definitions advanced by the American Therapeutic Recreation Association (ATRA) and the National Therapeutic Recreation Society (NTRS) (see **Table 4.1**, p. 54). This broad scope of practice has been outlined in six different TR practice models that reflect diverse roles and functions of TR practitioners. **Table 4.2** (p. 56) describes each of these TR practice models, their theoretical constructs, and the basic purpose of TR according to each. Since issues like health, psychosocial adaptation, and quality of life are complex, there is a need for a wide range of services that promote health and life quality through play, recreation, and leisure.

It is beyond the limits of this text to adequately explain all aspects of practice and corresponding functions of practitioners. Therefore, we focus the remainder of this text on clinical TR practice. In essence, *TR clinical practice refers to deliberate and purposeful use of an intervention process aimed at helping people with illnesses and disabilities improve their health and increase their capacity to use play, recreation, and leisure for ongoing health and life quality*. An underlying assumption of TR clinical practice is that clients have conditions, both internal and external to themselves, that diminish optimal health and well-being. Therefore, a thoughtful and careful intervention process must be used to help clients restore, achieve, or maintain health and well-

being. Furthermore, clinical practice targets both clients and their environments so that functioning improves and external resources support coping, adaptation, and the pursuit of health and life quality through leisure.

This chapter provides an overview of TR clinical practice. We describe a 5-phase process to help clients *learn, adapt,* and *grow* and have a greater sense of *competence* in maintaining health and life quality through play, recreation, and leisure. Forthcoming chapters will describe in greater detail processes and procedures introduced in this chapter. Before we begin with a definition of clinical practice, it is important to dispel two false assumptions about the word "clinical."

First, people frequently confuse the term *clinical* with a place. It is a mistake to assume that services provided by recreation therapists are clinical merely because they are associated with an agency that has a mandate to provide care. Rather, *clinical practice involves a dynamic process of change*. This process transcends the place. Therapeutic recreation can be clinical during a community outing to the mall with clients recovering from head injuries, or during a backpacking trip with clients recovering from substance abuse, or in a community recreation center with older adults at risk for depression and social isolation, just as much as it could be with these same people in a hospital or rehabilitation center.

Second, it is a mistake to assume that TR services are clinical merely because practitioners refer to them as therapeutic or therapy (as in recreation therapy). Labeling something clinical does not make it so. To understand clinical practice is to understand what occurs between clients and recreation therapists when they share a commitment to reaching mutually desirable goals.

Defining Clinical Practice

The clinical practice of therapeutic recreation is the *systematic and planned use of recreation and other activity interventions and a helping relationship in an environment of support with the intent of effecting change in a client's attitudes, beliefs, behaviors, and skills necessary for psychosocial adaptation, health, and well-being.* Key elements contained in this definition capture the essence of clinical TR (see **Figure 4.1**). First, clinical practice is systematic and planned out. This means that clinical TR services are organized, with sufficient thought and consideration given to factors that will influence the actual benefits derived by clients. For instance, recreational activities and other learning experiences are carefully selected so they match the needs, interests, and abilities of clients and serve as a source of motivation. A *supportive environment* is created to enhance needed and desired changes. Also, *clear intentions* guide clinical practice. Typically, purposeful intentions are specified as client goals; however, specifying goals is not enough. Goals must be monitored and adjusted as needed. This also means that recreation therapists are expected to exercise some *control* over the actual methods or strategies that are used with clients in an effort to be accountable for the intended outcomes. The changes that clients experience are expected to be influenced by deliberate use of TR interventions.

While recreation therapists must exercise control over methods they use to help clients achieve intended outcomes, they do not dictate everything that occurs. They develop and maintain a therapeutic alliance or *helping relationship* with their clients. Within these relationships, therapists and clients share both the responsibility for selecting *targets for change* and the credit for reaching targeted goals. Ultimately, the aim of this process is to facilitate change in clients' thoughts, feelings, and behavior that will enable them to maintain their health and well-being with as much self-direction as possible.

The defining characteristic of clinical practice is that recreation and other related activities are used as a *means* for achieving outcomes. While recreation therapists make an effort to use recreational activities that are of interest to and appropriately challenging for clients, they are also careful to use activities that can be a means for clients to benefit beyond the activities themselves. A game of cards, for example, may be selected because it can be used to stimulate thinking, provoke the use of fine motor skills, or serve as the basis for maintaining socially appropriate behaviors, while also being of interest and enjoyable for the client. Most importantly, card games may be a vehicle for meaningful activity. For instance, card games were an important part of the care plan for Leonard, an 80-year-old with Parkinson's disease in an adult day care center. Not only did the card games require him to exercise cognitive and motor functioning, but also he enjoyed playing Uno and Crazy Eights with his grandchildren on weekends.

Facilitating Learning, Adaptation, and Growth

Clinical practice should be individualized according to the needs, hopes, and aspirations of each client. When you consider the range of clients served, it is easy to

Table 4.1: Definition of TR from professional organizations (ATRA, 2000 and NTRS, 2000)

Professional Organization	Definition of Therapeutic Recreation
American Therapeutic Recreation Association (ATRA)	The provision of Treatment and Recreation Services to persons with illnesses or disabling conditions. The primary purposes of Treatment Services, which are often referred to as Recreational Therapy, are to restore, remediate or rehabilitate in order to improve functioning and independence as well as reduce or eliminate the effects of illness or disability. The primary purposes of Recreational Services are to provide recreation resources and opportunities in order to improve health and well-being.
National Therapeutic Recreation Society (NTRS)	Treatment, education and recreation services to help people with illnesses, disabilities and other conditions to develop and use their leisure in ways that enhance their health, functional abilities, independence, and quality of life.

imagine an infinite number of goals that can be addressed in clinical practice. Generally, clinical practice is aimed at helping individuals deal with illnesses or disabling conditions so that they can lead satisfying lives. Clients are helped to *learn, adapt*, and *grow*, so they can maximize the potential for health and well-being through play, recreation, and leisure.

When used to facilitate *learning*, clinical practice focuses on a teaching/learning process that results in new knowledge, skills, and insights. For example, clients can be assisted to learn about the value and utility of play, recreation, and leisure in improving their health and reducing the chances of further health complications. This can happen through leisure education or other variations of health promotion programs. For some clients this may represent the first time they have ever considered the role and function of leisure in their lives. Of course, this would also involve learning about the nature and scope of one's illness or disabling condition. Clients may learn or relearn physical, social, and cognitive skills needed for participating in their preferred recreation and leisure activities. Clients can also learn about the availability and use of assistive devices. Newly learned skills, combined with new knowledge about opportunities and resources, provide an essential base for changing behavior and maintaining a healthy lifestyle that includes physically and socially active leisure.

The clinical practice of TR also involves helping clients *adapt* to their present health status and any functional limitations they are experiencing now or may experience in the future. For some clients the adaptation process involves acquiring cognitive, physical, or social compensatory strategies that maximize independent and self-directed action. Adapting to limitations imposed by an acute health crisis or chronic disabling conditions can also expose feelings and issues related to clients' attitudes, beliefs, and motivations. For example, the performance component inherent in TR intervention programs (doing an activity) often evokes a variety of emotional responses. Recreation therapists assist clients in their process of adaptation by acknowledging, exploring, and reconciling feelings and attitudes evoked when clients recover and rehabilitate. Likewise, recreation therapists facilitate the adjustment process by providing opportunities to explore feelings that arise when clients attend community outings and encounter attitudinal and/or architectural barriers or experience limitations in their performance because of changes in their functional status. Clinical interventions are also used to help clients adapt to changes involved in

reintegration back into their home environments, or adapt to new living conditions (e.g., moving into a nursing home).

When facilitating client *growth*, TR clinical practice helps clients to see the possibilities for a satisfying and meaningful life. The relationship between recreation therapists and their clients is critical to fostering hope and a sense of empowerment. "Most therapists come to realize that the ideas they communicate to patients about what is possible for them are also important. These ideas help patients to change their worldview and to consider ways they might find fulfillment and satisfaction" (Morris, 1994, p. 6). While clinical interventions that focus on learning and adaptation can lead to improvements in a client's physical, psychological, cognitive, or social functioning, the motivation to apply these functional gains are perhaps most important. Consequently, clinical practice ought to assist clients in determining the sources of meaning in their lives (e.g., friendships, creative expression) and realizing the possibilities for fulfillment. If the client chooses to pursue these growth experiences, the role of the TR professional is to ensure opportunity.

Paradoxically, facilitating growth may be of greatest importance for those clients beyond any hope for a cure or in the very last stages of life. Such is the case with individuals who have advanced dementia or terminal illnesses like cancer and AIDS. Growth in these instances relates to spiritual challenges such as making sense of or finding meaning in life's circumstances—even in the presence of impending death. Facing one's mortality can be a growth experience and an important part of the spiritual journey. Hospice care is one context where recreation therapists can support the spiritual growth of another human being.

Characteristics of TR Clinical Practice

- Systematic
- Intentional
- Change oriented
- Controlled

Components of TR Clinical Practice

- Helping relationship
- Recreation activity as a means
- Supportive environment

Figure 4.1: Key characteristics and components of clinical practice

Table 4.2: Summary of TR practice models

Practice Model	Theoretical Basis/Construct	Purpose of TR
Health Protection/ Health Promotion Model (Austin, 1998)	Humanistic psychology, high-level wellness, stabilization, and actualization tendencies	TR assists persons to recover following threats to health and to achieve as high a level of health as possible. Through the use of activity, recreation, and leisure TR helps people to deal with barriers to health so they can achieve their highest level of health and wellness.
Leisure Ability Model (Stumbo & Peterson, 1998)	Various theoretical constructs, such as locus of control, learned helplessness, intrinsic motivation, causal attribution, and flow	TR assists persons to develop, maintain, and express a freely chosen, appropriate, and enjoyable leisure lifestyle. Barriers to leisure involvement are minimized through functional interventions, leisure education, and the provision of recreation opportunities.
Aristotelian Good Life Model (Widmer & Ellis, 1998)	Aristotelian ethics and the "good life"	TR increases client freedom and responsibility to attain human happiness (the "good life"). TR focuses on helping clients achieve more than "primary goods" (e.g., biological and mobility needs). TR also focuses on "secondary goods" (e.g., learning, meaningful loving friendships/relationships, wisdom). Ultimately leisure and intellectual virtues are sought.
Self-Determination and Enjoyment Enhancement Model (Dattilo, Kleiber & Williams, 1998)	Motivation and self-determination (Deci, 1980, 1995)	TR sets the stage for people to enjoy themselves. Because people seek challenges commensurate with their competencies, therapists help clients to gain a realistic sense of the degree of challenge inherent in an activity and the needed adaptations to maximize enjoyment. If enjoyment occurs, people may push beyond their present ability, thereby improving functioning.
TR Service Model (Van Andel, 1998)	Leisure, work typology, freedom, and intrinsic motivation (Neulinger, 1974, 1981)	TR provides services that empower the client to achieve his or her desired goals and experience a sense of fulfillment, satisfaction, mastery, and well-being.
TR Outcome Model (Van Andel, 1998)	Developmental theories	TR provides opportunities for play, recreation, and leisure experiences that contribute to a person's development.
Optimizing Lifelong Health and Well-Being Model (Wilhite, Keller & Caldwell, 1999)	Developmental theory of human aging and adaptation (Baltes & Baltes, 1990)	TR provides educational opportunities and designs and/or facilitates supports that will enable clients to optimize experiences through compensation, resulting in healthy leisure lifestyles.

Facilitating learning, adaptation, and growth for clients often depends on modifications to the physical and social environment. Without such changes, clients can lack opportunities and support to improve and maintain functioning and experience satisfying lives through recreation and leisure. **Exhibit 4.1** illustrates this point.

☆• • •Thinking Trigger

Which of these three terms—learning, adaptation, or growth—best reflects your understanding of TR's value?

• • •☆

Five Phases of the Clinical TR Process

When clinical practice promotes learning, adaptation, or growth, TR practitioners use a systematic 5-phase process to guide the delivery of clinical services. There is an organized methodology to the work. It follows a logical, step-by-step progression from the beginning formulation of a working relationship with a client to discharge or termination of services. Austin (1996) stated "the therapeutic recreation process is a systematic problem-solving procedure used by therapeutic recreation specialists to help clients improve their levels of health by meeting identified needs" (p. 45). He contends that there are four phases to this process—*assessment, planning, implementation,* and *evaluation.* These same four phases serve as a framework for professional standards of practice issued by TR professional organizations. However, since we place significant emphasis on the therapeutic relationship as a necessary and integral part of the clinical change process, we have designated a fifth phase to this process—*termination.*

While the clinical process used in TR involves a systematic application of each phase, a point of clarification is warranted. The clinical process is not necessarily linear. It does not always follow a singular path from beginning to end. Practitioners must be prepared to move in and out of each phase as needed, depending on the client and the situation (see **Figure 4.2**). For instance, the assessment phase never really ends since, throughout your working relationship with a client, you are always searching for information that is relevant to clinical decision making. Likewise, once goals are set they may need to be altered or discarded and others developed based on new information. The process is also far from being linear when unexpected circumstances necessitate an early termination of services. Nevertheless, this 5-phase process largely defines the clinical TR process used with clients. The following overview provides a general sense of the process and how it is integrated.

Exhibit 4.1: Modifying the environment

Larry's individualized transition services plan (part of his special education IEP) included a TR intervention program designed to help him learn community travel skills. He was taught to identify the correct bus stop and bus number that would take him from school to home. His recreation therapist always accompanied him when he practiced. One day, he decided to do it on his own, without permission. He appeared at his front door with a proud smile on his face and a bag of chips and a soda in his hands. (He had learned how to buy things at the store, too.) His mother was furious and went directly to the principal demanding that Larry's recreation program cease. Barriers to Larry's independent functioning had less to do with his potential competence and more to do with his mother's overprotectiveness. In retrospect, the intervention plan failed to address a critical environmental factor—his mother's fears and concerns.

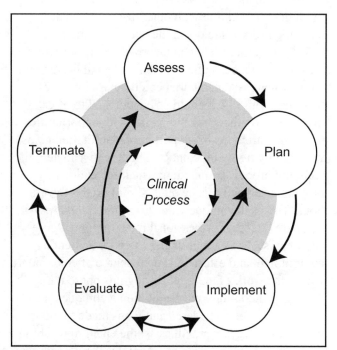

Figure 4.2: Clinical process

Phase 1: Assessment

Gathering relevant information about a client and making judgments about this information begins the clinical process. This becomes the basis for all other phases and is the key indicator for deciding whether to proceed in a helping relationship with a client. It is most important to have an idea of the information you want and to know what you will do with the information once you get it. Otherwise your time and the client's time is wasted. Good assessments involve multiple methods of gathering information. Along with standardized methods, you must use observation to find some confirmation between what the client says and what other professionals and family members say about the client. Develop sensitivities to the situational context of the client—how the environment affects the client as well as his or her perceptions about the situation. Finally, the assessment process should focus on strengths as well as client limitations. Strengths can be used to compensate for deficits and provide a balanced perspective about the person. Chapter 7 provides a detailed explanation of fundamental approaches used in assessing clients.

Phase 2: Planning

Deciding on a helpful course of action is predicated on the information gathered during an assessment and a prioritization of needs. This course of action is reflected in intervention or care plans. These plans are created with an awareness of a client's overall care, often in collaboration with other disciplines. The planning process factors in the client's strengths as well as limitations and can incorporate various strategies. For instance, a client's interest in nail design and employment as a manicurist could be used in care planning. This client could be encouraged to offer manicures to others, providing her with opportunities to use her strengths to support her rehabilitation goals while enjoying social contact. Clients can also help the planning process by deciding which recreational programs and activities would be preferred interventions. This is the unique value of *recreation therapy* as compared to other professional interventions. Recreation can serve as a motivating force for a client's commitment and effort and add a degree of enjoyment within the work of therapy. During this phase the variety of modalities and facilitation techniques available can be considered and plans made to incorporate them in ways that will assist the client in reaching intended outcomes. Chapter 8 explains the procedures used in this phase.

Phase 3: Implementation

During this phase, recreation therapists exercise innovative and creative approaches to helping clients by using systematic and planned interventions that incorporate the use of activities. Some interventions require specialized training, such as aquatic therapy and adventure-based counseling. Yet activities are not the only element that must be used in the implementation phase of clinical TR practice. When practiced as a clinical intervention, therapeutic recreation involves three essential and interrelated elements: activities, the environment, and a helping relationship (Mobily, 1985). Each element can be used to facilitate psychosocial adaptation.

While it is interesting to discuss the relative merits of activities, the environment, and therapeutic relationships as they pertain to TR clinical practice, none alone is enough to work effectively with clients. There can be variations in the amount of attention each element receives, relative to the others. Seasoned therapists know how to find the right blend among these three elements, always using all three when implementing interventions.

Activities

Recreation therapists use almost any activity considered recreation or leisure. These include traditional activities such as games, sports, expressive and creative arts, crafts, social activities, aquatics, music, drama, and horticulture. Of course, activities classified as recreation reflect social and cultural norms and may not appear to be recreation to every client, or they may carry certain meaning and restrictions in some cultures. According to Austin (1996) recreation activities hold the potential to be therapeutic if they are goal-directed and carefully selected by therapists to match needs and capabilities. Additionally, activities are more likely to produce therapeutic outcomes if they have meaning to the client, require active participation, and offer the potential for feelings of mastery, pleasure, and satisfaction. Chapter 9 presents information about the nature and scope of activities used in clinical practice, including criteria for selecting activity modalities. Note that clinical TR practice uses activity primarily as a means to facilitate learning, adaptation, and growth. Consequently, recreation therapists will often utilize action-oriented experiences not necessarily considered recreation in the traditional sense. These activity-based interventions help clients to improve functional skills and to meet various psychosocial needs. In these instances, the activities serve as a catalyst for change. Examples of such interventions include animal-assisted therapy, stress management, adventure-based counseling programs (e.g., ropes courses, group initiatives), community reintegration, and leisure education and counseling. Beyond this, preferred recreational activities ought to be used with clients as much as possible. Motivation is usually heightened, and there is greater potential for enjoyment and meaning to be derived from the experience.

Environment

The second essential element of clinical TR practice is the physical and social environment. As described earlier, a person's environment has a direct bearing on attitudes, beliefs, and behavior. Therefore, recreation therapists structure the environment to help motivate clients to engage in behaviors that contribute to their health and quality of life. Chapter 10 describes ways in which recreation therapists humanize care environments to facilitate learning, adaptation, and growth. This includes manipulating the physical environment so that, for example, traditionally sterile long-term care environments become attractive spaces filled with opportunities for pleasant activities that give messages of life and vitality. Environments such as restaurants, parks, and shopping malls present realistic learning situations for clients to confront obstacles. Clients apply their skills and abilities in negotiating and navigating through these environments, and are provided with opportunities for learning and adapting. Additionally, the social environment is structured in ways that promote support and companionship, thereby increasing feelings of belonging and a sense of community. Increasingly, recreation therapists also modify physical and social environments in clients' homes and communities so that their potential for health and life quality is increased.

Therapeutic Relationships

The third essential element of clinical practice is the relationship therapists have with their clients. Therapeutic relationships involve an ability to use oneself as an effective tool in helping people change. A positive, working relationship or therapeutic alliance with a client is adjusted throughout the process according to the needs of the client and the specific goals of the intervention. This relationship creates conditions necessary for clients to learn, adapt, and grow. Chapter 11 describes the nature and scope of therapeutic working relationships. Compassion and respect for the

client and a mutual commitment to and a shared responsibility for achieving outcomes characterize these relationships (Gelso & Carter, 1994).

Phase 4: Monitoring, Adjusting, and Evaluation

This phase of the TR process is essentially concerned with making sure that the plan is being implemented as intended and determining any need to make adjustments. While evaluation is a distinct phase itself, the basis for evaluation is actually set during the planning phase when goals and time frames for evaluating progress are specified. Care plans or intervention plans typically designate a time to evaluate progress (e.g., 2-week intervals). Writing a progress note in the client's chart usually completes the evaluative phase. Yet, despite this formal evaluation period, therapists continuously monitor and evaluate the clinical process during every encounter with a client. They are also alert to other indicators of change such as conversations with other staff in care plan or team meetings, or in informal reports about a client's situation. Chapter 13 describes the role of documentation in monitoring and evaluating services.

Phase 5: Termination

The evaluation phase is typically considered to be the final phase in the TR clinical process. It often culminates in a written discharge plan signaling the end of services. Sometimes a TR intervention plan terminates even if there is no discharge from the facility. Goals may have been met, warranting an end to services, or perhaps circumstances such as a change in the conditions of the client or even their own lack of willingness to comply with interventions may be cause for termination. Beyond this, there is another important dimension to termination—bringing closure to the working relationship between the recreation therapist and the client. Whatever the reason for ending TR interventions, there ought to be a time to say goodbye and to reflect on the experience of working together. In some instances it may be very hard for a client to say goodbye to a therapist who has invested so much time and effort. It can also be emotionally difficult for a therapist to say goodbye. Both client and therapist deserve an opportunity to acknowledge the emotional as well as practical aspects of their work together, and to bring the relationship to an appropriate ending. This is discussed further in Chapter 11.

Enhancing Competence

When TR clinical practice is used to help clients learn, adapt, and grow, they are being assisted with psychosocial adaptation. As explained in Chapter 3, successful psychosocial adaptation means that people contending with illnesses and disabling conditions find an optimal fit between their needs and aspirations and the resources and opportunities in their environment. Consequently, clients have greater capacities to interact with their environments and to be actively involved in social, vocational, and leisure pursuits. In essence, this restores their sense of competence.

Restoring and promoting client competence is fundamental to TR clinical practice. All human beings have a desire to interact effectively with their physical and social environments and to view themselves as competent in their quest for a happy and fulfilling life. White (1959) labeled this need *competence-effectance motivation*. Restoring competence generally requires changes in a person's thoughts, beliefs, attitudes, and behavior. Thoughts and beliefs about personal competence will have a direct influence on motivation and goal-directed behavior. Thus, TR clinical practice helps to restore competence by assisting clients to change self-perceptions as they improve functioning, learn and use coping skills to manage stress, adapt to changes brought on by illnesses or disabling conditions, and incorporate recreation and leisure as an essential part of health and life quality.

Clinical Practice beyond the Individual Level

Note that the description of clinical practice in this chapter was limited to that which occurs between a therapist and an individual client. In practice, the clinical change process is also facilitated through group work. Therapeutic groups are designed and implemented so that several clients can share experiences intended to stimulate learning, adaptation, and growth. The elements used when implementing clinical practice discussed earlier (e.g., activity, environment, relationships) are now used in the context of a group. Perhaps the most significant factor associated with therapeutic groups is the relationship group members have with one another. Through their interaction, clients can help each other meet common needs. In Chapter 12 we discuss the nature and scope of therapeutic groups as a part of clinical practice.

Clinical practice, whether delivered individually or through group work, also reflects effective programming in response to needs of the agency. Peterson and Stumbo (2000) advocate a systematic approach to programming that begins with comprehensive planning. This involves an analysis of system needs, resources, and limitations (e.g., mission of the agency, staff, facilities) as well as client needs. If done properly, comprehensive planning would lead to specific programs designed not only to facilitate relevant client outcomes, but also to complement the broad array of services provided by other professionals within the system. Consequently, clinical TR services would make a value-added contribution to the system of care. Consider, for example, leisure-time management planning groups run by recreation therapists for individuals preparing for discharge from a substance abuse treatment program. Another example would be family support programs intended to help families have more meaningful visits with loved ones who live in nursing homes because of Alzheimer's disease. Conceptualizing, designing, and implementing such programs are additional parts of clinical practice discussed further in Chapter 12.

Summary

The clinical practice of TR is a systematic and planned process intended to facilitate change in a client's health and well-being. This process, while not limited to any particular setting, must be organized and systematic. Therapists follow a progression of interrelated phases in their clinical work with clients including assessing, planning, implementing, evaluating, and terminating. These phases do not always occur in a precise orderly progression, although the process always starts with an assessment of needs. Clinical practice utilizes activity-based interventions, supportive and responsive environments, and a therapeutic relationship to facilitate a client's learning, adaptation, and growth. While client needs and circumstances vary widely, a fundamental focus of TR clinical practice is psychosocial adaptation. Whether delivered individually or through group work, clinical practice involves purposeful and deliberate interventions aimed at enhancing clients' sense of personal control and competence. However, helping clients restore and maintain competence is complex, requiring theoretical knowledge about human behavior and the change process. Such knowledge is essential for planning and implementing services that promote psychosocial adaptation, health, and life quality. The next chapter provides an overview of some theories that recreation therapists can use to plan and to implement effective clinical services.

References

American Therapeutic Recreation Association. (2000). Definition statement. Available online: http://www.atra-tr.org/definition.htm

Austin, D. (1996). *Therapeutic recreation: Processes and techniques* (3rd ed.). Champaign, IL: Sagamore Publishing.

Austin, D. (1998). The health protection/health promotion model. *Therapeutic Recreation Journal, 32*(2), 109–117.

Baltes, P. and Baltes, M. (1990). Selective optimization with compensation. In P. Baltes and M. Baltes (Eds.), *Successful aging: Perspectives from the behavioral sciences* (pp. 1–34). New York, NY: Cambridge University Press.

Dattilo, J., Kleiber, D., and Williams, R. (1998). Self-determination and enjoyment enhancement: A psychologically based service delivery model for therapeutic recreation. *Therapeutic Recreation Journal, 32*(3), 258–271.

Deci, E. (1980). *The psychology of self-determination.* Lexington, MA: Lexington Books.

Deci, E. (1995). *Why we do what we do: Understanding self-motivation.* New York, NY: Penguin Books.

Gelso, C. and Carter, J. (1994). Components of the psychotherapy relationship: Their interaction and unfolding. *Journal of Counseling Psychology, 41*, 296–309.

Mobily, K. (1985). A philosophical analysis of therapeutic recreation: What does it means to say "we can be therapeutic?" Part I. *Therapeutic Recreation Journal, 28*(1), 14–26.

Morris, J. (1994). Some cautions when using functional assessment scales. *Topics in Geriatric Rehabilitation, 9*(3), 2–7.

National Therapeutic Recreation Society (2000). NTRS Definition—Therapeutic Recreation. Available online: http://www.nrpa.org/department

Neulinger, J. (1974). *Psychology of leisure: Research approaches to the study of leisure.* Springfield, IL: Charles C. Thomas.

Neulinger, J. (1981). *The psychology of leisure* (2nd ed.). Springfield, IL: Charles C. Thomas.

Peterson, C. and Stumbo, N. (2000). *Therapeutic recreation program design: Principles and procedures* (3rd Ed.). Needham Heights, MA: Allyn & Bacon.

Stumbo, N. and Peterson, C. (1998). The leisure ability model. *Therapeutic Recreation Journal, 32*, 82–96.

Van Andel, G. (1998). TR service delivery and TR outcome models. *Therapeutic Recreation Journal, 32*(3), 180–193.

White, R. (1959). Motivation reconsidered: The concept of competence. *Psychological Review, 66,* 297–333.

Widmer, M. and Ellis, G. (1998). The Aristotelian good life model: Integration of values into therapeutic recreation service delivery. *Therapeutic Recreation Journal, 32*(4), 290–302.

Wilhite, B., Keller, J., and Caldwell, L. (1999). Optimizing lifelong health and well-being: A health enhancing model of therapeutic recreation. *Therapeutic Recreation Journal, 33*(2), 98–108.

Chapter 5
Understanding Theories That Guide Practice

Guided Reading Questions

After reading this chapter, you should be able to answer the following:
- What is a theory?
- How does theory help with planning and providing clinical TR services?
- How does the clinical practice of TR mesh with a social psychological perspective?
- What is the role of cognition (perceptions and beliefs) in coping with stress and changing health behaviors?
- What is self-efficacy and how can it be changed?
- What does self-efficacy have to do with learning and adapting recreation and leisure behaviors?
- What role does the environment have in shaping self-efficacy beliefs, maintaining or changing health behaviors, and coping with stress?

Introduction

In the last chapter we explained that TR clinical practice involves the deliberate and purposeful use of interventions to help clients to achieve psychosocial adaptation, health, and life quality. Recreation therapists facilitate change in clients' attitudes, beliefs, and behaviors through a combination of three essential ingredients: *activity-based interventions*, *supportive and responsive environments*, *and therapeutic relationships*. Together, these ingredients help clients learn, adapt, and grow in ways that support using play, recreation, and leisure for health and life quality.

Helping clients change attitudes, beliefs, and behaviors is a complex endeavor. Clients can experience both internal and external barriers to using recreation and leisure for their health and well-being. For instance, clients' physical and psychological states influence how competent they feel to affect their health and happiness. Additionally, environmental factors often affect their sense of competence and the opportunities they have to achieve and maintain health and life quality. Therefore, the change process used in clinical practice must have a framework for understanding how people change attitudes, beliefs, and behaviors. We look to theories to provide this framework.

What Is a Theory?

A *theory* serves multiple functions. It provides a framework that combines, organizes, and synthesizes concepts that form a body of knowledge. This theoretical framework gives meaning to observed facts and provides a logical basis for explaining and predicting a phenomena, such as human behavior and experiences (Wiersma, 1991). Theories also provide a basis for developing and testing new knowledge, which is critical to advancing clinical practice in the health professions. Furthermore, theories provide a conceptual base from which to plan interventions that promote lifestyle change. For these reasons, understanding theoretical foundations that guide TR practice is critical.

This chapter provides a theoretical framework that TR practitioners can use to guide their clinical practice. We have selected only a few theories relevant to clinical practice. These include Social Cognitive Theory and the concept of self-efficacy (Bandura, 1977a, 1986), theoretical work on stress and coping (Lazarus and Folkman, 1984), and three applied health theories—the Health Belief Model (Hochbaum, 1958; Rosenstock, 1990) and the Theories of Reasoned Action and Planned Behavior (Ajzen & Fishbein, 1980).

Status of Theory in Therapeutic Recreation Practice

Therapeutic recreation practice has been viewed as lacking a strong and consistent theoretical framework. Various professionals in the field, including Peterson

(1989), Sylvester (1989), and Malkin (1993) have expressed concern about the limitations this poses for advancing the discipline. For example, a review of TR research published in the *Therapeutic Recreation Journal* between 1986 and 1990 found that few of these studies had a defined theoretical framework (Bedini & Wu, 1994). Lack of a theoretical base defeats a primary purpose of research—to build and test theory. It also reduces the ability to communicate with other health-related disciplines. "This lack of conceptual and theoretical explication also interferes with the ability of other groups to understand how TR services relate to a larger cadre of health care and human service professionals" (Shank, Coyle, Boyd & Kinney, 1996, p. 180).

TR professionals need theories to inform selection and use of interventions and provide a basis for testing and expanding clinical practice (Shank, Coyle & Kinney, 1993). In the past few years, there have been significant efforts made by professionals to articulate the conceptual and theoretical assumptions influencing TR practice. Recent issues of the *Therapeutic Recreation Journal* presented and critically examined six distinct models of TR practice (see Table 4.1, p. 54). As part of his review and synthesis of these six TR practice models, Mobily (1999) identified common theoretical concepts consistently used when explaining TR practice. He included perceived freedom, attribution theory, perceived control, competence, effectance motivation, learned helplessness, and flow experiences (see **Table 5.1**).

These concepts are associated with each theory presented in this chapter. Since we only present five theories, we begin with a brief discussion of the assumptions that guided our selection.

Assumptions Influencing Theory Selection

Clinical practice is about helping clients learn, adapt, and grow in ways that improve and maintain health and quality of life. We contend that TR practice operates from the holistic health and wellness paradigm (see Chapter 2), which is pertinent to both health care and human services. TR has the specific intention of promoting play, recreation, and leisure as a means to health and quality of life. Following are three additional assumptions behind our selection of theories pertinent to TR practice. With these assumptions in mind, we have selected several theories commonly used in health promotion, research, and practice.

TR is an Applied Discipline Using Borrowed Theory

While the theories presented in this chapter encompass most of the concepts contained in the various TR practice models, they are not unique to therapeutic recreation, nor have they been developed through the discipline's own research and practice. Like other TR authors, we borrow theories from other fields (e.g., social psychology, health psychology) since we believe that TR is an applied discipline. Some may find fault with this, yet we fully agree with Mobily (1999) when he addressed this issue in his critique of the six TR practice models:

> All of the theoretical knowledge that TR now claims as its own originated within other disciplines such as social psychology, psychology, and sociology, to name a few. If anything is needed, it is the acquisition of more theoretical knowledge from related fields and its application to the practice of TR. As an applied profession, TR need not apologize about the use of theoretical knowledge from other fields, but instead exercise wisdom in the selection of what is borrowed and care in its application to TR. (p. 178)

We also recognize that no single theoretical model can adequately explain and guide all TR practice. TR practice is too diverse, as are the needs of the clients. Furthermore, the direct application of the theories presented in this chapter to TR practice remains to be tested empirically. Yet the theories presented embrace many basic assumptions that operate in TR practice, especially practice designed to be clinical.

TR Practice Can Be Guided by a Social Psychological Perspective

While numerous theoretical explanations for human behavior exist, those theories that have emerged from social psychology are most relevant to TR clinical practice. The relevance of social psychology to clinical practice stems from social psychology's focus on understanding the interrelationships between individual behavior and the social environment (Iso-Ahola, 1980). The application of a social psychological approach also makes sense to TR given that human behavior is explained in terms of dynamic interplay between prior behavior, personal factors (including cognitions), and environmental conditions. As a theoretical perspective, it is easily integrated with the client–system approach and with the process of psychosocial adaptation.

Why Use a Social–Psychological Perspective?

Mannell and Kleiber (1997) reviewed the historical origins of the social psychology movement in North America from its early focus on theories about attitude and attitude change to its more contemporary focus on social cognition. Because social psychology explains individual behavior, it is often applied to a variety of fields. "The value of social psychology for understanding contemporary life has been recognized by psychologists and nonpsychologists alike" (Mannell & Kleiber, 1997, p. 34). Researchers and practitioners from many different fields (e.g., business, education,

health, social work, recreation) utilize a social psychology perspective since it extends "the boundaries of traditional psychology into the realms vital to contributing solutions for real-world problems—the areas of health, ecology, education, law, peace and conflict resolution" (Zimbardo, 1992, p. xiv).

While the broad social psychological perspective focuses on understanding the processes that explain human behavior across all types of settings and situations, a number of specialized applications of the social psychology framework have developed. A social psychology perspective has been applied to the two areas of primary importance to therapeutic recreation: leisure (Iso-Ahola, 1980, 1995) and health (Rotter & Quine, 1994). "In these subfields, not only have major social psychological theories been applied to understanding the issues of interest, but also theories specific

Table 5.1: Common terms used in TR practice models

Term	Definition
Perceived freedom	Perception that one has the freedom to make choices, engage in an activity, or embark on a course of action of his or her own choosing.
Attribution theory	Theoretical perspective that attempts to show the relationship between the causal explanations a person gives to events in their life and their subsequent behavior (see Weiner, 1985).
Perceived control	Perception that the outcome of a situation is directly under the influence of the person and their behavior. Distinctions are often made between internal and external locus of control. Individuals with an internal locus of control believe that the outcomes of a situation result from their behavior. Individuals with external locus of control believe that outcomes of a situation are determined by luck, fate, powerful others, chance or other reasons independent of the individual (see Rotter, 1990).
Competence	Intrinsic drive that encourages individuals to interact effectively (i.e., producing desired outcomes and avoiding undesirable ones) with their environment. Skinner (1995) states that competence is synonymous with effectance.
Effectance motivation	Intrinsic drive that motivates individuals to engage in transactions with their environment and to experience themselves as capable of effecting change through the transaction (see White, 1959).
Learned helplessness	Pattern of responding to a situation by giving up and not trying. This response arises from repeated experiences in which the individual has not been able to successfully affect the outcome of a situation. Such thinking results in low motivation and pervasive sense of pessimism (see Seligman, 1975).
Flow experiences	Subjective experience reported by individuals that occurs when they have been involved in an activity in which there is an optimal match between demands inherent in the activity and skills used to meet the demand. This matching results in an experience in which the individual is totally absorbed. Flow experiences can occur in leisure/recreation experiences (see Csikszentmihalyi, 1990).

to these subfields have been developed" (Mannell & Kleiber, 1997, p. 35). Thus, the use of a social psychological perspective within clinical TR practice makes sense given the direct application of social psychology to understanding leisure and health behavior.

TR Practice Must Recognize the Role of Cognition in Changing Behavior

Change relies heavily on a client's cognitive functioning. Iso-Ahola (1980) explained in *The Social Psychology of Leisure and Recreation* that cognitions are critical determinants of human behavior. "Several cognitive mechanisms (e.g., processes of person perception, causal attribution, and decision making) mediate all human responses to a varying degree. Thus cognitions, emotions, and motives play a central role in energizing and directing behavior" (p. 17). He went on to explain that recreation therapists need to know about clients' cognitions to remove psychological barriers that hinder satisfying recreation and leisure involvement.

In a recent interview regarding his current views on the relationship between theory and TR practice (Mobily, 2000), Iso-Ahola maintained that a primary focus of TR practice is to enhance client self-perceptions and feelings of control since these cognitions affect motivation and goal achievement. "Therapeutic recreation will make a huge difference if it can make people believe in themselves (e.g., self-efficacy) on the one hand and make them motivated about life and various activities on the other" (p. 302). He offered the following example:

> When stroke victims begin their rehab program, involvement in recreation activities drastically and permanently changes their perceptions of themselves and their future in a positive way. Subsequent involvement will reinforce these perceptions and thus become intrinsically rewarding. Activity involvement that readily enhances one's sense of competence and self-determination is more likely to lead to functional improvement than activity involvement that is psychologically less meaningful. (p. 304)

The theories presented in this chapter emphasize the role of clients' cognitions in behavioral change. They assume that a client has at least a moderate capacity to learn from observing others, anticipating outcomes, reflecting on experiences, and expressing preferences in terms of choices. In particular, a client's beliefs about personal control related to regulating behavior have a prominent role in theories used to guide behavior change.

An emphasis on cognition is nothing new for therapeutic recreation; it has been implied in all of the primary concepts and theoretical bases claimed to guide TR practice. For example, the Self-Determination and Enjoyment Enhancement Model (Dattilo, Kleiber & Williams, 1998) and the Optimizing Lifelong Health and Well-Being Model (Wilhite, Keller & Caldwell, 1999) assume that clients can appraise their motives and the level of challenge inherent in leisure experiences. Likewise, Stumbo and Peterson's Leisure Ability model (1998) identifies intrinsic motivation and self-determination as theoretical anchors for TR practice. These anchors involve cognitive mechanisms.

Some might wonder whether an emphasis on a client's cognitive capacities might preclude using a clinical change process with many clients who ought to receive TR interventions. Recent discussion of proposed TR practice models raised this issue. Widmer and Ellis (1998) acknowledged that their Aristotelian Good Life model may be inappropriate for clients with cognitive limitations (e.g., developmental disabilities, Alzheimer's disease) because this model assumes that clients would have the ability to make decisions based on values and personal meaning of happiness. Nichols' (1998) critique of the model expressed similar concerns. We raise this issue because we are aware that our approach to the clinical practice of TR, particularly as it is presented in this text, uses very explicit cognitive-behavioral processes and techniques. Some readers may find that this framework would not apply to clients with severe cognitive limitations or in situations where there is little time to use cognitive-behavioral interventions. Certainly, clinical processes need to be modified to fit the abilities of each client and other practice constraints, but the change process advocated here clearly involves understanding and engaging a client's thoughts, perceptions and beliefs.

Social Cognitive Theory

Social Cognitive Theory (SCT) is one of the most widely used theories in research on health-related interventions. In particular, the concept of self-efficacy (Bandura, 1977a, 1977b, 1982, 1986) has been used in a variety of research studies on phobic behavior, pain (including chronic pain), depression, substance abuse, cancer, and social anxiety. SCT incorporates the environment into a framework for understanding human behavior. Behavior is explained in terms of a reciprocal interaction between personal factors and the environment. In SCT a complete understanding of the environment and its influence on an individual's beliefs and behavior requires an understanding of how the individual interprets the environment. This interpretation can vary since it is influenced by the person's cognitive perceptions of the environment, including real, distorted, or imagined factors. Thus, from a social cognition perspective, helping clients change behaviors requires attention to two things:

1. The extent to which the environment offers opportunity and support for change
2. The situation as cognitively constructed by clients.

Social cognition is concerned with what information individuals select, how it is used, and how it is combined to make judgments about oneself and others.

Self-Efficacy

At the heart of SCT is the construct of self-efficacy. *Self-efficacy describes a person's belief about whether or not he or she can successfully engage in and execute a specific behavior.* It affects how much effort an individual applies to a task. SCT, and in particular the construct of self-efficacy, focuses on the individual's conviction that she or he can successfully perform the behavior needed to produce the desired outcome.

SCT focuses on the interaction among three constructs: outcome expectancies, self-efficacy beliefs, and outcome expectations. The value or degree of importance that a person attributes to a particular outcome is labeled *outcome expectancy*. Individuals use outcome expectancies to help them determine if they should engage in a particular behavior. Self-

efficacy beliefs are also used in this manner. *Self-efficacy beliefs* are the judgments an individual makes regarding his or her ability to perform a particular behavior. Finally, *outcome expectations* refer to an individual's beliefs that when the particular behavior is performed by him or her, it will result in the valued outcome. While efficacy beliefs and outcome expectancies influence whether a behavior will be engaged in, it is important to note that the outcome of the behavior subsequently influences self-efficacy beliefs (**Figure 5.1**).

The distinctions between self-efficacy beliefs, outcome expectancy, and outcome expectations allow therapists to understand a client's motivation for engaging or not engaging in a task. For instance, consider a person involved in a community program for people with developmental disabilities. This client refuses to attend the center's monthly dances. When discussing his lack of involvement, the recreation therapist discovers that the client believes that being at the dance would be fun (high outcome expectation). The client also states that having fun is important to him (high outcome expectancy). Despite the client's statements that he knows how to dance (high self-efficacy beliefs), he still refuses to participate. Further discussion reveals that the client is uncomfortable in social settings and feels that he doesn't have the ability to engage anyone (particularly a girl) in a conversation (low self-efficacy beliefs). This belief is his primary reason for not attending the dance. The therapist can now use this knowledge to target a more appropriate goal of social skill development. Typically, people who have high self-efficacy beliefs are more likely to feel that they have personal control (i.e., competence) over situations and therefore are more willing to engage in action.

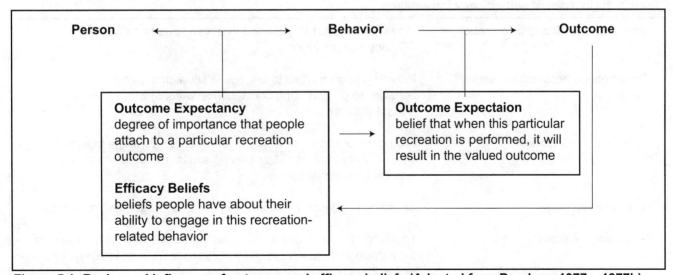

Figure 5.1: Reciprocal influence of outcome and efficacy beliefs (Adapted from Bandura, 1977a, 1977b)

Research has suggested that self-efficacy can be influenced through four sources of information: performance accomplishments, vicarious experiences, persuasion, and physiological arousal (see **Table 5.2**). Individuals selectively process and combine these diverse sources of information to make self-efficacy judgments about themselves and others. The process by which each of these sources of information affects self-efficacy is individualized and dependent on the individual's cognitive processing of the experience.

Performance accomplishments refer to prior experiences or current experiences in which the client actually performs the action and derives the desired outcome. Performance accomplishments are thought to have the strongest influence on self-efficacy beliefs, as repeated success builds one's sense of competence. When people believe they are capable of performing the task, they are much more willing to engage in it and to persist at it when they encounter obstacles. The difficulty of the task, how much effort individuals think they have expended on the task, and the amount of assistance received when performing the task influence the degree to which performance experiences affect self-efficacy judgments. In the previous example, the client begins to attend a social skills group and participates in role-play exercises where he has to initiate and sustain conversations with other group members (male and female) for five minutes. His self-efficacy beliefs in this area will be enhanced if he believes that the role-play exercises are relevant and challenging (like talking to people at the community dance), if he succeeds in the task, and if the therapist does not need to offer any prompts during the role-play exercises.

Vicarious experiences are those situations where a person observes another (i.e., a role model) doing the activity. They also influence self-efficacy beliefs. In terms of the cognitive processing of vicarious experiences, self-efficacy judgment will be affected by how similar the individual feels he or she is to the role model, the diversity among the models seen performing the behavior, and the strategies used by the model. Let's return again to the example. If, during the social skill training group, the client sees a number of different peers able to engage others in conversation, he is more likely to think "If they can do it, so can I."

Persuasion is the most commonly used method in clinical practice to influence self-efficacy beliefs. Unfortunately, it is also the least effective of the four methods. In the example we have been using, suppose the recreation therapist's response to the client's beliefs about his conversation skills was to suggest that "Having conversations is really easy! Besides, you're a smart guy. You have a lot of things to talk to people about. Look, you're talking to me now." Most likely, the client would remain resistant to attending the monthly dances despite this verbal persuasion. Research has indicated that persuasion is least effective at changing self-efficacy beliefs. Furthermore, the effectiveness of persuasion is influenced by the credibility of the persuader. Most likely, the client would not see the therapist as similar to himself. For this reason, peer mentoring is a common approach used in many agencies.

Physiological arousal refers to the internal state of the individual when performing the action and the degree of comfort or discomfort the action provokes in the client. The situational factors that the person attends to and their prior experiences with the effects

Table 5.2: Sources of self-efficacy information

Sources of Efficacy Information	Ways To Use Activity-Based Interventions to Influence Efficacy Information
Performance accomplishments	Providing opportunities to engage in situationally relevant behavior (e.g., practicing social conversations) with and/or without support.
Vicarious experiences	Arranging for clients to view similar others perform the task either in person or on video. Having similar others discuss their successful experiences.
Verbal persuasion	Providing suggestions, verbal support, encouragement, and praise.
Physiological arousal	Teaching clients to recognize physiological responses and manage them through the use of relaxation exercises, visual imagery, and biofeedback.

of physiological arousal on their performance affect the cognitive processing of physiological information. Once again, let us return to the example. When discussing how he felt during the role-play, the client reports that he could feel his heart pounding and his palms sweating. The recreation therapist would be wise to point out to the client that he was successful in his performance even with those physiological responses and recommend that he use deep breathing to help himself relax. In this way, the therapist helps the client begin to associate the physiological response with a successful outcome and reinforces a self-efficacy belief that "I can do well even if I feel a little scared."

Implications for Therapeutic Recreation Practice

Social Cognitive Theory, and in particular the concept of self-efficacy, has significant relevance for TR practice. Understanding the sources by which self-efficacy expectations can be influenced is fundamental to helping clients change their behavior. Designing and implementing interventions that utilize varied sources of efficacy information is imperative. Table 5.2 contains some common ways that different sources of efficacy information can be incorporated into interventions.

Likewise, TR practitioners need to be aware that the activity-based nature of their work provides ample opportunities for clients to experience performance accomplishments that can enhance self-efficacy beliefs. Therapists should design activity-based interventions that utilize realistic, short-term goals (e.g., breaking large goals into smaller, more manageable subgoals). From a SCT perspective, realistic, short-term goal setting is preferred because it offers psychological advantages. For instance, such goals enhance motivation because they seem achievable, allowing clients to focus their energy on the here and now. They also provide immediate incentives and guides for evaluating performance. If goals seem unachievable, clients have a reason to not try (e.g., "Why bother, I'll never be able to take a girl out on a date. I would have to talk to her all night long."). Realistic, short-term goals also provide a standard by which clients can make positive self-efficacy judgments.

Research has indicated that self-efficacy beliefs do generalize to other areas. However, generalization most likely occurs to activities similar to those in which self-efficacy was restored by treatment (Bandura, 1977a, 1977b). Understanding the contexts in which self-efficacy beliefs can be generalized helps practitioners design viable intervention options and environments that promote such generalization. From a SCT perspective it makes little sense to take clients with developmental disabilities on an outing using a facility van if the intent is to have the client use community facilities independently. The gains that may be attained in terms of self-efficacy beliefs would not generalize due to the dissimilarity in the environments (e.g., van vs. public transportation). Furthermore, the degree of assistance provided might hamper any self-efficacy development (e.g., "The staff ran the trip, I couldn't do it myself.").

The final and most important application of SCT to TR practice is to avoid thinking about change from a unidirectional perspective. While it is easy to think that all a person has to do to feel healthier or happy is change a particular behavior (e.g., be more socially active), SCT reminds therapists that the particular behavior that is a target for intervention is influenced by the person (especially his or her cognitions and beliefs about his or her ability to perform the behavior) *and* the physical and social environments. A change in any one component influences the other component. Likewise, either component can inhibit change in the other. For instance, a person who decides that he or she would like to be more socially active could be inhibited by lack of social support in the environment or by perceptions that no social support existed (e.g., cognitive distortions such as "No one ever wants to go anywhere with me. The things I want to do would bore them.").

Theoretical Perspectives on Stress and Coping

Stress and coping have been two of the most frequently examined factors in health and health behavior. *Stress* has been defined as a both a *stimulus* and a *response*. For instance, the demands inherent in recovering from a stroke (e.g., dealing with motor or communication limitations and pressure from a rehabilitation professional to engage in activities to improve functioning) can be unwelcome stimuli. Such stimuli can provoke a response that some might label as stress. The response may be manifested physiologically as an upset stomach or other glandular activity (e.g., sweating). It can also be manifested psychologically as in withdrawal, anxiety, or depression.

Seyle's *General Adaptation Syndrome* (1976a, 1976b)—whereby the body's mechanisms prepare to "fight" or take "flight" in the face of stress—was a significant theoretical advancement in the study of stress. However, Seyle concentrated on physiology alone, to the exclusion of myriad psychological factors. During the last half of the 20th century, stress researchers concluded that any conceptualization of stress would have to take into consideration cognitions, personality, and social factors that mediate perceptions and responses to stress. These factors figured prominently into studies of resiliency exhibited by children and adults when faced with the stress associated with chronic illnesses and disabling conditions.

The process of dealing with stress, whether viewed as a stimulus or a response, has been labeled *coping*. Stressed individuals can engage in behavior associated with play, recreation, and leisure to cope with stress. For instance, play and recreation activities can be used as a source of distraction from anxiety and tension. Recreation and leisure activities may also be used to enhance a person's psychological sense of being in control, thereby decreasing feelings of stress. Therapeutic recreation services frequently assist clients with coping and adapting to their illness and disability-related conditions. Play and recreation can represent coping resources for the individual to use in tolerating, managing, or resolving stress.

The contemporary view of stress considers it to be a transaction between the person and environmental stimuli. This view acknowledges the importance of an individual's perception in defining the stressor, its potential to cause harm and the perceived abilities and other external resources that can be used to cope with the stressor. Lazarus and Folkman (1984) have advanced the view of stress that emphasizes individual perception and interpretation. They defined *psychological stress* as "*a particular relationship between the person and the environment that is appraised by the person as taxing or exceeding his or her resources and endangering his or her well-being*" (p. 19; emphasis added). Their theory postulates that cognitive appraisal and coping responses are the two pivotal mediating factors in the person-environment transaction. Lerman and Glanz (1997) have utilized much of the theoretical work completed on stress and coping (Lazarus & Folkman, 1984; Lazarus, 1991) and applied it specifically to health. Their model, the *Transactional Model of Stress and Coping*, reflects the role of cognitive perceptions, coping efforts, and general health outcomes —all of which have applicability to clinical TR practice.

Figure 5.2 illustrates how stress and coping interrelate. Imagine how this might occur, given some

source of stress. First, when stress is perceived, people engage in a cognitive appraisal process at two levels:

1. Appraising the risk or threat posed by the stressor
2. Appraising options for responding

Next, these perceptions influence the response to the stressor, which is labeled "coping." The response is also shaped by other factors such as general coping style and the degree of social support perceived. Generally, a person's coping efforts result in outcomes that affect emotional well-being, functional status, and general health behaviors. We now examine the components of the model more closely.

Cognitive Appraisals

Cognitive appraisals involve a process in which individuals evaluate a situation with respect to its significance for their well-being. Lazarus and Folkman (1984) identified three types of cognitive appraisals: primary appraisal, secondary appraisal, and reappraisal.

Primary appraisal occurs first when an individual encounters stress. The individual evaluates the stressor as *threatening*, *harmful*, or *challenging*. This appraisal permits anticipatory coping. "*Threat* concerns harms or losses that haven't yet taken place but are anticipated" (Lazarus & Folkman, 1984, p. 32, emphasis added). *Harms* or *losses* are the perceptions that some damage has already occurred, perhaps due to an injury or illness, damage to self-esteem, or the loss of a loved one. "The most damaging life events are those in which central and extensive commitments are lost" (Lazarus & Folkman, 1984, p. 32). An example might be the loss of one's home resulting from placement in a nursing home. This placement may produce perceived losses associated with control (e.g., "I can no longer go where I want or do what I want."), memories (e.g., "This home is my life. I raised my children here."), and perceptions of a future that threatens one's social life, independence, and spirituality (e.g., "I'll lose contact with my friends and my church."). Finally, primary appraisal can deem the stressor as *challenging*, which means that there is a perceived potential to gain or grow as a result of the encounter (e.g., "Maybe being here will help me with my arthritis."). A situation is more likely to be appraised as a challenge when the person has some sense of control over his or her emotions and behavioral responses to the situation.

Secondary appraisal involves a cognitive evaluation of what can be done about the stressor. According to Lazarus and Folkman (1984), secondary appraisal "is a complex process that takes into account which coping options are available, the likelihood that a given coping option will accomplish what it is supposed to, and the likelihood that one can apply a particular strategy or set of strategies effectively" (p. 35). Secondary appraisals involve a set of expectancies for the coping response and the outcome. In this way, they are similar to the cognitive processes articulated in Bandura's (1982) concept of self-efficacy. For instance, in the prior example, the woman who entered the nursing home might wonder whether recreation is among her options for coping with the isolation she anticipates at the nursing home. She might wonder if there is a way to stay connected with friends by telephone or through letter writing (which she immediately discounts due to the crippling arthritis that contributed to the placement in the first place). She might also worry about not being able to go to morning mass, which she did regularly as a source of emotional comfort and companionship.

Reappraisal is the third type of appraisal. (This is not depicted in Figure 5.2.) Reappraisal refers to changed views that result as new information is received from the environment. For instance, the nursing home resident may change her appraisal of the situation once she is taken on a tour of the facility by the recreation therapist and shown the chapel. She might also feel better about staying in touch with friends after learning that adaptive computer equipment is available that will allow her to dictate her letters and that the recreation therapist will teach her how to use it. However, as explained in the section on self-efficacy, this woman's appraisal would be most strongly influenced if she actually had the chance to attend religious services or use the computer. While there is little real distinction between appraisal and reappraisal, the interaction between primary appraisals ("What are the threats to my well-being?") and secondary appraisals ("What can be done about it?") determines the degree of stress and the extent of one's reactions or coping responses.

Factors Influencing the Cognitive Appraisal Process

Certain personal factors influence a person's cognitive appraisals. Specifically, the greater the degree of commitment to someone or something, the greater the vulnerability to threat of loss. In the case of the person placed in a nursing home, fear of abandonment, isolation, and dependency increases the vulnerability this person feels as a result of stress. Beliefs, in terms of defining reality and in terms of personal control to change or alter the stressful situation, also play a key role in the appraisal process. Beliefs about personal control can be a general disposition that an individual carries into all situations. They can also be situational or context specific. Lazarus and Folkman (1984) contend that situational control appraisals "are products of the individual's evaluations of the demands of

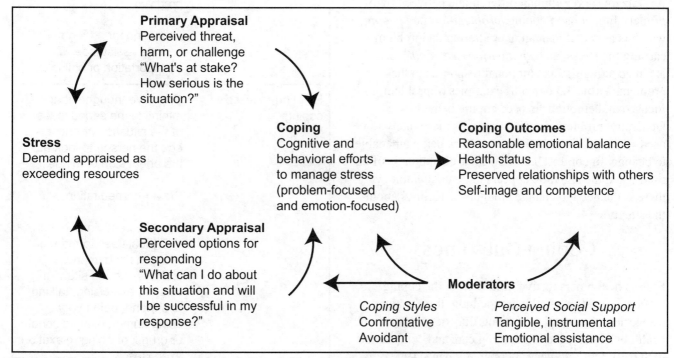

Figure 5.2: Transactional model of stress and coping (Adapted from Lerman & Glanz, 1997)

the situation, as well as his or her coping resources and options and ability to implement the needed coping strategies" (p. 69). Consider, for instance, the person with a chronic illness such as multiple sclerosis. Managing frequent bouts of chronic fatigue by relying on the support of others is much easier to do once an individual has some experience using this form of coping assistance at particular times in the course of the illness.

Responding to Stress: Coping

Once an individual appraises a situation as stressful, he or she responds to it in some way. This response has been labeled as coping. *Coping* has been defined by Lazarus and Folkman (1984) as "*constantly changing cognitive and behavioral efforts to manage specific external and/or internal demands that are appraised as taxing or exceeding the resources of the person*" (p. 141; emphasis added). Coping is theorized as being a process that is situation-specific and responsive to constantly changing demands and conflicts that a person experiences. Coping is also considered to be a deliberate effort rather than an automatic adaptive behavior, and it is not necessarily dependent on successful resolution of the problem. In essence, coping is any effort that is aimed at managing (not mastering) stressful conditions. Generally, the intent of coping is to restore a sense of balance or psychological equilibrium such that the individual can continue to function in a relatively stable manner.

Lazarus and Folkman differentiate between two primary functions of coping: *problem-focused coping*, which is aimed at managing or altering the problem causing the stress, and *emotion-focused coping*, which is aimed at regulating emotional responses to the problem. **Table 5.3** contains examples of problem-focused and emotion-focused coping behaviors. Generally, problem-focused coping is more likely to be used when the situation is appraised as being amenable to change. In contrast, emotion-focused coping is often used when the situation appears to be unalterable, yet there is the need to change thoughts or feelings about the situation.

Coping Outcomes

From a health perspective, results from the coping process can ultimately be grouped into three main categories: emotional well-being, functional status, and health behaviors, such as seeking care and compliance with treatment regimens (Lerman & Glanz, 1997).

According to Taylor (1999), coping efforts are judged successful if they reduce physiological and psychological states of arousal and permit the individual to return to prestress activities. In health crises, coping outcomes are associated with specific targets of adaptation pertinent to the experiences of illness, treatment, and hospitalization. These include dealing with pain and incapacitation, dealing with the hospital environment, and developing adequate relationships with professional staff. General outcomes include preserving a reasonable emotional balance and satisfactory self-image, maintaining a sense of competence and mastery, and preserving relationships with family and friends (Moos & Schaefer, 1986). It has been demon-

Table 5.3: Problem-focused and emotion-focused coping

Type of Coping	Sample Behaviors
Problem-focused coping	Seeking information about one's medical condition or disability
	Planning problem-solving strategies, such as making lists of questions to ask or reading about adaptive equipment
	Cooperating with health care professionals in prescribed health care program
	Arranging for a friend to provide assistance with transportation or childcare
Emotion-focused coping	Cognitive thoughts that minimize the seriousness of the situation or encourage the person to look at the bright side of things
	Prayer or meditation
	Specific behaviors that an individual uses to manage emotions and improve feelings about a situation, such as exercising, talking to a friend, doing yoga, using humor, using alcohol or drugs, or doing relaxation exercises

strated that recreation activity can be used with hospitalized clients to achieve these adaptive tasks and thereby increase their sense of coping abilities (Shank, Coyle & Kinney, 1991).

Factors Influencing the Coping Process

A person's general coping style and a person's perception of social support moderate and influence a person's coping effort (see Figure 5.2, p. 71). TR practitioners must understand the roles of these mediating factors when designing interventions focused on assisting clients in the process of coping.

Coping Styles

In contrast to situation-specific coping efforts (problem-focused or emotion-focused), individuals also develop more enduring coping styles considered to be relatively stable characteristics or dispositions of that person (Lazarus, 1993). Two common coping styles are the *avoidant style* and the *confrontative* or *vigilant style* (Taylor, 1999). Neither style is necessarily better than the other; however, the avoidant style seems to work better with short-term stressors whereas the confrontative style reflects cognitive and behavioral strategies suitable for long-term threats. The avoidant coping style finds particular value in activities that help divert or distract attention away from sources of stress, including boredom. Thus, *diversional activities* can be a valuable part of clinical TR when they are used purposefully to help people cope.

Recall the concept of hardiness (Exhibit 2.6, p. 26) advanced by Maddi and Kobasa (1984). Hardiness emerged from research on executives who despite highly stressful work conditions had unusually high resistance to stress-related illnesses. These individuals tended to have a disposition whereby they viewed stress as a *challenge* rather than a threat, strong *commitments* to things of value in their lives, and a high degree of perceived *control* in their lives. In essence, hardy individuals may appraise stressful situations more favorably than others under similar circumstances.

Another frequently examined personality trait or disposition related to coping styles is optimism. *Optimism* is a reflection and extension of other qualities such as hope, hardiness, and personal control. Optimists are people who believe that good rather than bad things will happen to them. Optimists tend to see the positive in situations, and because they anticipate favorable outcomes, they are inclined to expend effort in changing situations to produce the outcomes they want. Positive attitudes and beliefs associated with optimism can boost the immune system and help maintain health (Hafen, Karren, Frandsen & Smith, 1996). Optimism is an effective stress-buffering disposition. Martin Seligman's (1990) research verified this view. He found that optimists show greater persistence in the face of stress, whereas pessimists tend to give up or disengage from the situation.

Social Support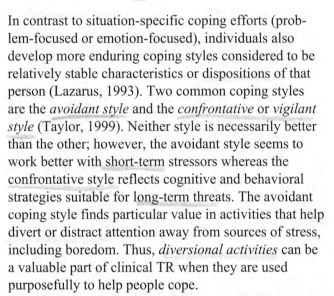

The coping process involves the transaction between the individual and the environment. As such this process is shaped by an individual's social context. The social ties a person develops throughout life serve as a significant moderator of negative effects of stress on health and well-being (Sarason, Sarason & Garung, 1997). Thoits (1986) conceptualized social support as *coping assistance*. Support from others enables a person to gain new perspectives, receive assistance, and vent feelings. Social support is generally understood as the tangible and intangible resources a person can count on as a result of his or her interaction with others. Social resources consist of one's *social network* (the size, density, durability, and frequency of social contacts), *social relationships* (the existence, number, and type of relationships), and *social support* (the type, source and quality of the resources). Support can be in the form of tangible, instrumental aid, as in the provision of money, information, and specific assistance with getting various tasks done. For instance, a person undergoing treatment for a medical condition may find it very helpful to gather information from someone else who had the same illness or treatment. Having friends or neighbors assist with transportation to and from medical appointments or grocery stores is another example of tangible assistance. Support also can be in the form of intangible emotional assistance through affection, acceptance, and comfort (Hafen et al., 1996). Such warmth and reassurance can fortify the individual's resolve to cope with greater confidence and self-assurance.

Social support plays an important role in protecting health in two primary ways. First, social support enhances health by increasing positive feelings and a sense of esteem, stability, and control over one's environment. Second, social support buffers the negative consequences of stress (Cohen & Syme, 1985). Strong social support also produces health benefits within the immune system as a result of confiding in others (Pennebaker, 1990). Confiding can be done in private intimate conversations with a friend, family member, or a health professional. Confiding is also a significant part of any social support group, such as those found in oncology programs. Having others to talk to about problems and concerns can help with accurate appraisal of risks or threats posed by the situation, as well as helping to realize the resources that can be drawn upon in this situation. At the very least, confiding in others who are accepting and reassuring can increase the chances of feeling validated and cared for. It is important to note, however, that confiding does not have to be exclusively verbal sharing or face-to-face. Self-disclosure can occur through keeping a diary or journaling (Murray, 1997), whereby an individual writes about traumatic past events or current stressful situations. For example, many patients, caregivers, or other people who share a particular disabling condition find relief in confiding in peers or professionals through Internet chats.

Implications for TR Practice

Since coping is considered to be a process dictated by a particular situation and the thoughts and actions of the person as the situation unfolds, coping processes are open to modification through education and counseling (Folkman et al., 1991). Coping processes are influenced by available resources that a person is aware of and can access, including personal skills and abilities, social resources, and psychological resources such as self-efficacy beliefs. Each of these can be changed, and coping training programs have been developed for diverse populations **Exhibit 5.1** contains two examples of coping skills training programs developed for persons with HIV/AIDS (Folkman et al., 1991) and individuals with mental health disorders (DeNelsky & Boat, 1986). Lazarus (1991) has emphasized that what a person wants to accomplish in a stressful transaction is an important principle of coping that underlies the choice of a coping strategy. Therefore, any attempt to help a client through coping training would depend on understanding what the client wants to accomplish in the particular situation. For example, if a client wants to find ways to take his or her mind off the situation, teaching assertiveness skills to meet the problem head-on will not work.

TR coping programs must be designed with a realization that whether people use recreation and leisure as a coping behavior depends on the perceptions they have about recreation and leisure. For instance, the cognitive appraisal process includes an assessment of whether the source of stress can be changed and the individual's coping resources and options. The *option to use* recreation to change the situation depends on an individual's knowledge and experience. Furthermore, beliefs about one's *ability to use* recreation effectively are also a matter of perception and experience.

Interventions aimed at helping clients cope should involve assistance and support to make accurate appraisals of their situations and reasonable assessments of their coping resources. An essential part of interventions is enhancing the personal and environmental coping resources. TR interventions can support problem-focused as well as emotion-focused coping strategies. For instance, play and recreation activities can be used as a means of distraction and distancing oneself from stressors. Clients can be assisted to obtain and use information through reading materials that are both informative and emotionally comforting. Similar outcomes can be derived from both formal and informal social activities. Furthermore, clients can be assisted and supported in their use of play and recreation as an active coping mechanism. This is clearly reflected in a wide variety of TR interventions, including medical play and preprocedural play activities used with children facing surgery or other invasive medical procedures. Children are assisted to work through their fears and apprehensions by pretending to be a doctor or nurse caring for a doll using medical play materials such as a stethoscope, needles, and bandages. Likewise, journaling, reminiscing, and relaxation training can be used to promote coping and adaptation in adults. **Exhibit 5.2** (p. 76) highlights two examples of clinical TR services based on coping theory. They show how theory can guide the delivery of TR services.

Health-Related Theories

The approach to TR practice presented in this text reflects the belief that play, recreation, and leisure can contribute to health. We take a broad view of *health* to be a *dynamic, multidimensional state of well-being comprised of physical, social, psychological, and spiritual manifestations that taken together reflect a balanced, positive state of well-being.* Thus, health is more than the absence of illness or disease. The existence of an illness (e.g., cancer) or a chronic disability (e.g., schizophrenia) would not preclude the individual from experiencing an overall state of health. Health involves a subjective interpretation, which is particularly relevant to people who have chronic illnesses and disabling conditions. Such individuals can be very healthy in terms of relationships with others and a positive outlook on life (Donatelle & Davis, 1999).

Therapeutic recreation practice can be considered a form of health promotion when practitioners assist people to achieve and express a healthy lifestyle. Ideally recreation behavior could become a health habit that reduces or prevents negative conditions associated with illness or disability. According to Taylor (1999) a "health habit is a health-related behavior that is firmly established and often performed automatically, without awareness" (p. 53). Of course, many behaviors considered to be recreation are not health promoting (e.g., excessive forms of passive entertainment, illicit drug use). Unhealthy behaviors can be pleasurable and thus resistant to change. Recreation therapists would work with clients to become aware of and use recreation behaviors that contribute positively to their personal sense of physical, social, psychological, and spiritual well-being. For example, physically and socially active recreation behaviors are associated with lower rates of skin ulcers, urinary tract infections, and depression among adults who have spinal cord injuries (Coyle, Shank, Kinney & Hutchins, 1993).

There are several theoretical models used to understand health behavior and to guide intervention programs. Brief descriptions of the *Health Belief Model* (Hochbaum, 1958; Rosenstock, 1990), the *Theory of Reasoned Action*, and the *Theory of Planned Behavior* (Ajzen & Fishbein, 1980) are presented here. These models have relevance to the clinical practice of TR when play and recreation are used to improve and maintain health status, functional capacity, and quality of life. Each of these models reflects the importance of attitudes, perceptions, and beliefs in shaping health behavior.

Health Belief Model

The most influential attitudinal theory used to understand health behavior is the Health Belief Model originally posited by Hochbaum (1958). This model is based on the premise that a person's health behavior is largely influenced by whether the person perceives a health threat and whether a particular behavior would be effective in reducing the threat. The general knowledge and beliefs an individual has about the illness or disabling condition shapes these perceptions, as well as whether the consequences of the condition are thought to be serious. Likewise, the knowledge and beliefs about the health behavior (e.g., recreation) is perceived in terms of the potential effectiveness of the behavior

Exhibit 5.1: Coping training programs

The ***Coping Effectiveness Training Program*** (Folkman et al., 1991) involves teaching persons with HIV/AIDS new appraisal and coping techniques. *Appraisal skill development* focuses on teaching clients to reduce large, global stressors into more specific parts. Simply put, this involves examining a situation in terms of what is most troubling and what can be done about it. *Coping training* involves learning to distinguish between problem-focused and emotion-focused coping and when to use each. Problem-focused training emphasizes decision-making skills. Emotion-focused training involves both cognitive and behavioral strategies, such as the use of spiritual and religious resources, humor, exercise, relaxation, meditation, and the pursuit of pleasant activities such as going to the movies, shopping, or listening to music. The final ingredient in this program includes social support training. This involves how to identify what kind of support is needed, from whom to seek it, and how to maintain it. This training program emphasizes skill development and the appropriate match of coping strategies to specific stressful situations.

The ***Coping Skills Model*** (DeNelsky & Boat, 1986) assists individuals with a variety of mental health disorders to develop general skills that would assist them in their efforts to remain in the community. They define coping skills as "the physical, emotional, and cognitive *components of adaptability* that an individual needs in order to manage life situations" (p. 323). Three categories of coping skills include:
1. *Interpersonal relationships* (including general and intimate social skills)
2. *Thinking and feeling* (including appropriate emotional arousal and awareness of feelings)
3. *Approaches to self and life* (including realistic self-expectations and the ability to experience healthy pleasure and satisfaction)

Recreation as a specific way to learn coping skills was related to each category, particularly social interaction, diversion, and relaxation training. This approach is consistent with the general view that recreation interests and skills are an important part of the entire set of coping skills needed by individuals with mental illness (Anthony, Cohen & Farkas, 1990; Kapelowitz, 1999; Liberman, 1988).

in reducing the health threat, and whether the costs (e.g., burdens and barriers) outweigh the benefits derived from the behavior (Rosenstock, 1990).

Consider the situation of a 38-year-old married mother of three who has a spinal cord injury resulting from a car accident. Part of her overall rehabilitation program includes recreation therapy, aimed at preparing her for resuming her premorbid lifestyle. This includes physically and socially active recreation for herself, as part of her relationship with her husband, and within the family. How would the Health Belief Model fit her situation? What are the implications for clinical practice? Theoretically one would begin with the perceptions this woman has of her current situation and her anticipated future. Presumably she would be concerned about the consequences of her injury and the extent to which her spinal cord injury will interfere with her abilities to function as a wife, mother, friend,

and perhaps employee. In the course of her rehabilitation, she may learn that she is susceptible to secondary health problems that may be physical (e.g., urinary tract infections, skin breakdown due to pressure sores), social (e.g., diminished activities with family and friends), and emotional (e.g., feelings of depression and loss). Assuming she values being a wife, mother, and friend, she may perceive her situation as serious and severe. She may also learn that committed, purposeful engagement in physically and socially active recreation and leisure pursuits can minimize the likelihood of any of these secondary health problems. According to the Health Belief Model, the final perceptions that would determine her health behavior have to do with barriers to engaging in physically and socially active recreation. The major implication for the TR practitioner is to provide interventions that enhance knowledge and change beliefs about the

Exhibit 5.2: Clinical TR services based on coping theory

Helping clients cope with the stress of illness and hospitalization is one of the fundamental functions of recreation therapy services at the Clinical Center of the National Institutes of Health in Bethesda, Maryland. Recreation therapy interventions are based on coping theory, beginning with an assessment of the client's primary and secondary appraisal process. Clients' perceptions of their situation are explored through interviews, including questions about the level of stress the client is experiencing and the degree to which they believe they are equipped to cope with the situation. A combination of standardized and in-house stress and coping inventories are used, including rating scales pertaining to optimism, boredom, pain, and relaxation. Intervention strategies are identified and selected so that they parallel the client's preferred coping style as well as other potential coping resources. An important part of the intervention plan involves the client and the therapist establishing target outcomes related to managing, tolerating, or alleviating stress. These may be an increased ability to relax, more frequent contact with a social support network, or reduced levels of anxiety and boredom. The *Art of Relaxation* program includes stress management and relaxation training, social activities, and myriad crafts, games, music, reading, and meditation activities. Interventions also include use of Vibro-acoustic chairs and mats that induce relaxation through music and gentle massage. Leisure education and exercise training are also used with clients who have longer hospitalizations. Outcomes are monitored through client ratings after each session and at discharge (Ballard, 2001; Patrick & Ebel, 1994).

Increasing clients' coping skills is also a primary focus of TR in addiction treatment. Carruthers and Hood (in press) developed a cognitive-behavioral coping skills program based on Shiffman and Wills' (1985) stress coping process model. The program is designed to teach clients how to reduce negative stress and increase positive aspects of their lives that bring resiliency and joy. For example, clients are taught to examine irrational thinking and increase positive thoughts and beliefs about their abilities to manage external pressures. Clients are also taught cognitive-behavioral methods for distracting themselves from worry, relaxing, and increasing "joy building behaviors" such as listening to music, getting a massage, or eating enjoyable food. This intervention program includes typical cognitive-behavioral strategies like role-plays, behavioral contracts, and homework. The program involves seven sessions, with each session having three distinct phases. During the session's instructional phase clients review coping skills information. During the application phase clients have one or two days to complete homework related to the session topic. Finally, the debriefing phase involves clients in a follow-up meeting to discuss their experiences with applying instructional materials. Carruthers and Hood field-tested this program in three hospitals. Evaluation data collected on more than 150 clients indicated that they perceived the goals of the program to be very relevant and that they improved or improved slightly in all goal areas. More research is needed to examine the effectiveness of this promising theory-based TR intervention program in helping clients recover and maintain sobriety.

relationship between recreation involvement and reduced susceptibility to health problems.

The Health Belief Model has been used in a variety of research studies that investigated health behaviors, including dieting, use of health screening programs (e.g., mammography), and safe sex practices (Taylor, 1999). Perceived barriers to engaging in a health behavior appear to be the strongest influential factor on health behaviors. Furthermore, while the Health Belief Model has been used widely, the best research appears to be conducted when the model is extended to include *personal intentions to behave* (Brannon & Feist, 2000). Taylor concurs, and goes one step further to stress the importance of self-efficacy. "The Health Belief Model leaves out at least one important component of health behavior change: the perception that one will be able to engage in the behavior" (p. 65). The Theory of Reasoned Action and Theory of Planned Behavior overcome this weakness in the Health Belief Model.

Theory of Reasoned Action and Theory of Planned Behavior

These two theories are presented together because one is an extension of the other. Both have been developed by Ajzen and represent the role of personal intentions in people's health behaviors. Ajzen and various colleagues (Ajzen & Fishbein, 1980; Ajzen & Madden, 1986) contended that people generally think about their goal-oriented behavior and consider the implications of their actions as part of their decision-making. According to Ajzen's Theory of Reasoned Action, behavior is a function of a person's *attitude* toward a particular behavior (which can be shaped by past experiences and by the expectations of others), and *beliefs* that the behavior will produce positive and valued outcomes. Together, one's attitude toward the behavior and the inclination to conform to the expectations of others shapes behavioral *intentions*. As a result of theoretical refinement, Ajzen extended the Theory of Reasoned Action to include *perceived behavioral control*. Thus, the Theories of Reasoned Action and Planned Behavior contain three essential parts: a person's attitudes toward a behavior, the social influence or subjective norm, and perceptions about one's ability to control outcomes of the behavior (see **Figure 5.3**, p. 78). Simply stated, the greater the ease with which a person believes he or she can perform the behavior, the more likely the person is to have behavioral intentions (Brannon & Feist, 2000).

Both of these theories have had widespread use and provide a foundation for understanding whether a person will practice a particular health behavior, including recreation and leisure behavior (Azjen & Driver, 1991, 1992).

Implications for Therapeutic Recreation Practice

The theories presented about health behavior have clear implications for TR clinical practice, especially when used to help clients change their level of health and well-being. In an effort to promote play, recreation, and leisure as health behaviors, practitioners need to increase clients' knowledge and understanding regarding the role of recreation and leisure in reducing immediate (e.g., managing pain) and long-term (e.g., physical deconditioning) health threats. These theories reflect the importance of others in establishing expectations and providing support and encouragement for positive health behaviors. Obviously this has implications for client education programs to be extended to family education. For instance, spouses have a critical role to play in the complete rehabilitation of clients recovering from strokes or cardiac conditions. They can be pivotal in encouraging and supporting a resumption of physically and socially active recreation if their knowledge and understanding has been increased as well. Finally, as indicated in these health theories, a client's perceived behavioral control seems to have the most influence on engaging in and maintaining health behaviors. Therapeutic recreation interventions need to emphasize actual recreation and leisure skill development in clients. Learning about the potential benefits of recreation and leisure coupled with adaptive skills and compensatory strategies that permit active recreation and leisure involvement increase the likelihood that health outcomes can be achieved. When TR is practiced as a clinical intervention aimed at improving health, the ultimate intention of the interventions is to increase clients' competence to use recreation and leisure as part of a healthy lifestyle.

Final Comments about Theory

No single theory is best for guiding TR practice. We have presented several theories that have been referred to in TR literature as being reflected in practice. These theories contain a social–psychological perspective that TR practitioners and educators claim to be part of practice; however, as with all possible theories, the ones presented in this chapter need to be tested empirically for their usefulness to TR practice. Brannon and Feist (2000) found that all the health-related theories were less than adequate in explaining and predicting health behaviors, in part because of the general difficulty in measuring peoples' attitudes and beliefs. They also point out that none of the existing theories is comprehensive enough to adequately cover health-seeking behaviors as well as prevention or adherence behaviors. That is, the process of initiating behavior change is not necessarily the same as maintaining the change. Finally, the existing theoretical models are limited in their ability to accurately reflect the various demographic, socioeconomic, and cultural influences on health behavior. Each model implies that individuals experience some type of barrier or obstacle, and tend to place significant emphasis on personal control of behavior. Brannon and Feist remind us that some barriers, such as racism and poverty, may be outside the individual's control and may constitute experi-

ences that are quite different than the life experiences of researchers and health care providers. Likewise, an unsupportive and resource-deficient environment can hamper a person's desire and intention to incorporate recreation and leisure into a healthy lifestyle. Thus, any attempts to explain health behavior and psychosocial adaptation, and any subsequent health promotion or intervention programs must give full consideration to such external influences on behavior.

Additionally, while each of the theories presented were slightly different, they share a set of testable assumptions about health and human behavior, which can serve as a foundation for clinical TR interventions. They are:

- Individuals' attitudes, perceptions, and beliefs directly influence their behavior. These "cognitions" are pertinent to the person's experience of stress and the meaning illness and disability holds for the

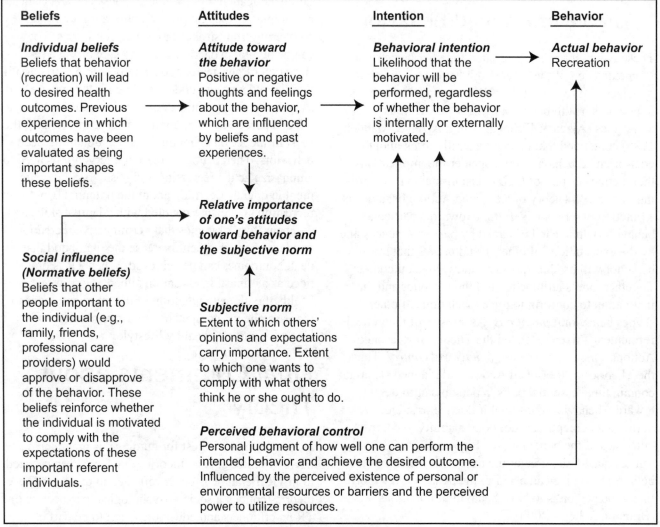

Figure 5.3: Theories of reasoned action and planned behavior (Adapted from Montano, Danuta & Taplin, 1997)

individual. Attitudes, perceptions and beliefs are also relevant to understanding the individual's view of recreation as an actual or potential aid in coping and adaptation and in understanding the person's perception of barriers associated with recreation involvement. They are pertinent to the efficacy expectations a person formulates about themselves and others in relation to desired outcomes, such as health and happiness. *Therefore, to help a person use recreation as a coping mechanism and as a means to improving and maintaining health and well-being, TR interventions must be aimed at altering the individual's thinking as it relates to their health-related behaviors.*

- Transactions between the individual and the physical and social dimensions of his or her environment, both past and present, provide input that is integral to formulating attitudes, perceptions, and beliefs. The environment is critical to either supporting or impeding positive health behaviors. Environmental cues help shape awareness of options and cues for action. *Therefore, TR interventions must incorporate the physical and social environment to aid in learning, adaptation, and growth.*

- Attitudes, perceptions, and beliefs are modified most effectively through actual action experiences, as long as the individual has the opportunity to alter their cognition by reflecting on the experience. Reflection is essential to changes in perceived control and personal competence, which increases the likelihood of an individual engaging in desired behavior in the future. *Therefore, TR interventions need to emphasize learning through experience, and utilize processing techniques to maximize change and generalization to life in the future.*

Summary

This chapter presented Bandura's Social Cognition Theory (Bandura, 1986), Lazarus and Folkman's (1984) theoretical work on stress and coping, the Health Belief Model (Hochbaum, 1958; Rosenstock, 1990), and the Theories of Reasoned Action and Planned Behavior (Ajzen & Fishbein, 1980). Each of these theories can be used to explain how experiences contribute to the construction of beliefs about health-related behavior and about one's abilities to use such behaviors for achieving and maintaining health and well-being.

They can be used to guide TR interventions designed to assist clients in changing their thoughts, beliefs, attitudes, and behaviors or managing environmental barriers related to health, leisure, and life quality. These theories, however, can seem abstract without application. Therefore, the next chapter focuses on applying theory to practice.

References

Ajzen, I. and Driver, B. (1991). Prediction of leisure participation from behavioral, normative, and control beliefs: An application of the theory of planned behavior. *Leisure Sciences, 13,* 185–204.

Ajzen, I. and Driver, B. (1992). Application of theory of planned behavior to leisure choice. *Journal of Leisure Research, 24,* 207–224.

Ajzen, I. and Fishbein, M. (1980). *Understanding attitudes and predicting social behavior.* Englewood Cliffs, NJ: Prentice-Hall.

Ajzen, I. and Madden, T. (1986). Prediction of goal directed behavior: Attitudes, intentions, and perceived behavioral control. *Journal of Experimental Social Psychology, 22,* 453–474.

Anthony, W., Cohen, M., and Farkas, M. (1990). *Psychiatric rehabilitation.* Boston, MA: Boston University Center for Psychiatric Rehabilitation.

Ballard, S. (2001, September). *Relaxation techniques and symptom reduction.* Paper presented at the American Therapeutic Recreation Association's Annual Conference, New Orleans, LA.

Bandura, A. (1977a). *Social learning theory.* Englewood Cliffs, NJ: Prentice-Hall.

Bandura, A. (1977b). Self-efficacy: Toward a unifying theory of behavioral change. *Psychological Review, 84*(2), 191–215.

Bandura, A. (1982). Self-efficacy mechanism in human agency. *American Psychologist, 33,* 122–147.

Bandura, A. (1986). *Social foundations of thoughts and action: A social cognitive theory.* Englewood Cliffs, NJ: Prentice-Hall.

Bedini, L. and Wu, Y. (1994). A methodological review of research in the *Therapeutic Recreation Journal* from 1986 to 1990. *Therapeutic Recreation Journal, 28,* 87–98.

Brannon, L. and Feist, J. (2000). *Health psychology: An introduction to behavior and health* (4th ed.). Belmont, CA: Wadsworth.

Carruthers, C. and Hood, C. (in press). Coping skills program for individuals with alcoholism. *Therapeutic Recreation Journal.*

Cohen, S. and Syme, L. (1985). *Social support and health.* London: Academic Press.

Coyle, C., Shank, J., Kinney, T., and Hutchins, D. (1993). Psychosocial functioning and changes in leisure lifestyle among individuals with chronic secondary health problems related to spinal cord injury. *Therapeutic Recreation Journal, 27*(4), 239–252.

Csikszentmihalyi, M. (1990). *Flow: The psychology of optimal experience.* New York, NY: Harper Perennial.

Dattilo, J., Kleiber, D., and Williams, R. (1998). Self-determination and enjoyment enhancement: A psychologically based service delivery model for therapeutic recreation. *Therapeutic Recreation Journal, 32*(3), 258–271.

DeNelsky, G. and Boat, B. (1986). Coping skills model of psychological diagnosis and treatment. *Professional Psychology: Research and Practice, 17*(4), 322–330.

Donatelle, R. and Davis, L. (1999). *Health: The basics* (3rd ed.). Boston, MA: Allyn & Bacon.

Folkman, S., Chesney, M., McKusick, L., Ironson, G., Johnson, D., and Coates, T. (1991). Translating coping theory into an intervention. In J. Eckenrode (Ed.), *The social context of coping* (pp. 239–260). New York, NY: Plenum Press.

Hafen, B., Karren, K., Frandsen, K., and Smith, L. (1996). Social support, relationships, and health. In B. Hafen, K. Karren, K. Frandsen, and L. Smith (Eds.), *Mind/body health: The effects of attitudes, emotions and relationships* (pp. 261–289). Boston, MA: Allyn & Bacon.

Hochbaum, G. (1958). *Public participation in medical screening programs* (DHEW Publication No. 572). Washington, DC: U. S. Government Printing Office.

Iso-Ahola, S. (1980). *The social psychology of leisure and recreation.* Dubuque, IA: Wm. C. Brown.

Iso-Ahola, S. (1995). The social psychology of leisure: Past, present, and future research. In L. Barnett (Ed.), *Research about leisure: Past, present and future* (pp. 65–96). Champaign, IL: Sagamore Publishing.

Kapelowitz, A. (1999, September). Psychiatric rehabilitation —An overview. Unpublished paper presented at the American Therapeutic Recreation Association Annual Conference, Portland, OR.

Lazarus, R. (1991). Foreword. In J. Eckenrode (Ed.), *The social context of coping* (p. ix). New York, NY: Plenum Press.

Lazarus, R. (1993). Coping theory and research: Past, present and future. *Psychosomatic Medicine, 55*, 234–247.

Lazarus, R. and Folkman, S. (1984). *Stress, appraisal and coping.* New York, NY: Springer

Lerman, C. and Glanz, K. (1997). Stress, coping and health behavior. In K. Glanz, F. Lewis, and B. Rimer (Eds.), *Health behavior and health education* (2nd ed., pp. 113–138). San Francisco, CA: Jossey-Bass.

Liberman, R. (1988). *Psychiatric rehabilitation of chronic mental patients.* Washington, DC: American Psychiatric Press.

Maddi, S. and Kobasa, S. (1984). *The hardy executive: Health under stress.* Chicago, IL: Dow Jones-Irwin Dorsey.

Malkin, M. (1993). Issues and needs in therapeutic recreation research. In M. Malkin, and C. Howe (Eds.), *Research in therapeutic recreation: Concepts and methods* (pp. 3–23). State College, PA: Venture Publishing, Inc.

Mannell, R. and Kleiber, D. (1997). *A social psychology of leisure.* State College, PA: Venture Publishing, Inc.

Mobily, K. (1999). New horizons in models of practice in therapeutic recreation. *Therapeutic Recreation Journal, 33*(3), 174–192.

Mobily, K. (2000). An interview with professor Seppo Iso-Ahola. *Therapeutic Recreation Journal, 34*(4), 300–305.

Montano, D., Danuta, K., and Taplin, S. (1997). The theory of reasoned action and the theory of planned behavior. In K. Glanz, F. Lewis, and B. Rimer (Eds.), *Health behavior and health education* (pp. 85–112). San Francisco, CA: Jossey-Bass.

Moos, R. and Schaefer, J. (1986). Life transitions and crises: A conceptual overview. In R. Moos (Ed.), *Coping with life crises* (pp. 3–28). New York, NY: Plenum Press.

Murray, S. (1997). *Patient's lived experience of acute rehabilitation and recovery contained in a creative journal.* Unpublished doctoral dissertation, Temple University, Philadelphia, PA.

Nichols, S. (1998). The Aristotelian good life model: A critique. *Therapeutic Recreation Journal, 32*(4), 309–312.

Patrick, G. and Ebel, J. (1994, September). *Coping through recreation therapy: A return to our roots.* Paper presented at the American Therapeutic Recreation Conference, Orlando, FL.

Pennebaker, J. (1990). *Opening up: The healing power of confiding in others.* New York, NY: William Morrow & Company.

Peterson, C. (1989). The dilemma of philosophy. In D. Compton (Ed.), *Issues in Therapeutic recreation: A profession in transition* (pp. 21–33). Champaign, IL: Sagamore Publishing.

Rosenstock, I. (1990). The health belief model: Explaining health behavior through expectancies. In K. Glanz, F. Lewis, and B. Rimer (Eds.), *Health behavior and health education* (pp. 39–62). San Francisco, CA: Jossey-Bass.

Rotter, D. (1990). Internal versus external control of reinforcement: A case history of a variable. *American Psychologist, 45*(4), 489–493.

Rotter, D. and Quine, L. (1994). *Social psychology and health: European perspectives.* Aldershot, UK: Avebury.

Sarason, B., Sarason, I., and Garung, R. (1997). Close personal relationships and health outcomes: A key to the role of social support. In S. Duck (Ed.), *Handbook of personal relationships* (pp. 547–573). New York, NY: Wiley.

Seligman, M. (1975). *Helplessness.* San Francisco, CA: W. H. Freeman.

Seligman, M. (1990) *Learned optimism.* New York, NY: Alfred A. Knopf.

Seyle, H. (1976a). *Stress in health and disease.* Woburn, MA: Butterworth.

Seyle, H. (1976b). *The stress of life* (rev. ed.). New York, NY: McGraw-Hill.

Shank, J., Coyle, C., Boyd, R., and Kinney, W. (1996). A classification scheme for therapeutic recreation research grounded in the rehabilitative sciences. *Therapeutic Recreation Journal, 30*, 179–196.

Shank, J., Coyle, C., and Kinney, W. (1991, September). *A comparison of the effects of clinical versus diversional therapeutic recreation involvement on rehabilitation outcomes.* Paper presented at the Benefits of Therapeutic Recreation in Rehabilitation Consensus Conference, Lafayette Hill, PA.

Shank, J., Coyle, C., and Kinney, W. (1993). Efficacy studies in therapeutic recreation research: The need, the state of the art, and future implications. In M. Malkin and C. Howe

(Eds.), *Research in therapeutic recreation: Concepts and methods* (pp. 301–335). State College, PA: Venture Publishing, Inc.

Shiffman,. S. and Wills, T. (Eds.). (1985). *Coping and substance abuse*. Orlando, FL: Academic Press.

Skinner, E. (1995). *Perceived control, motivation, and coping*. Thousand Oaks, CA: Sage Publications.

Stumbo, N. and Peterson, C. (1998). The leisure ability model. *Therapeutic Recreation Journal, 32*(2), 82–96.

Sylvester, C. (1989). Impressions of the intellectual past and future of therapeutic recreation: Implications for professionalization. In D. Compton (Ed.), *Issues in therapeutic recreation: A profession in transition* (pp. 1–20). Champaign, IL: Sagamore Publishing.

Taylor, S. (1999). *Health psychology* (4th ed.). New York, NY: McGraw-Hill.

Thoits, P. (1986). Social support as coping assistance. *Journal of consulting and clinical psychology, 54,* 416–423.

Weiner, B. (1985). An attributional theory of achievement motivation and emotion. *Psychological Review, 92,* 548–573.

Wiersma, W. (1991). *Research methods in education*. Boston, MA: Allyn & Bacon.

White, R. W. (1959). Motivation reconsidered: The concept of competence. *Psychological Review, 66,* 297–333.

Widmer, M. and Ellis, G. (1998). The Aristotelian good life model: Integration of values in therapeutic recreation service delivery. *Therapeutic Recreation Journal, 32*(4), 290–302.

Wilhite, B., Keller, J., and Caldwell, L. (1999). Optimizing lifelong health and well-being: A health enhancing model of therapeutic recreation. *Therapeutic Recreation Journal, 33*(2), 98–108.

Zimbardo, P. (1992). Foreword. In S. Brehm (Ed.), *Intimate relationships* (pp. XIV–XVI). New York, NY: McGraw-Hill.

Questions

following:

process in TR clinical practice?

ctions between their thoughts, feelings, and

a client's involvement with TR interventions?

tion reflections influence learning, adaptation,

ed in TR clinical practice?

- Individuals' attitudes, perceptions, and beliefs directly influence their behavior.

- Transactions between individuals and the physical and social dimensions of their environment, both past and present, provide input that is integral to formulating attitudes, perceptions, and beliefs.

- Attitudes, perceptions, and beliefs are modified most effectively through actual action experiences, as long as individuals have opportunities to reflect on these experiences.

At the core of these theoretical assumptions is an appreciation of the interrelatedness of *thinking*, *feeling*, and *behaving*, which is fundamental to helping people recover from illness, cope, and adapt to disabilities, and ultimately achieve and maintain quality of life. There is a reciprocal interaction between cognition and behavior. That is, cognitions (perceptions and beliefs) influence behavior, and behavior in turn alters or reinforces cognitions. TR practice is based on an additional assumption about human behavior, which contends that a primary motivating force for human beings is personal control and an innate drive to feel competent (Skinner, 1995). Thus, when recreation therapists use activity-based interventions clinically, they operate from the premise that the client's behavior and experience with TR interventions can alter thoughts and feelings and ultimately establish positive beliefs about competence and control. If the client's competence system is positively impacted, then increases are likely to be seen in the client's use of recreation in achieving and maintaining health.

The end result of this learning, adaptation, and growth is a greater sense of competence needed to maintain health and life quality through play, recreation, and leisure. In Chapter 5 we discussed several theories that guide clinical work. However, theory can seem abstract unless applied to situations that reflect TR practice. Therefore, this chapter links theory and practice by integrating Chapter 4 and Chapter 5. We begin with an explanation of a theory-based cognitive–behavioral change process that can occur in TR practice. To help illustrate this change process, we present three distinct applications or cases, followed by an explanation of various cognitive–behavioral procedures and techniques commonly used to help clients achieve their intended outcomes.

Therapeutic Recreation and the Cognitive–Behavioral Change Process

A cognitive–behavioral approach to TR practice is informed by a set of common assumptions derived from the theories presented in Chapter 5. These assumptions can be summarized as follows:

The Cognitive–Behavioral Change Process in TR Practice

Figure 6.1 illustrates the change process that occurs when therapeutic recreation is practiced clinically using a cognitive–behavioral approach. It reflects an interrelatedness of social–psychological theory, client behavior change, and the clinical TR process facilitated by a recreation therapist. The underlying theoretical assumption is that human behavior is shaped and maintained by an interaction between one's thoughts, feelings, past behavior, and any environmental influences that might suggest, encourage, or reward certain behaviors. From a theoretical perspective (the double-lined circle area in Figure 6.1), the motivation to act is influenced by thoughts and feelings a person has about oneself, the situation at hand as well as similar past experiences, environmental influences, and the desire to feel competent (antecedents). These thoughts, feelings, and environmental factors ultimately shape behavior (action), and behavior, in turn, produces further thoughts and feelings (consequences) that either confirm or disconfirm previously held cognitions and emotions. The consequences of one's action most directly shape behavior change, and so consequences have a pivotal role in the development and maintenance of healthy and satisfying behavior.

At the client level (bounded by the square box in Figure 6.1), the elements labeled appraisals, client behaviors, and client reflections parallel antecedents, action, and consequences. Specifically, the client's decision to take action (behavior) is influenced by antecedents, such as an appraisal of the challenges inherent in the situation, the resources or supports in the environment, and beliefs about one's personal control and competence. The client's experience with the consequences of this behavior (reflection) either helps maintain the behavior or discourages it from occurring again.

Also illustrated in Figure 6.1 is the behavior of the recreation therapist (bounded by a single circle). The therapist is engaged in a systematic process of helping clients achieve outcomes associated with learning, adaptation, and growth. Recreation therapists use their understanding of human behavior and theories of

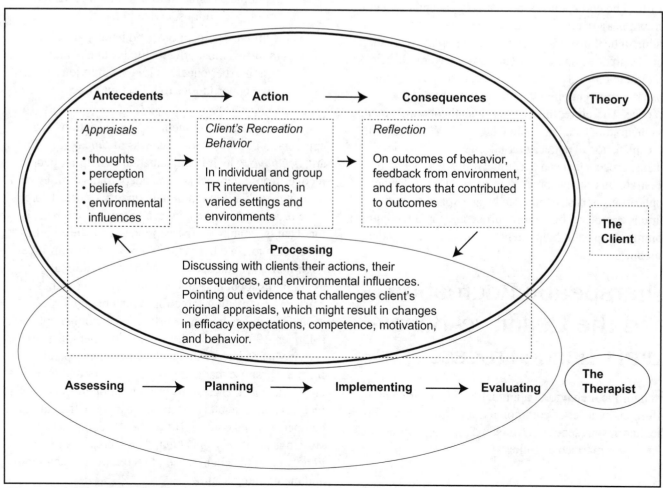

Figure 6.1: Overlay of theory and practice

behavior change to guide them as they engage in the clinical process of assessing, planning, implementing, and evaluating. For instance, understanding antecedent perceptions and beliefs that subsequently influence client behavior is a critical part of the assessment process. Recreation therapists also take care in planning and implementing interventions that involve activities, the environment, and a helping relationship. Finally, with the support of the recreation therapist, clients reflect on the consequences of their action, allowing them to make interpretations that can result in new appraisals of themselves and their situation. This reflective process (known as *processing*) is critical to fostering changes in client motivation, confidence, and competence to use recreation to achieve and maintain health and well-being.

Figure 6.1 illustrates an integration of theory and practice. To make this cognitive–behavioral change process more concrete, a brief summary of the interrelated parts—antecedents (appraisals), action (recreation behavior), and consequences (reflection)—will be presented.

Antecedents

Prior to engaging clients in TR interventions, recognize that individuals have a variety of thoughts, perceptions, and beliefs that will influence their readiness and motivation to get involved. Recreation therapists are particularly interested in clients' perceptions of themselves, others (including the recreation therapist), their health condition, their situation, and the role and meaning of recreation in their life, generally and in times of stress. Additionally, recreation therapists are interested in clients' perceptions of what it means to be a patient or client, and whether they see themselves as active or passive partners in their pursuit of health and wellness. Clients' existing self-efficacy and sense of competence (i.e., their beliefs that they can manage their situation or successfully interact with their environment) may be threatened or diminished by their health condition or circumstances. Such perceptions would influence their motivation to act. Thus, a recreation therapist strives to understand the client's appraisal of their situation and how these perceptions might shape their needs, expectations, and goals related to health and life quality. These thoughts and feelings are *antecedents* to any action that might be taken. Since every client is unique, these perceptions will also be influenced by developmental stage, past experiences, culture, and the meaning and significance clients attach to the situation or goal. A thorough assessment

ought to include examining the client's perceived threat or vulnerability created by their situation as well as the perceived benefits and barriers associated with recreation involvement and its relevance to meeting their needs.

Action

In this model *action* refers to the actual behavior of the client. This behavior can occur as a result of a client's own choosing during discretionary time. It is also associated with structured TR interventions designed to facilitate change. Thus, a client's action is influenced by the various TR interventions used to help the client achieve mutually agreed upon goals. These interventions include carefully selected activities suitable to the client's needs and interests, provided either individually or through structured intervention groups. Throughout the interventions, the recreation therapist monitors client behaviors and provides reassurance, encouragement, and support. (See Chapters 9–12 for more detail on each element of the intervention process.)

Consequences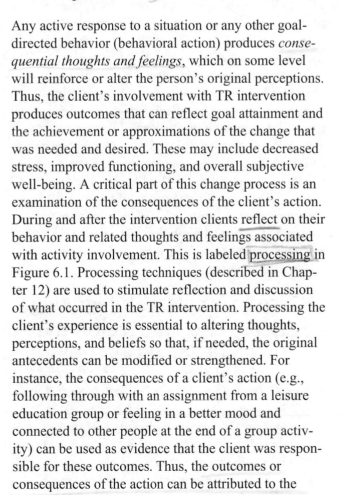

Any active response to a situation or any other goal-directed behavior (behavioral action) produces *consequential thoughts and feelings*, which on some level will reinforce or alter the person's original perceptions. Thus, the client's involvement with TR intervention produces outcomes that can reflect goal attainment and the achievement or approximations of the change that was needed and desired. These may include decreased stress, improved functioning, and overall subjective well-being. A critical part of this change process is an examination of the consequences of the client's action. During and after the intervention clients reflect on their behavior and related thoughts and feelings associated with activity involvement. This is labeled processing in Figure 6.1. Processing techniques (described in Chapter 12) are used to stimulate reflection and discussion of what occurred in the TR intervention. Processing the client's experience is essential to altering thoughts, perceptions, and beliefs so that, if needed, the original antecedents can be modified or strengthened. For instance, the consequences of a client's action (e.g., following through with an assignment from a leisure education group or feeling in a better mood and connected to other people at the end of a group activity) can be used as evidence that the client was responsible for these outcomes. Thus, the outcomes or consequences of the action can be attributed to the client, thereby positively affecting control beliefs. The intended end result of this change process is improved or strengthened self-definition, motivation, confidence, and competence.

• • •Thinking Trigger

Apply the concepts of *antecedents, actions,* and *consequences* to an experience you have had with making changes (e.g., losing weight or learning a new skill).

What were your thoughts, perceptions, or beliefs before you did anything?

How did your thinking change after you took action?   **• • •**

Case Illustrations

The application of a cognitive–behavioral change process to the clinical practice of TR can be illustrated in the following case examples. The first case example focuses on the change process as it occurred with a CTRS and one client. The second case example illustrates how theoretical perspectives regarding behavioral change were integrated into an intervention protocol designed for inpatient rehabilitation settings. This protocol, while developed for a physical medicine and rehabilitation population, is also applicable to clients receiving behavioral health care. The third example illustrates the integration of theory into a community-based health and wellness program for women with physical disabilities. The variety in these examples serve as a reminder that clinical practice is a process, not a place.

Case Example 1: Integrating Theory and Practice on the Individual Level

Sal is a 29-year-old single male recently admitted to a rehabilitation hospital for a T-6 spinal cord injury resulting from a motor vehicle accident. He is engaged to be married, and he expects to serve as best man at his friend's wedding in a month. Sal has a degree in finance, and has maintained active involvement in

sports beyond his competitive days in high school and college. He's the captain of his company's basketball and bowling teams, and along with his fiancée is an avid skier. There is a physician order for a TR assessment.

A critical part of engaging Sal clinically is to recognize the importance of the cognitive antecedents to his involvement in recreation therapy: *What is his appraisal of the situation?* Sal's mind is filled with thoughts of what is happening to him and the challenges that lie ahead. His perceptions of hospitals are colored by his memories of visiting his grandfather, who eventually died in the hospital, and of the very sick and debilitated people he has seen since being hospitalized. He is afraid to admit his fear of never walking again. He believes one thing: only a doctor and maybe a physical therapist can help him. Sure, he's heard about people breaking their backs before, but who ever thinks it will happen to them? What will become of his career that was going so well? And what about his fiancée and his plans for marriage? Will he ever be a real man again?

When Sal meets Carol (his recreation therapist) for the first time, he is factoring her into his appraisal of the entire situation. He has to fit Carol into his cognitive scheme of rehabilitation along with all the other therapists he has met and is expected to work with. Sal obviously has some perceptions about what will be helpful to him, and may wonder about the relative value of recreation in his rehabilitation routine. It is up to Carol to understand as best she can Sal's thoughts, perceptions and beliefs as she tries to engage him in the TR clinical process. Certainly he needs to cope with his health crisis and the arduous task of rehabilitation. His appraisal of this situation and the role that recreation can play in his coping and adaptation is shaped by thoughts, perceptions, and beliefs he has of himself and the meaning of disability, rehabilitation, and recreation.

Carol begins the clinical process with an assessment of Sal's physical and psychosocial needs. This includes an attempt to discern the thoughts, perceptions, and beliefs that will shape his role in the rehabilitation process. In collaboration with Sal, Carol sets goals to guide his intervention plan, and utilizes a variety of activity-based interventions to aid in his coping, adaptation, and recovery. This is labeled action in Figure 6.1. These TR interventions can be individual and group oriented, and can occur both inside and outside the hospital. For example, Sal would receive a combination of individual and group interventions focusing on leisure time management, wheelchair mobility, physical fitness, and socialization through adapted sports and community reintegration. His involvement in clinical TR creates a context for recovery and adaptation. Through appropriate TR interventions, Sal maintains his existing skills and abilities and develops new skills and compensatory strategies, thereby improving his functional independence. The intention is that Sal will be motivated and competent enough to continue to use recreation and leisure involvement in maintaining his health and quality of life.

An important question to ask is: *What will Sal take away from his experience in TR?* Successful rehabilitation is really only evident 12–18 months after discharge. Therefore, it is often up to the individual to prevent secondary health problems. In Sal's case, maintaining a physically and socially active lifestyle will reduce the chances of pressure ulcers, urinary tract infections, social isolation, and depression. How he thinks about himself, his disability, and the role of recreation in his health and well-being will be shaped by the experiences he has in rehabilitation. Rehabilitation in this regard is more than functional mechanics—it is a *learning* and *adapting* experience.

Each TR intervention Sal engages in can be used for feedback and reflection about his real abilities, his feelings about himself, his effort to reach his goals, and his hope for recovery. His performance in activities provides concrete evidence that Carol can use to reinforce adaptive behaviors and strategies, and confront faulty thinking and misperceptions. For example, the involvement of Sal's family, friends, and fiancée can help him come to terms with his notion of what it means to be independent, and how to ask for assistance without feeling helpless. Carol helps Sal reflect on and digest this feedback (i.e., *processing* the experience). This helps to confirm or disconfirm his antecedent thoughts and beliefs, and to attribute goal attainment and any other related change to his effort and persistence. The end result of this therapeutic change process is an increased sense of mastery, competence, and self-efficacy. Ultimately Sal will have learned to manage his disability, acquired adaptive strategies to function as independently as possible, and believed more strongly in his capacity to use recreation and leisure to experience renewed meaning and purpose in his life.

Case Example 2: Integrating Theory with Practice: A TR Psychosocial Rehabilitation Protocol

A clinical TR protocol focusing on psychosocial functioning, skill acquisition, and feelings of competence was developed as part of a federally funded project[1]. The protocol served as a cognitive–behaviorally oriented intervention guide that used activity-based interventions to address three major psychosocial themes: competence/mastery, relationships with others, and independence (see **Table 6.1**, p. 88). The primary rehabilitation themes apply to diverse client populations and settings, including physical rehabilitation and behavioral health care. Each psychosocial rehabilitation theme translated into generic TR goals, which were then individualized as TR rehabilitation outcomes for each client. Examples of three individuals involved in the protocol include:

Jake, a 30-year-old man with schizophrenia, had constant difficulties living in a group home. His issues included managing free time, maintaining social involvement with his housemates, and making use of adult education classes at the YMCA.

Martha, a 58-year-old grandmother, suffered a stroke (CVA), which caused many complications for her favorite role in life—caring for her two grandchildren. Restoring her sense of competence and her hope for continued enjoyable relationships with her grandchildren were primary concerns for her rehabilitation. Her interest in music was the key.

Kahlil, a 44-year-old salesman struggling with alcoholism, had a rehabilitation plan that centered on staying sober. His TR intervention focused on substance-free leisure activities, alone and with others. His personal goals involved resurrecting old interests in woodworking and gardening, finding others to share these interests with, and connecting with community resources that would support these behavior changes.

Each client received five 30-minute individual TR sessions to address each theme as it related to clients' cognitive appraisals, behaviors during intervention sessions, and emerging skills. During the *first session* for each theme, the recreation therapist and the client discussed the relationship between the theme and the client's notion of successful rehabilitation. Discussion focused on how recreation and leisure involvement related to the theme. This provides an opportunity to explore the client's antecedent thoughts related to personal control beliefs and motivation to change.

Table 6.1: TR intervention model

Primary Rehab Theme	TR Psychosocial Goals	Focus of Intervention	Intervention Process *same for all 3 stages*	TR Outcomes
Stage 1: Mastery and Competence	• Increased sense of positive self-image • Adjusted sense of self in relation to disability • Increased sense of control • Increased sense of self-efficacy • Ability to set concrete, limited goals	Leisure skill development	Session 1 • Discuss importance of the recreation opportunities theme in rehabilitation • Discuss how theme relates to recreation and leisure • Help client identify TR outcomes relative to TR focus • Help client choose one or more outcomes relative to TR focus	• Identifies and utilizes diversional recreation • Makes decisions regarding the structure/use of free time • Demonstrates ability to perform components of chosen activities • Plans, follows through, and completes chosen activities • Identifies personal benefits of recreation involvement • Indicates sense of confidence in maintaining leisure involvement
Stage 2: Relations with Others	• Ability to identify benefits of social involvement • Increased awareness of social involvement • Increased ability to show support for others • Increased awareness of social supports • Ability to maintain relationships with family and friends • Increased sense of social competence • Increased understanding of the role of recreation and leisure in establishing, maintaining, and improving social relationships	Leisure interactions and social support	Sessions 2–4 • Conduct appropriate activities to facilitate TR outcomes • Verbal discussion (processing) to relate client functioning in activities relative to TR outcomes (expectations, success, problems, possible solutions, feelings about performance, alternatives) • Continue with the same or add new activities • Continue discussion and probes	• Identifies interests and skills that can be shared with others • Identifies existing and potential leisure partners • Identifies times and places available for social contact • Arranges for social contact • Initiates contact with family, friends, acquaintances • Demonstrates ability to engage others in social situations • Indicates awareness of benefits of social contact • Indicates awareness of how leisure can be used for social relationships
Stage 3: Assertiveness and Independence	• Increased sense of independence • Increased ability to problem solve • Increased willingness to take risks • Positive sense of future preparedness • Increased sense of self-efficacy • Increased ability to identify strategies	Discharge planning and reintegration	Session 5 • Review sessions 2–4 • Help client verbalize and think about TR outcomes in terms of TR goals • Help client process TR goals in terms of rehab theme • Discuss importance of continuing to address thematic issues and ways recreation can help • Prepare for next rehab theme or termination and discharge	• Identifies leisure barriers and institutes alternative strategies • Identifies scenarios involving recreation involvement that are causes of concern and offers possible solutions • Identifies leisure pursuits for after discharge • Develops plan to access leisure resources upon discharge • Identifies and accesses support services needed to engage in leisure involvement in the community • Indicates confidence in ability to manage leisure time after discharge

Next, the client collaborated with the therapist to set recreation-related outcomes. For example, the issue of mastery and competence was often addressed through a broad goal of increasing feelings of personal control, along with the TR outcome of making decisions regarding the use of free time while hospitalized.

Sessions two through four focused on having the client engage in recreation activities to facilitate the achievement of the previously established goals related to the theme. The most critical part of these sessions was processing thoughts, feelings, and behavior related to activity performance. During the sessions the therapist assisted each client to reflect on expectations, problem-solving strategies, and feelings evoked by the activity, always encouraging clients to make accurate appraisals of their abilities. Often, individualized "homework" was discussed and mutually agreed upon for the client to complete in between sessions. For instance, Kahlil had to research community gardening opportunities and woodworking classes available back home, while Martha had to make a tape recording of activity ideas she could most easily do with her grandchildren despite her left-side paralysis. Homework presented opportunities for clients to practice skills or continue exploring issues raised in sessions.

Finally, *session five* was devoted to a discussion about the connections between TR goals, the psychosocial theme, and the client's overall rehabilitation experience. The goal of this session was to integrate all other sessions and to transition into the next theme. The session was also used to reinforce the use of recreation and leisure activities and experiences to address ongoing social and psychological needs created by hospitalization and adjusting to life after discharge.

Case Example 3: Integrating Theory with Practice: A Community-Based Health and Wellness Protocol

The *Women with Physical Disabilities Health and Wellness Project* was an NIH research project[2] developed by faculty in Temple University's Therapeutic Recreation Program. Unlike the other case illustrations, this program represented a community-based application of clinical practice with women with physical disabilities at risk for secondary health problems such as fatigue, poor muscle strength and endurance, depression, and social isolation. This program's design utilized a variety of cognitive–behavioral techniques to assist women with physical disabilities to make lifestyle changes that would enable them to live a healthier and more physically and socially active life. Delivered in a group format to women who resided in the community, the program was composed of three 90-minute workshops, three individualized in-home sessions, and the development of a peer-driven support group for workshop participants. Components of the program follow:

Workshop I

In the first workshop, women with physical disabilities were invited to explore a wellness framework and to apply it to their personal life. Particular emphasis was placed on:

- Understanding the women's personal beliefs about health and wellness
- The relationship between being physically and socially active and one's physical and psychological health and well-being
- Their sense of control and competence regarding health and well-being

At the end of this workshop, participants completed a lifestyle self-assessment covering six areas: leisure, physical activity, stress, nutrition, relationships, and their knowledge and attitudes about secondary conditions related to their disability.

Workshop II

By design, the project intended to facilitate an increase in health behaviors in at least two areas. In this workshop, participants focused on physical activity as a distinct component of a healthy lifestyle, and were assisted to develop an individualized action plan for lifestyle change. A number of salient topics were discussed in an effort to uncover their current attitudes and beliefs about physical activity, which would influence behavioral change. After discussing their past and present experiences with being physically active, they discussed societal norms and images about physically active women, and the particular benefits they experienced (or anticipated) from being physically active. They were then asked to develop for themselves a realistic image of what it would mean to be physically active. Barriers to physically active lifestyles were brainstormed and discussed. Women were taught exercise routines using elastic Thera-Bands for strength and flexibility. These exercises were individualized to accommodate each woman's abilities. Participants also brainstormed ways to increase physical activity using a variety of recreation-related alternatives. Following this, each participant developed a personal "physical activity action plan" incorporating the Thera-Band exercises. Action plans were developed with the following points in mind:

- Setting realistic goals that identified small steps and indicators of success

- Monitoring behavior (e.g., participants were asked to keep a journal and to comment on their experience with following their plan)

- Rewarding targeted behaviors (participants were encouraged to identify a reward for themselves when they complied with their personal plan)

Following the development of their action plan, participants discussed a variety of factors that could influence their adherence to an action plan. The focus was on positive sources of motivation. This included environments conducive to exercising (e.g., parks, shopping malls), the role of social support (both for companionship and encouragement), and the issue of pleasure and enjoyment. For example, one participant found that exercising with a friend while watching and talking about a TV program was a strategy that was both productive and enjoyable.

Individualized In-Home Sessions

During the weeks between Workshops II and III, each woman received several home visits for follow-up and personalized guidance. The initial follow-up visit focused on the physical activity action plan and any personal or environmental factors that could support or impede the change process (e.g., daily schedule, routine responsibilities, existing or potential support of others). Particular emphasis was placed on recreation and leisure interests that complemented the goals of the action plan. Women were asked to explore other preferred leisure options that would also increase their level of physical activity (e.g., rowing, swimming, gardening). All visits provided consultation, guidance, and assistance in reviewing and refining the action plan. This included discussions about control beliefs and the perceived consequences of the participant's behavior relative to the desired lifestyle change. Often these processing discussions led to modifications of the action plan by incorporating new strategies and supports needed to overcome obstacles and reach reasonable goals. The end result was reinforced feelings of competence and control in their ability to be physically active.

Workshop III

Project participants reassembled to reflect together on their efforts at making lifestyle changes. Workshop facilitators used group work strategies to promote a sense of group identity among the women. Women shared with each other the status of their action plans and the factors that influenced adherence, compliance, and success as well as behaviors/actions that helped or interfered with their efforts to make lifestyle changes. They discussed their experiences with using a journal (diary) for monitoring compliance and the role of rewards in their action plans. Within the safety of this group women were able to support each other if they felt frustrated with slow progress, and they were able to serve as models for each other and resources for suggestions. During this workshop participants were asked to select another target for change (e.g., leisure, nutrition, stress management) and were assisted in developing a new action plan in this area.

Peer Support Groups

At the second and third workshops the women were encouraged to make plans for their own follow-up and support. Participants were encouraged to get together with each other around a recreation activity, like attending the movies, going out to dinner, or shopping. Phone numbers and email addresses were shared at the second workshop to facilitate contact and the development of this peer support group. During the third workshop, participants agreed upon a recreation activity to do as a group. When gatherings occurred, the participants experienced a continued sense of support and companionship, which all expressed was an essential ingredient in their healthy lifestyles.

Commonly Used Cognitive–Behavioral Procedures

Each of the preceding case examples highlighted the integration of theory with practice. In each case behavioral change was facilitated because therapists were attentive to both the cognitive and behavioral aspects involved in learning, adaptation, and growth. Cognitive factors such as perceived personal control and competence were addressed, both as antecedents and consequences of behavior. A combination of activity-based interventions, supportive environments, and a therapeutic relationship contributed to the TR clinical change process. Also incorporated into each case example were common cognitive–behavioral procedures used by recreation therapists to facilitate behavioral change. These procedures focus on target behaviors, and the personal beliefs that people hold about their behavior and their ability to act in ways that lead to health and well-being.

Using cognitive–behavioral procedures to change behavior is not unusual in TR clinical practice—it has an established acceptance. For instance, Bullock and Luken (1994) developed a leisure education program for individuals with mental illness based on cognitive–behavior modification principles. Following the guide of Meichhenbaum (1986), they incorporated the following five principles of behavior change:

1. Enable clients to define problems and set goals
2. Help clients learn and use self-monitoring strategies regarding their thoughts, feelings, and behaviors
3. Develop and practicing coping skills
4. Evaluate progress
5. Modify personal action plans to promote progress and success

The most important part of their leisure education program was gradual exposure to increasingly more difficult tasks in natural environments so that clients could apply and practice skills in an effort to maintain and generalize them. Kastrinos and Malkin (1997) identified a number of cognitive–behavioral techniques that recreation therapists can and should use in their work with individuals with depressive episodes. Deiser and Voight (1998) developed a relapse prevention program based on cognitive therapy principles. More recently, Carruthers (1999) found a strong parallel between cognitive–behavioral models of addictions treatment (such as pathological gambling) and procedures used in TR modalities like stress management, self-esteem, leisure education, and communications and relationship training programs.

The activity-based nature of TR practice is a natural arena for using cognitive–behavioral procedures. Many of the common cognitive–behavioral procedures described by psychologists Thase and Beck (1993) are easily incorporated into TR practice. These include a *schedule of activities* to counteract loss of motivation, hopelessness, and rumination on negative thoughts; *behavioral rehearsing* (including modeling and coaching) to help individuals practice and master each step leading to completion of a task; and the *use of diversion* through physical activity, exercise, social contact, and play to temporarily reduce most forms of anxiety, anger, and depressed affect.

Wright, Thase, Ludgate, and Beck (1993) explained that many of the objectives and procedures used by activity therapists (e.g., recreational therapists, horticulture therapists) embrace cognitive–behavioral principles useful in promoting behavioral change:

> The activities therapist can be resourceful and creative in trying to set up success experiences for the patient by breaking tasks down into small steps (e.g., graded task assignments). Group feedback is another useful tool in activity therapy. Discussions of therapeutic activities in a group setting may provide valuable information to challenge patients' erroneous conclusions that they performed poorly, accomplished little, or looked foolish. (p. 79)

Wright and colleagues highlighted two common cognitive–behavioral techniques used by recreation therapists in their work with clients: graded task assignments (breaking tasks down into small steps), and reality-checking or confronting cognitive distortions (group feedback on performance). These and other cognitive–behavioral techniques were embedded in each of the previous case examples. What follows is an explanation of a variety of cognitive–behavioral procedures typically incorporated into TR interventions. Whenever possible, we discuss how the cognitive–behavioral procedure was included in the prior case examples.

We have placed different techniques into three broad categories related to assisting clients with goal attainment: *information management, behavior management, and support management.* While each category is presented separately, various techniques could be placed in more than one category. For instance, while journals and diaries are presented as a self-monitoring technique related to information management, they can also be used as a behavior management technique for clients to track their personal progress and change in physical activity, socializing, or time management. It is also likely that therapists will incorporate more than one cognitive–behavioral technique.

Information Management

As its name implies, information management provides clients with information and assists them to process information in ways that promote behavioral change. Knowledge and self-awareness are prerequisites to behavioral change, and both are increased through relevant information. A variety of cognitive–behavioral procedures and techniques are concerned with helping clients manage the wealth of information provided to them. Those particularly relevant to TR follow.

Client Education

While not typically identified as a specific cognitive–behavioral technique, client education is included here since it is the primary means by which clients receive information and because it addresses both cognition and behavior. According to Falvo (1999), client or patient education should be "directed not only toward the patient's understanding of his or her condition and treatment but also toward adaptation and behavioral changes that will produce positive health outcomes" (p. 4). Recreation therapists use client education to provide information about adaptive devices, symptom management, self-advocacy, recreation and leisure resources, and health promotion. The premise is that accurate information produces knowledge, and that knowledge is power. Thus, accurate and relevant information helps clients feel empowered to behave in ways that contribute to their health and well-being.

In each case example, recreation therapists provided clients with information to help them understand the purpose of TR and the role of recreation in health promotion and rehabilitation. The recreation therapist involved Sal in educational activities that provided him with information about the value of physical activity in the prevention of secondary conditions that often occur with spinal cord injury. The women's health and wellness program focused on educating the women about wellness and the role of a physically and socially active lifestyle in promoting health and well-being. Particular emphasis was placed on the use of recreation as a means to be physically and socially active and as a reward for changed behavior. Generally, the focus of client education within TR is on the provision of information that assists clients in understanding their conditions, the rehabilitation process, and the role of recreation in helping them regain and maintain their health and life quality.

Cognitive Restructuring and Retraining

As presented throughout this chapter and the preceding chapter, client cognitions (perceptions and beliefs) influence behavior. Therefore, it is important to discern the amount and type of information clients can and choose to take in. Sometimes certain information is overlooked, especially when a person is under stress or feels threatened by particular circumstances. Sometimes information is distorted in ways that reinforce

negative self-image or feelings of helplessness. Internal monologues (e.g., thoughts a client might have such as "I'll never be able to do that." "I've tried and I just fail.") often stop an individual from attempting behavioral change. In these instances therapists use a technique called *cognitive restructuring*, which helps to challenge distortions. One of the primary ways that recreation therapists challenge cognitive distortions is through reality checks (Kastrinos & Malkin, 1997). *Reality checks* involve asking the client to describe concretely what occurred in a TR session, or to restate what had been discussed. The therapist and the client then have an opportunity to discuss whether the thoughts and perceptions are accurate and they can then "reframe" the situation with missing information and an alternative perspective.

Confronting cognitive distortions, especially when clients are depressed and feeling helpless is often necessary in clinical practice. In the case of Sal, the therapist may tell him that he will learn activities such as cycling, skiing, weightlifting, and swimming in his TR groups. These activities, Sal is told, will help him get stronger and, in the long run, can help him avoid secondary health problems. However, Sal's antecedent thoughts and perceptions can interfere with his ability to benefit from these TR interventions. For example, his all or nothing thinking (e.g., "My life is ruined—if I can't walk or run, I can't be happy.") must be confronted with reality checks to help him find reasonable and realistic expectations for his future. This may be done in a variety of ways, including conversation, modeling, and involvement in the activities. Similarly, in the women's health and wellness program, perceptions and beliefs about one's control and competence in modifying current lifestyle behaviors was a primary focus in workshops and in-home sessions. Addressing a variety of immobilizing thoughts through group discussions and individual sessions was complemented by other behavioral techniques and were pivotal in facilitating behavioral change. Kastrinos and Malkin (1997) stress the importance of training and supervision when using cognitive restructuring techiniques in TR pracitice.

Cognitive retraining is another cognitive–behavioral technique often used in rehabilitation. Cognitive retraining is used primarily with clients who have experienced a neurological injury that impairs their cognitive abilities. Its purpose is to teach the client, through a variety of techniques, compensatory strategies that will allow them to function more effectively. For instance, individuals with brain injuries often have problems with short-term memory. Cognitive retraining would teach them to use a variety of compensatory strategies, such as a memory book and telememo watches. These watches can store phone numbers, names, dates, appointment times, and brief reminder messages to help with memory deficits. The memory book would contain their daily appointments, medication lists, and other pieces of information that they have difficulty remembering. Parenté and Herrmann (1996) describe these and a number of other strategies and external aids that can be used in cognitive retraining programs.

Self-Observation C

Self-observation involves a set of techniques, such as journals, diaries, and videotapes, used to help clients obtain accurate information about behaviors and accompanying thoughts and feelings. Clients are asked to keep a log of specific behaviors and the external and internal events, thoughts, and feelings that immediately preceded and followed the behavior. For example, women in the health and wellness program were asked to complete a self-assessment of their behavior in six areas related to wellness. They were also encouraged to keep a journal about their thoughts, feelings, and actual behavior related to their action plans. Journal entries were often shared during group and individual sessions. Journal entries helped the women examine relationships between their thinking and behavior and the influence this had on achieving their goals for lifestyle modification. In the case of Sal, the therapist requested that he use a log when he wasn't involved in an intervention group to record when he did weight shifts. Weight shifts are one way individuals with SCI can minimize their risk for getting pressure ulcers. This log provided Sal and his therapist with data about how well he was incorporating this health behavior.

2 Behavior Management

Numerous cognitive–behavioral techniques focus on helping clients manage specific behaviors and subsequently increase their feelings and beliefs about personal control and competence. TR intervention programs almost always include a structured set of activity options for clients to participate in, thereby counteracting isolation, rumination, and inactivity. In essence, there is a constant invitation to engage in activity and have opportunities for learning, adaptation, and growth. Other specific procedures and techniques used in TR practice follow.

Skills Training A

In skills training therapists teach the behavioral components of necessary or desired skills and create situations where clients can practice these skills. An important part of skills training is attending to thoughts and feelings that clients have immediately before and after engaging in training sessions. Social skills, including assertiveness training, recreation activity skills, and relaxation techniques are a common focus of skills training.

For example, in the inpatient rehabilitation protocol presented earlier, skills training was primarily used to address the first theme of mastery and competence. Recreation activities developed particular skills or adaptive strategies needed for improved physical and cognitive functioning. For some clients, assertiveness training was included so that they would have the confidence to be self-advocates and to resume active roles in their families and community. Some were taught to use relaxation skills to manage the anxiety they experienced during hospitalization. Skills training was also incorporated into the women's health and wellness project to teach the women new exercise routines using therabands. In the case of Sal, the TR intervention plan included training in wheelchair mobility skills and adaptive sports.

Modeling B

Modeling is a common cognitive–behavioral technique used within TR practice. Modeling refers to a technique in which clients are influenced to change their behavior by viewing others perform the behavior, either in person or on video. Specifically, modeling is a technique that is used to increase a client's self-efficacy through vicarious learning. Carol had Sal view a video on wheelchair sports that showed other individuals with spinal cord injury engaging in recreational behaviors that Sal thought he could never do again. Through group discussions and peer support meetings in the women's health and wellness project women served as models for each other as they discussed their progress at making lifestyle changes.

Homework and Behavioral Assignments C

Success in clinical practice is often dependent on what happens in between intervention sessions. A common technique used to encourage continuity past the end of a particular session is assigning homework. Homework can be any type of assignment that the therapist and the client decide should be done before the next session. These assignments reinforce topics discussed or skills addressed in the session. Research has indicated that homework assignments are best if they produce some tangible evidence of accomplishment, such as a written assignment. It is also helpful if homework assignments are identified for both the client and the therapist. For instance, clients involved with the inpatient rehabilitation treatment protocol were taught relaxation techniques; however, these skills take practice. Therefore, clients were asked to keep a record of when they practiced. Meanwhile, the therapist assumed responsibility for obtaining audiotapes that the clients preferred to use during relaxation practice.

Another example of using homework occurs when clients complain of boredom and disinterest in leisure activities. After individual intervention sessions focus on discussing the potential benefits of leisure involvement, a homework assignment can be to keep a log of what the client does for recreation over a specified period of time, and how he or she feels prior, during, and immediately after participating in a recreation activity. The therapist's homework might be reading articles on leisure boredom or consulting with a colleague regarding available leisure options in the client's community. The identification of specific homework tasks for each party conveys an awareness of and an ongoing commitment to the behavioral change process on the part of both client and therapist (Taylor, 1999).

In the women's health and wellness program, clients were asked to complete worksheets focused on leisure awareness, interests, and attitudes following the first workshop session. These worksheets were then discussed at the first in-home follow-up meeting and used to add recreation options to the women's physical activity action plans. Recreation therapists also had their homework. They researched physically active recreation resources in the women's home community prior to the first in-home visit.

Self-Reinforcements and Contracting Techniques

This category of cognitive–behavioral approaches includes a wide variety of techniques that focus on the use of reinforcement to elicit particular behaviors. Self-reinforcements involve systematically rewarding oneself to increase or decrease a particular behavior. Taylor (1999) identifies four types of self-reinforcements: positive and negative self-rewards and positive

and negative self-punishment. *Positive self-rewards* involve reinforcing oneself with something desirable or pleasurable when a targeted behavior is performed. *Negative self-rewards* are the opposite, reinforcing the targeted behavior by giving oneself something undesirable. *Negative self-punishment* involves the administration of some unpleasant stimulus to punish an undesirable behavior. *Positive self-punishment* involves withdrawing some desirable reinforcer in the environment each time an undesirable behavior is performed, such as giving up viewing a favorite TV program. Reinforcements in the form of rewards play an important part in behavioral change action plans, as was the case in the women's health and wellness project. Each participant had an action plan that specified personal rewards and criteria for earning them. The rewards were identified as part of the goal setting/action planning process. The rewards were used to reinforce efforts at lifestyle change.

Research has also indicated that using *behavioral contracts* in conjunction with rewards is an effective approach to facilitating behavior change (Taylor, 1999). Behavioral contracts are written statements designed collaboratively between a therapist and a client detailing what rewards and punishments are contingent on the performance or nonperformance of a behavior. They clarify expectations associated with intervention plans and verify or affirm commitments to meeting these expectations.

A behavioral contract could be incorporated as an intervention strategy in the inpatient rehabilitation protocol. For instance, suppose a client resisted coming to recreation therapy sessions. His or her inconsistent participation was blamed on feelings of depression and loneliness. The client preferred to stay in his or her room and watch daytime soaps on television. The recreation therapist could establish a contract with the client stipulating that in exchange for attending TR intervention sessions the therapist would provide the client with a videotaped recording of the TV show. The contract would call for an even exchange of intervention session minutes for TV minutes.

Token Economies

Often behavioral contracts are used jointly with token economies. Most often used in behavioral healthcare systems, token economies provide clients with a specific positive reward when particular behaviors are consistently displayed. Unlike behavioral contracts, token economies are typically preestablished as a routine part of the care process. **Exhibit 6.1** contains more information about token economies and a sample token economy used in a summer camping program.

⟨ Support Management

Cognitive–behavioral approaches recognize the role of the physical and social environment in promoting or inhibiting change. A final category of techniques used in clinical practice involves helping clients use supports within the physical and social environment. Two approaches that have particular relevance to TR are stimulus control and social support.

Stimulus Control ⟨

Understanding environmental influences on behavior and modifying them is at the heart of stimulus control. Usually stimulus control procedures modify a specific health behavior. Clients are taught to develop ties between stimuli in the environment and specific behaviors. For example, the in-home follow-up meetings that were part of the women's health and wellness project focused on environmental barriers in the home that prohibited the women from following through with their action plan. Some participants modified their

home so that they would have space conducive to exercising. Some used visual reminders, such as leaving their Thera-Bands tied to a doorknob.

Other examples of stimulus control often used in treatment are acronyms, pictures, or personal items displayed in the environment to prompt certain behavior. For instance, women in the wellness project were encouraged to place inspirational stickers and sayings in various spots in their home and work environment to remind them of their commitment to changing their behavior. Another example of stimulus control is when staff use display boxes with adults with Alzheimer's disease who are having difficulty with finding their way around a facility. These boxes are placed at the entrance to a resident's room and filled with personal artifacts. This display becomes an environmental cue that the marked room belongs to them.

Social Support ⟨

Helping clients recognize and manage the social support available to them is a vital aspect that must be considered in clinical practice. The involvement of families and significant others is critical to successful rehabilitation. Engaging family and significant others

Exhibit 6.1: Token economies

"The basic idea behind the token economy approach to behavioral change is to create an effective way to increase and strengthen socially desirable and adaptive behaviors primarily within institutional settings" (Vondracek & Corneal, 1995, p. 81). The theoretical foundation for token economies is found in learning theory and in the principles of operant conditioning. In a token economy, desirable target behaviors displayed infrequently by the client are identified and then rewarded when displayed. The assumption underlying token economies is that the positive rewards (tokens) will result in increases in the desired behavior. Occasionally, token economies will also employ negative reinforcement. In such economies, clients are fined (i.e., they lose tokens) when they display specified undesirable behaviors (e.g., cursing or fighting). The tokens, which a client earns after a specified time period, are tallied and exchanged for some type of backup reinforcer. Care must be taken to make certain the backup reinforcers are attractive enough to clients that they will be motivated to try and attain them. Token economies require specific exchange rules regarding the number of tokens needed for a particular back up reinforcer and careful monitoring to verify that clients only obtain tokens in accordance with program rules. That is, tokens can not be transferred from one client to another. Clients must not be allowed to share, steal, or barter for tokens. A major concern with token economies is that the desired behaviors will not continue once the token economy program has ended or the client leaves the facility. To overcome this limitation, therapists who utilize a token economy in their work with clients need to make certain that the economy is implemented in a variety of environments, that its use is gradually faded or substitute with social reinforcers, and that the client is taught self-reinforcement techniques. By doing so, it is more likely that the client will be able to continue to display the target behavior (Vondracek & Corneal, 1995).

Recreation therapists at Elwyn Institute in Media, Pennsylvania, use a token economy in a summer day camp for youth with severe emotional disorders. Youth attending the day camp are awarded "points" at the end of each activity period if they displayed the desired target behaviors during the activity related to task participation and peer interaction. At the end of the camp day, points are totaled and exchanged for "camp bucks." This camp currency can then be used at Elwyn's canteen for purchasing supplies, food, soda, or candy.

in the intervention program—enlisting their support and helping them modify negative responses to specific client behaviors (e.g., responses that might inhibit the clients' efforts at behavioral change and/or independence) are examples of social support management. Social support was an explicit theme addressed in the inpatient rehabilitation protocol described in Table 6.1 (p. 88). Spouses and other members of the clients' social support network were involved in various TR programs. Likewise, in the case of Sal and in the women's health and wellness project, the importance of social support was stressed. Women were encouraged to form their own support group that would naturally encourage them to be more socially active.

Often in behavioral healthcare settings clients must learn new ways of interacting with family and significant others. Cognitive–behavioral techniques such as role-playing are often used to assist them. In other settings, recreation therapists might be involved in helping clients assess their support especially as it relates to friends and leisure involvement. Certainly this would be a focus in Sal's rehabilitation program.

However, managing social support is not just focused on family and friends. It also involves helping clients recognize and manage the support available from staff in the care environment. For example, recreation therapists make sure that clients are aware that members of the clergy are available to them. Also, an important cognitive–behavioral approach that facilitates the development of staff support for clients is to have staff routinely review the client's progress and provide positive reinforcement for the client's effort at behavioral change (Tunks & Bellissimo, 1991). In her role as a recreation therapist, Murray (1997) creatively used journaling to encourage the explicit use of this technique in a physical rehabilitation setting. Murray helped clients make a journal of their rehabilitation experience. As part of this process, she placed into each client's journal worksheets entitled "Today in _____ therapy" (e.g., physical therapy). Clients were asked to use the page to rate how hard they felt they had worked that day in a specific therapy. Staff were also encouraged to write their perceptions of the client's work effort and progress on this page. (A completed worksheet is provided in **Exhibit 6.2**). Murray demonstrated that journaling, as a novel recreation therapy intervention, successfully engaged the client and the rehabilitation team in a routine evaluation of the client's efforts at behavioral change and promoted supportive interactions among each. She indicated that team members enjoyed conveying progress to clients in their own language along with drawing and doodling (e.g., stick figures of a person learning to stand and walk). Participants reported that it made them feel important to carry their own journal about their rehabilitation that they could circulate among clinical departments for input.

Final Thoughts about a Cognitive–Behavioral Approach to Practice

Using a cognitive–behavioral framework in clinical practice has both strengths and limitations. Certainly it is not the only way to work with clients. Yet, it does offer a way to individualize care and at the same time assist clients to use play, recreation, and leisure to support their health and well-being. It is also a process that has to be collaborative for clients to benefit.

According to Hart and Morgan (1993) clinical practice that is based on a cognitive–behavioral framework recognizes the *legitimacy of the individual's cognition*. Therapists must realize that clients' perceptions and appraisals are accurate from the individual's perspective. They cannot be dismissed as irrational or nonsensical. Yet they are open to change through experience since *cognition and behavior reciprocally influence one another*. The concrete, tangible nature of activity-based modalities used in TR practice is particularly suitable for this reciprocal exchange. Thus, helping clients to meet their needs and achieve their goals by addressing both cognition and behavior can be an effective approach to clinical TR practice. In addition, a cognitive–behavioral framework is very educational and therefore excellent for structured health promotion and disease prevention services.

A cognitive–behavioral approach also has some limitations. The procedures and techniques presented in this chapter require training and supervision. Integrating theory with practice comes with experience; it cannot be accomplished through an academic program alone. Experience is often only as good as the supervision a practitioner receives. Opportunity to discuss issues as they arise in practice is pivotal to gaining understanding and competence in using this approach. Accessing a client's perceptions and beliefs depends on a therapeutic relationship anchored in trust and respect, as well as a keen sensitivity to nonverbal communication. This is especially true with clients who have minimal abilities to verbalize their feelings but still communicate through their eyes, facial expressions, and body language. While some clients may have cognitive limitations that preclude using some of these techniques, others may have personal or cultural reasons for rejecting this approach. Appreciate the influence of the environment on a person's perceptions, beliefs, and behavior. It might be more important in some instances to focus your efforts on modifying the environment. In some instances there is just not enough time to explore fully the individual's thoughts, perceptions, and beliefs related to change. Thus, a good deal of thought, insightfulness, and sensitivity is required when using a cognitive-behavioral approach in clinical practice.

Summary

This chapter built on the explanation of clinical TR practice and its applied theoretical base presented in Chapters 4 and 5. Specifically this chapter offered an opportunity to understand how theory can inform and direct practice. Drawing from the theoretical perspective presented in Chapter 5, which emphasized the interrelatedness of thinking, feeling, and behaving, this chapter contained a cognitive–behavioral explanation of the clinical change process as it can occur in TR practice. Several examples illustrated its application with clients. In each case various cognitive–behavioral procedures were used to assist clients with learning, adaptation and growth so that they could improve and maintain health and well-being.

This chapter also included a description of common cognitive–behavioral strategies that can be incorporated into clinical practice with a wide range of clients in diverse settings.

Exhibit 6.2: Staff's entry in client's rehabilitation journal (Murray, 1997)

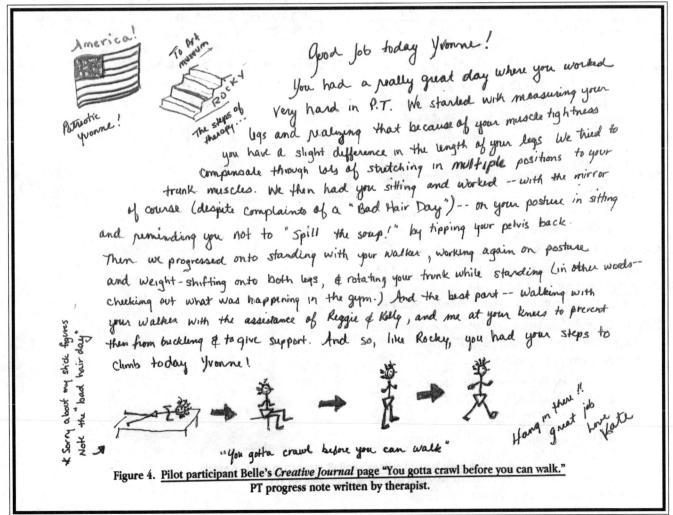

Figure 4. <u>Pilot participant Belle's *Creative Journal* page "You gotta crawl before you can walk."</u>
PT progress note written by therapist.

References

Bullock, C. and Luken, K. (1994). Reintegration through recreation: A community based rehabilitation model. In D. Compton and S. Iso-Ahola (Eds.), *Leisure and mental health.* (pp. 215–231). Park City, UT: Family Development Resources, Inc.

Carruthers, C. (1999). Pathological gambling: Implications for therapeutic recreation practice. *Therapeutic Recreation Journal, 33*(4), 287–303.

Deiser, R. and Voight, A. (1998). Therapeutic recreation and relapse prevention intervention. *Parks & Recreation, 33*(5), 78–83.

Falvo, D. (1999). *Effective patient education: A guide to increased compliance.* Gaithersburg, MD: Aspen.

Hart, K. and Morgan, J. (1993). Cognitive–behavioral procedures with children: Historical context and current status. In A. Finch, W. Nelson, and E. Ott (Eds.), *Cognitive–behavioral procedures with children and adolescents: A practical guide* (pp. 1–19). Needham Heights, MA: Allyn & Bacon.

Kastrinos, G. and Malkin, M. (1997). Integration of cognitive therapy techniques with recreational therapy. In Compton, D. (Ed.), *Issues in therapeutic recreation: Toward the new millennium* (2nd ed., pp. 445–460). Champaign, IL: Sagamore Publishing.

Meichhenbaum, D. (1986). Cognitive behavior modification. In F. Kanfer and A. Goldstein (Eds.), *Helping people change.* New York, NY: Pergamon Press.

Murray, S. (1997). *Patient's lived experience of acute rehabilitation and recovery contained in a creative journal.* Unpublished doctoral dissertation, Temple University, Philadelphia, PA.

Parenté, R. and Herrmann, D. (1996). *Retraining Cognition: Techniques and applications.* Gaithersburg, MD: Aspen.

Skinner, E. (1995). *Perceived control, motivation, and coping.* Thousand Oaks, CA: Sage Publications.

Taylor, S. (1999). *Health psychology* (4th ed.). New York, NY: McGraw-Hill.

Thase, M. and Beck, A. (1993). An overview of cognitive therapy. In J. Wright, M. Thase, A. Beck, and J. Ludgate (Eds.), *Cognitive therapy with inpatients: Developing a cognitive milieu* (pp. 3–34). New York, NY: Guilford Press.

Tunks, E. and Bellissimo, A. (1991). *Behavioral medicine: Concepts and procedures.* New York, NY: Pergamon Press.

Vondracek, F. and Corneal, S. (1995). *Strategies for resolving individual and family problems.* Washington, DC: Brooks/Cole Publishing.

Wright, J., Thase, M., Ludgate, J., and Beck, A. (1993). The cognitive milieu: Structure and process. In J. Wright, M. Thase, A. Beck, and J. Ludgate (Eds.), *Cognitive therapy with inpatients: Developing a cognitive milieu* (pp. 61–87). New York, NY: Guilford Press.

Endnotes

[1] This protocol was part of grant funded by the U.S. Department of Education, National Institute on Disability and Rehabilitation Research (NIDRR), cooperative agreement #H133B80048.

[2] This intervention was part of a research grant from the National Center on Medical Rehabilitation Research, a division of the National Institutes of Health (NIH). Grant # R01 HD35059.

Part 3

The TR Clinical Process

Chapter 7
Assessing Clients

Guided Reading Questions

After reading this chapter, you should be able to answer the following:

- What is the purpose of assessment?
- What methods of data gathering can be used in the assessment process? What are the benefits, disadvantages, and issues associated with each?
- What factors influence assessment interviews?
- What is meant by the concepts of validity, reliability, and usability? How do these concepts affect the assessment process?
- What standardized assessment tools are available for gathering data related to individuals' leisure lifestyles?
- With what types of interdisciplinary assessment might a recreation therapist be involved?

Introduction

Thus far in the text, we have been talking generally about clinical practice, a 5-phase process that includes assessing, planning, implementing, evaluating, and terminating. This 5-phase process begins with the gathering of data to identify "targets" for change within the individual or the physical and social environment. The client–system perspective, discussed in Chapter 3, is the foundation for this 5-phase process. Thus, this perspective is the cornerstone from which the assessment process should proceed. The client–system perspective highlights key areas that recreation therapists should consider in the assessment process, including information about the client's biological, psychological, and social functioning, spirituality, and lifestyle. It also highlights developmental, cultural, and environmental influences. Assessment procedures that allow data to be obtained in each of these areas are crucial for recreation therapists who work from a holistic perspective. The information gathered allows therapists to obtain a realistic picture of their clients. This includes information about clients' wants, needs, aspirations, and hopes in addition to information about client functioning and environmental constraints or barriers that inhibit lifestyle change.

The Data Gathering Process: TR Assessments

In Chapter 4 we defined clinical practice as a systematic and intentional process using play, recreation, and other activity-based interventions as a means to helping clients achieve and maintain a sense of competence, health, and quality of life. Clinical practice focuses on change in the environment or in the clients' attitudes, beliefs, or behaviors. Data gathering or "assessment" is the cornerstone of clinical practice. *Assessment* involves the use of systematic procedures for gathering *def.* select information about an individual for the purpose of making decisions regarding that individual's program, intervention plan, or clinical services. These data provide information about the individual's functioning and about the client's desires and goals. It assists with decision-making—determining not only which courses of action are most likely to deliver valued outcomes, but also which courses of action are most likely to facilitate clients' sense of competence, health, and well-being. Assessment data is combined with clinical judgment to determine relevant client outcomes that can be met through clinical TR programs.

Methods of Data Gathering

For recreation therapists to conduct successful assessments they must understand the techniques used to gather data and the issues that affect the accuracy, truthfulness, and usability of the data. Assessment data is collected through *self-report, observation, performance testing,* and *secondary data sources.* Most likely, you will use a combination of these four data gathering methods in your assessment procedures, regardless of the service delivery setting in which you work.

Self-Report Methods

Self-report methods supply information about the client's situation and self-perceptions. Self-report methods involve collecting data directly from clients, either through an interview or by having them complete some type of self-administered questionnaire. Many assessment instruments used in TR are self-report measures. For instance, the short form of the Leisure Diagnostic Battery—Version A (Witt & Ellis, 1989) asks clients to indicate the degree to which they agree or disagree to 25 statements using a Likert scale. Client responses reflect individual perceptions at that particular moment and may or may not be totally objective. The same can be said for information collected through interviews. Self-report data reflects the client's worldview. Despite the subjective nature of this data, interviews and self-report questionnaires provide recreation therapists with useful information that reflects a client's perception of their situation, including their disabling condition.

Interviews

Interviewing is the predominant method by which recreation therapists collect self-report data for assessments. Interviews allow therapists to collect information about a client's ability to communicate both verbally and nonverbally, the client's cognitive ability to generate, elaborate, and organize responses to questions, and the client's perceptions of their life situation.

Therapists who excel in interviewing recognize the influence that their physical presence has on the process. Gender, age, racial group, and physical appearance elicit differing reactions from clients. Your cultural, religious, political, and personal history will influence your ability to "hear" your client. Knowing yourself and recognizing the biases that your worldview creates is critical to successful interviewing. For example, a therapist's unfounded fears about working with persons with acquired immune deficiency syndrome (AIDS) may hinder his or her ability to respond to the client's need for physical contact. You must also understand the effect of your own emotional state on your ability to listen. How you are feeling, your preconceptions about

a client or a certain diagnosis, or your ability to focus your attention influences how well you can listen to clients, and in turn, how sensitive your care will be. Clients are more likely to respond and elaborate on questions if they feel as if you are truly listening. Good *attending skills* are needed to elicit this feeling in clients. Attending skills refers to behaviors that together "let the client know you are interested in him or her and are paying attention to what he or she has to say" (Austin, 1991, p. 234). It includes behaviors associated with eye contact, body language, and vocal qualities. **Table 7.1** defines each of these behaviors and highlights their purpose during an interview.

Using the Interview Environment. Good interviewers also understand how the environment influences the interview process. Distractions like ringing phones, overhead announcements, or the location of chairs, desks, or tables are examples of environmental issues that impact an interview. Consider the environment when conducting an assessment interview. Each setting has different advantages. Taking clients to the recreation room or on a tour of the facility while interviewing them can hasten the formation of a therapeutic relationship. Some clients will welcome the opportunity to move about the facility; however, others may prefer the familiarity of their room. Your selection of an interview environment should be guided by your client's desires and the ability of the setting to be private and distraction-free. These environmental elements are prerequisites to establishing a sense of trust and openness in the interview process.

Recording Data. Beginning therapists are also uncertain about how to handle note taking during an interview. If you want to record your clients' responses, you should ask permission. Care should be taken so that your note taking does not short-change the verbal exchange. In addition to verbatim or general notes about your client's responses to your questions, you may also want to record your observations about your client's nonverbal body language, eye contact, and openness. Be aware of the potential for cultural biasing in your observations. Notes should be recorded in such a way that you would be comfortable allowing your client to examine them.

Determining Interview Content. To be competent at interviewing, therapists must gather information from clients in a systematic, thorough, useful, and economical manner. The client–system perspective is useful in developing content for an interview guide. In addition, because we advocate that recreation therapists utilize a cognitive–behavioral approach in their clinical practice, interview content should also focus on clients' overt behaviors, cognitions (e.g., thoughts, beliefs, attitudes), and physiological responses. During the interview, you need to pose questions that allow clients to elaborate on the difficulties they are having (e.g., "I can't get along with my family"), what their thoughts are about these difficulties (e.g., "Each time before I talk with my dad, I think 'Here we go again, he never listens to what I'm saying.'"), and how these difficulties make them feel physically and emotionally (e.g., "It gets so that my heart is pounding and my stomach is in knots every time I see him!"). By focusing interview content on the cognitive thoughts and physiological responses that accompany behaviors, you are better able to identify appropriate intervention targets. Of course, there will be times when clients will not be able to respond to questions, or when verbal content will be less useful than nonverbal data. In these circumstances, observational data collection methods are most effective.

A portion of the interview should also focus on identifying environmental influences that support or hinder behavioral change. This discussion should not be limited to an exploration of the client's previous living environment. Rather, it should also include questions that explore the effects of the current environment as well as the impact anticipated living arrangements will have on the client's health, functioning, and life quality.

Asking Questions. Questions or probes are used to gather information during an interview. Skilled therapists phrase their questions using a variety of different formats so that clients do not feel interrogated. Examples include open, closed, and indirect/implied questions. *Closed questions* can usually be answered with a single word. Most frequently used by beginning therapists, closed questions are least effective for gathering information because they require limited client responses. Closed questions are effective, however, when you are interested in confirming information that is already known like date of birth, area of residence, or marital status. They are also effective in situations when clients' cognitive or communication skills limit

Table 7.1: Attending behaviors

Behavior	Definition	Purpose
Eye contact	Refers to the amount of time that passes before an individual averts his or her gaze from another person's face. It should be steady and nonthreatening.	Conveys interest in what the client is saying and that you are paying attention.
Body language	Refers to the therapist's physical appearance and use of body movements (e.g., hand gestures) as well as how personal space and environmental barriers are used. It typically should be perceived as open.	Indicates interest in and comfort level with a conversation. Therapist uses hand and body gestures to accent verbal statements or to indicate understanding of something the client has said without use of the spoken word (e.g., head nods).
Vocal qualities	Refers to the loudness, rate, and fluency of the therapist's speech patterns.	Serves to regulate and control the conversation. Speaking loudly is a way to gain control; however, it can detract from the interview process by causing the client to withdraw. Speaking too quickly can result in misunderstandings because the client does not have time to comprehend what was said. Fluency of speech (e.g., no stammering or halting speech) indicates assuredness and comfort with the topics being discussed.

their ability to respond. *Open questions* require a more elaborate response from the client. Open questions often begin with "How," "What," or "Why." However, "Why" questions can be threatening to a client, as they tend to challenge a client's behavior. Open questions require clients to generate thoughts, organize ideas, and respond to the therapist with information. Therefore, they have the potential to be more revealing than closed questions. *Indirect or implied questions* are really statements that suggest you need more information. Statements like "You must be really upset with your friends." or "I wonder what you were thinking when you started fighting?" are examples of implied questions. This type of questioning is most effective when the interviewer wants to obtain information about a client's feelings. There are numerous other communication skills that therapists use during interviews (see Chapter 11).

✴ • • •Thinking Trigger

How would your friends describe your mannerisms when engaged in a conversation? Do you think these mannerisms would help or hinder interviews with clients?   • • •✴

Structuring an Interview. Most interviews follow a particular pattern. Typically, they pass through various levels of information exchange. Initially, the exchange involves topics that are perceived by both parties as safe and nonthreatening. At this level, questions are usually superficial, socially acceptable, and comfortable. As clients and therapists feel more at ease with one another, they progress to the next level of exchange where areas of inquiry and responses become

more intimate. **Table 7.2** details the basic structure of an interview.

Observation

Observations are another way to gather information during an assessment. For instance, during interviews careful attention must be paid to the client's general appearance, body language, and comfort level (Shipley & McNulty Wood, 1996). In addition to "listening" during an interview, you should also observe the client's nonverbal behaviors, interaction style, speech patterns (e.g., halting speech), the amount of congruence between verbal and nonverbal messages, as well as the effects of the environment on the client's behavior. These observations are stored for later analysis. Similar observations are also made when you ask clients to engage in a task as part of the assessment process.

In the assessment process, observations involve more than causally watching a client; rather, they are systematic and structured. Observations can be unobtrusive (i.e., the client is unaware that they are being observed) or obtrusive (i.e., the client is aware of the observation). "The primary reasons for conducting observations is to record the client's behavior (not perceptions of behavior as in interviews) in as real-life situations as possible" (Peterson & Stumbo, 2000, p. 231). Some recreation therapists use systematic procedures for recording their observations. These procedures are used when *specific behaviors* (e.g., activity attendance, obscene language, fighting, time on task, self-stimulating behaviors, time spent out of one's room) have been identified as intervention targets. *Tally recordings* indicate how frequently a specific behavior occurs. In this type of recording, you record each time a client displays the behavior. When you are interested in

Table 7.2: Structure of an interview

Phase	Focus of Conversation	Purpose
Introduction	Ritual, small talk	Educate client about confidentiality, purpose of interview Put the client at ease by establishing genuine interest
Opening	Nondirective, exploratory	Determine client's awareness of issues, goals, desires for therapeutic relationship, and intervention outcomes
Body	Directive, exploratory	Information gathering on client's areas of interest, concerns, abilities, and goals
Closing	Summarizing, supportive	Reassure the client, instill hope, tie up loose ends, clarify expectations for future interactions

how long a behavior occurs, you record the amount of time that the client displays the behavior. This is called *duration recording. Interval recording* indicates how frequently a behavior is displayed during a specified time interval.

A wide variety of behaviors lend themselves to observational methods such as interpersonal interactions, task skills, problem-solving skills, activity level, and leisure involvement, to name a few. Therapists must remember, however, that observations never explain clients' motives for the behavior. To obtain an understanding of motive, you must couple your observations with interviewing.

Performance Tests

The third method available for use in assessments is performance testing. Performance testing involves the development of a testing condition and the identification of performance criteria for the skill being tested (Lasko-McCarthey & Knopf, 1992). For instance, a therapist interested in assessing a client's static balance would first identify the condition for displaying the skill. The therapist might ask the client to stand on one foot, with hands on hips, eyes opened and the opposite foot knee flexed. Next, the therapist must identify the criteria for success (e.g., the client remains standing for 10 seconds without falling). Typically, the criteria for success are based on "normal" abilities. Numerous criterion performance tests using recreation activities to assess client functioning can be developed. For instance, the OHIO Functional Assessment Battery (Olsson, 1994) identifies performance criteria for recreation-related tasks (see **Exhibit 7.1**). Assessment ratings are then derived based on the client's performance in these tasks.

Using Secondary Data Sources

Secondary data sources are the fourth data gathering method available for use when conducting assessments. They include any information you gather that is not obtained directly from the client. For example, important information can be obtained from family members, significant others, or available client records. All of these are considered secondary data sources.

Family members or significant others are a valuable secondary data source. These individuals can confirm or disconfirm information provided to you by the client. They can also offer you insight into the client's role

Exhibit 7.1: Sample tasks in OHIO Functional Assessment Battery

Sample Task	Functional Skills and Performance Criteria
Domino Patterns	*Cognition*
Task: Clients are asked to recreate four domino patterns that the therapist shows them for 10 seconds	New Learning: Scoring is based on the number of patterns that the client can recreate without visual cues
	Attention Span: Scoring is based on the percentage of time that the client is distracted and off task
	Retention Span: Scoring is based on the number of instructions that the client can restate to the therapist
Sporting Goods Shopping Trip	*Cognition*
Task: Clients are given a shopping list of sports equipment to buy, money, a blank check, and a worksheet. They are asked to: • Count and record the total amount of money provided to them • Read the shopping list of items and prices • Determine the total cost of their purchase if they get everything on the list • Determine if they need additional money, and if so write a check to the store in the correct amount	Money Management Skills: Scoring is based on the number of factors (e.g., money identification, addition, subtraction, check writing) successfully performed Attention Span: Scoring is based on the percentage of time that the client is distracted and off task

within the family. Reviewing client records provides you with abundant information about the client's medical status, medical precaution, medications, and general health status. Some therapists caution against record reviews prior to the assessment process, arguing such reviews may bias you. On the other hand, there are a number of sound reasons for reviewing records prior to conducting assessments. First, they provide information that has already been confirmed as accurate, including background information you may find useful. Secondly, you can avoid asking clients to repeat information that has already been gathered (unless there is a specific reason for doing so). Finally, record reviews alert you to any special precautions—such as dietary restrictions, the use of eyeglasses, ambulating restrictions, or suicide precautions—that must be considered before working with a client.

Special Considerations in Data Gathering

Therapists need to be cautious that they do not unwittingly focus their data collection exclusively on client problems and deficits. Use of the client–system perspective allows therapists to identify client strengths during the assessment process. Client strengths are resources that need to be used in planning as they reinforce clients' competence and abilities as oppose to disabilities and limitations. Focusing on client strengths facilitates client empowerment and competence.

It is also imperative that recreation therapists have confidence in their data gathering procedures. The results of data gathering must represent a valid baseline from which client progress and intervention effectiveness can be judged and documented. Such confidence is obtained when therapists are confident in the technical and practical aspects of their assessments.

Technical Evaluation

Technical evaluation is concerned with the statistical and research processes used in the development of interviews, observations, or performance testing. Technical evaluation is focused on validity and reliability issues. Sometimes labeled psychometric properties, technical evaluations appraise the accuracy and consistency of the data gathering procedures.

Evaluating the technical aspects of assessment instruments is a difficult task. In addition to understanding the various types of validity and reliability, therapists must also understand the statistical procedures used to measure these constructs. A detailed discussion of the statistical procedures used to establish validity and reliability is beyond the scope of this text. However, a brief overview of validity and reliability issues related to assessment procedures is described to more fully acquaint you with the concepts.

Before using an assessment instrument, especially if it is available commercially, examine the administration guide to check whether information about its validity, reliability, and usability is available.

Table 7.3: Types of validity

Type of Validity	Definition
Content	Degree to which experts or literature agree that the items and methods used to measure a skill or concept accurately represent it.
Criterion-related	Degree to which assessment findings relate to another objective rating of the skill or concept (i.e., the criterion). There are two forms of criterion-related validity: concurrent and predictive. In concurrent validity the criterion is obtained at about the same time as the assessment data. In predictive validity the criterion is obtained some time after the assessment data.
Construct	The degree to which the scores or ratings obtained from the assessment procedures are representative of the underlying theoretical construct being assessed, such as functional independence, depression, or leisure behavior.
Clinical	How useful an instrument is for specific clinical purposes. The instrument's use should be beneficial in the planning and evaluating of interventions (Kloseck & Crilly, 1997).

Validity

Validity refers to the accuracy of the assessment methods. For instance, if the assessment were to yield information about a client's leisure involvement, valid data would ascertain that you actually gathered information about the client's leisure involvement and not something else such as the client's leisure interests. At the minimum, assessment procedures should have *face* or *content validity*. This means that other therapists would agree that the assessment procedures are likely to yield the types of information for which they were designed. Other types of validity include *criterion validity*, *construct validity*, and *clinical validity* (see **Table 7.3**). When examining the validity of assessment procedures, you must realize that validity is a matter of degree and not an all-or-nothing property. "Numerous studies are needed, using different approaches, different samples, and different populations to build a body of evidence that supports or fails to support the validity …" of assessment procedures (Benson & Schell, 1997, p. 4).

Reliability

Reliability is concerned with replication. You are focused on ascertaining how confident you can be that another therapist would reach the same conclusions as you using the same data gathering procedures. Reliability indicates whether the results derived from the procedures were influenced by time, test anxiety, or environmental conditions. **Table 7.4** defines different ways to assess reliability.

When observational methods are used recreation therapists must be concerned with *intrarater* and *interrater* agreement. When only one rater is involved with client observations, you are concerned with the rater's consistency from one observation to the next. This is considered intrarater reliability. When two or more raters are conducting client observations, information is needed on both intrarater agreement and interrater agreement. Interrater agreement determines the consistency with which two or more raters agree when observing the behaviors of the same client.

Practical Evaluation

The practical evaluation of assessment procedures is equally important. Practical evaluation is concerned with usability and addresses the likelihood that the data gathering process is relevant to the agency mission and constraints such as clients' length of stay. Practical evaluation is focused on the ease with which the procedures can be used, the length of time it takes for data collection, the clarity and ease of scoring self-report forms, observations, or performance testing, and the appropriateness of the procedures for clients and clinical decision-making. This common-sense evaluation ascertains whether assessment procedures are appropriate for a given agency or group of clients given the realities of the setting.

Targets in the Assessment Process

Whether self-report, observations, performance testing, secondary data sources, or some combination of these methods are used, recreation therapists use the client–system perspective as a guide during data gathering.

Table 7.4: Types of reliability

Type of Reliability	Definition
Stability	Attempts to quantify the degree to which a variable, trait, or area of interest (e.g., quality of life) remains unchanged over time. Measures of stability are typically obtained by repeating the same assessment procedures on the same group of clients (e.g., test–retest). Use of this type of reliability is dependent on the assumption that the variable, trait, or area of interest is theoretically supposed to remain relatively stable in a normal population.
Equivalency	Attempts to estimate the degree of similarity among multiple forms of the same assessment tool. Changes in an individual's score are theoretically due to testing error as items in the tool are thought to measure the same content domain.
Internal consistency	Used with assessment measures that are identifying traits. This form of reliability attempts to ascertain how items relate to one another. All items in the measure are thought to be highly related as they are measuring the same construct.

Specific areas of interest include:

- Biological functioning, including physical functioning and health status
- Psychological functioning, including cognitive and emotional functioning
- Social functioning
- Spiritual functioning

In addition, you are also interested in collecting information about the client's current lifestyle, including recreation and leisure involvement, and environmental concerns related to the client's home, community, and social support network. Consider Mr. Murphy, a 55-year-old single man who reports during an assessment interview that he is quite unhappy, that he typically stays at home, and does not socialize with friends for pleasure. He also tells you that he believes this social isolation will increase due to the recent amputation of his leg. While the assessment interview has yielded useful information, it fails to provide a comprehensive picture.

As can be seen in **Table 7.5**, a number of additional potential intervention "targets" emerged for Mr. Murphy, other than the social isolation and impaired emotional well-being that were apparent during the first interview. By using the client–system perspective, additional needs associated with educating Mr. Murphy about his health condition and lifestyle, including using recre-

ation to prevent secondary complications were identified. Furthermore, a number of environmental issues related to social support also became apparent. As you can see, use of the client–system perspective provides you with an extensive range of information to consider in the data gathering process. However, you need to target your data collection efforts. Ultimately, the information you choose to gather should be determined by the mission of the agency, the role of TR in overall client care, the amount of time available to work with clients, and unique client needs and concerns.

The next sections provide a comprehensive overview of data that recreation therapists gather when using the client–system perspective. This overview will acquaint you with the areas of functioning that can be assessed. Note that recreation therapists do not primarily assess all of these areas due to lack of training, qualification, or professional boundaries. Other aspects of functioning may not be assessed by recreation therapists to avoid duplicating data already gathered by colleagues. Ultimately recreation therapists at each agency make decisions about which areas of functioning are most relevant for their TR assessment procedures. Just because you will narrow your focus, however, does not imply that you do not need to understand the range of functioning discussed in this section. Rather, this knowledge is imperative to understanding the range of influences that impact leisure behavior.

Table 7.5: An example of concerns identified using the client–system perspective

Client–System Area	Possible Needs and Concerns
Biological	Impaired mobility skills Complications from diabetes
Psychological	Impaired cognitive skills associated with planning and decision making Social anxiety Depressed mood
Social	Impaired abilities to initiate and maintain conversations
Spiritual	Sense of hopelessness and despair Unable to find meaning in life or make sense of current situation
Developmental	Difficulties adjusting to changes in self-image related to aging process
Lifestyle	Lack of knowledge about recreation and social opportunities within home and community Lack of knowledge about sedentary lifestyle and health impairments
Environmental	Changing social constellation within home environment (e.g., friends have moved) Transportation difficulties related to inability to continue driving

This knowledge also allows you to provide other professionals with additional information or perspectives about your client's functioning.

Assessing Biological Concerns

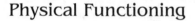

The biological aspect in the client–system perspective is concerned with the client's physical functioning and health status. Abundant information about clients' medical needs, health status, and precautions already exist in their records. Including a record review as part of your assessment procedures provides you with a solid preliminary understanding of relevant health-related issues and concerns. However, other areas of physical functioning are not as readily assessed via a record review. Discussion follows regarding the skills and abilities associated with physical functioning, including a definition of common terms and assessment methods that are most relevant to recreation therapists.

Physical Functioning

Areas of physical functioning of interest to recreation therapists include mobility, muscle strength and endurance, flexibility, cardiovascular endurance, perceptual motor skills, and visual and auditory perception. While some of these areas of physical functioning are of most interest to recreation therapists employed in physical rehabilitation, long-term care, and pediatric settings, clients' endurance and fitness levels are relevant to all recreation therapists, regardless of service delivery setting. This is because endurance and fitness levels are critical to maintaining and facilitating physical and emotional health and preventing secondary conditions. They are also prerequisite abilities for an active leisure lifestyle.

Typically, assessing physical functioning lies in the purview of physical therapists. However, in some settings, recreation therapists supplement the physical therapists' data. For instance, in physical rehabilitation settings, recreation therapists often facilitate community reintegration activities. Therefore, they must also supervise, assist, and *assess* a client's physical functioning in the community. **Table 7.6** (p. 110) contains definitions and assessment methods typically used to assess mobility, muscle strength and endurance, flexibility, and cardiovascular endurance. Definitions and assessment options for perceptual-motor functioning,

including the subskills in this area of balance, kinesthetic awareness, fine motor skills and motor planning are presented in **Table 7.7** (p. 111). **Table 7.8** (p. 112) contains definitions and assessment methods for visual and perceptual functioning. Each of these areas of physical functioning is explained in the following section.

Mobility. Mobility refers to the client's ability to move from one location to another. Clients are considered independent if they can move from one position to some other desired position (including the ability to move into a bed, move with a wheelchair, and transfer/ambulate with prescribed mobility devices), and if they can use their mobility techniques and devices in a variety of community settings (burlingame & Skalko, 1997). Recreation therapists are not typically involved in assessing basic mobility skills. Mobility assessment in clinical TR services is typically very applied and relates to advanced mobility issues that occur in recreation activities (see Table 7.6). For instance, recreation therapists would be involved in assessing whether clients can transfer from their wheelchairs to a swimming pool deck or whether clients can navigate their wheelchairs on uneven surfaces such as those found in backyard gardens or movie theaters. In addition, recreation therapists frequently assess mobility skills in community settings. Clients often display different functional abilities as a response to the environment, and so a community-based assessment of physical functioning may yield valuable information about a client's performance that is not as accurately assessed in the clinical environment. For example, newly injured clients may struggle to propel their wheelchairs up inclines or on uneven sidewalks. They may have difficulty initially navigating curb cuts. These challenges do not exist within the facility where handrails are in use and floors are level. Community reintegration activities allow recreation therapists to assess clients' physical functioning in naturalistic settings. Such information is valuable when determining consistency between in-center and community-based performance.

Muscle strength and muscle endurance. Muscle strength and endurance are important essentials in facilitating independence in activities of daily living, preventing disuse syndrome, and preventing some secondary complications that often accompany disability (e.g., chronic back pain). Most recreation therapists are not typically involved in formally assessing muscle strength and endurance. However, applied assessment in which clients are asked to perform a task that is part of their leisure repertoire can be used to assess muscle strength and endurance needed for recreation activities (e.g., Can a client carry a full watering can to water his houseplants?). In addition, recreation therapists may be involved in formally assessing muscle strength if they are directing a wheelchair sports program or weight-training program. Possible assessment techniques are described in Table 7.6. Assessing muscle strength and endurance independently or in conjunction with another rehabilitative therapist depends on the agency and the technical skills of the recreation therapist. While not always assessed by recreation therapists, muscle strength and muscle endurance are often targets for TR interventions as they are prerequisite skills needed for independence in a variety of life activities, including recreation and leisure.

Flexibility. Flexibility refers to the ability to move a joint through its typical range of motion (ROM). Ways of assessing flexibility are described in Table 7.6. Typically assessed by a physical therapist or exercise physiologist, functional abilities or movement patterns that can be compromised due to difficulties with the ROM in a joint or series of joints are of interest to recreation therapists. Flexibility is especially an issue when the focus of TR intervention is skill instruction related to premorbid or new recreation activities (e.g., a golf swing).

Table 7.6: Physical functioning skills and sample assessment methods

Physical Skill	Definition	Assessment
Mobility	Ability to move from one location to another	Recreation therapists are sometimes involved in assessing advanced mobility skills, such as the identification of transportation options, the ability to adapt mode of locomotion to compensate for changes in terrain and situation, and the ability to plan ahead when necessary to ensure the accessibility of the proposed route. These skills are not usually evaluated during an initial assessment, rather evaluation occurs later in the rehabilitation process. Performance testing and interviews are the typical assessment methods used.
Muscle strength	Maximum amount of force that can be elicited in a single muscle contraction.	Performance testing, such as manual muscle testing, the break test, and grip strength dynamometers.
Muscle endurance	Ability to perform submaximal muscle contractions repeatedly.	Performance testing with weight repetitions or isokinetic testing.
Flexibility	Ability to move a joint through its range of motion (ROM).	Performance testing in which the client is asked to move various joints through their normal ROM. Data is usually recorded as either within normal limits (WNL) for the joint or with limitation of motion (LOM) observed. Performance testing should be done bilaterally for comparison purposes and may be active, where the participant is asked to move the joint, or passive, where the therapist moves the joint through ROM.
Cardiovascular endurance	Ability of the heart and lungs to move oxygen to muscle groups in a manner that allows for normal activity with reasonable endurance over time (burlingame & Skalko, 1997).	Assessment of cardiovascular endurance is typically done via some form of submaximal stress testing, such as using arm crank or leg cycle ergometry, the step-test, or the 12-minute run–walk test. Expert training and medical supervision is required to assess cardiovascular endurance in individuals with disabilities or chronic illness.

Table 7.7: Perceptual motor skills and sample assessment methods

Perceptual Motor Skill	Definition	Assessment
Balance	Ability to maintain a posture against the pull of gravity. *Static* balance refers to the ability to maintain posture when the body is at rest. *Dynamic* balance refers to the ability to maintain posture when moving. *Sitting* balance refers to the ability to maintain an erect posture when in a seated position. *Standing* balance refers to the ability to maintain an erect posture when in an upright position.	Assessment usually involves development of criterion testing procedures that include performance testing of the client in a variety of positions and movements requiring static and dynamic balance. Recreation therapists can use table tennis as functional performance assessment for static and dynamic balance.
Kinesthetic Awareness	Awareness of one's body in space. Kinesthetic awareness includes body awareness, laterality, and bilateral coordination	Assessment usually involves development of criterion-based performance testing of a client during a recreation activity.
Body awareness	Ability to integrate sensory information to appreciate tactile sensation, the relationship of body parts to the whole, and the orientation of the body in space. This is necessary to follow structured exercise routines.	Typically assessed through observation of a client in a recreation activity.
Laterality	Ability to discriminate right and left. This skill involves verbal, sensory, conceptual, and visual–spatial components. The skill is a prerequisite for direction following and other tasks, such as map reading or adapted sports.	Formal testing procedures are typically not needed, as a client's response to right–left directions can be observed during a variety of tasks.
Bilateral coordination	Ability to coordinate the use of a right and left extremity (e.g., arms, legs). The skill is a prerequisite for many recreation tasks, like catching and throwing a ball, riding a bike, and exercise routines.	Typically assessed through observation of a client in a recreation activity.
Fine motor	Ability to use the hands and fingers. Typically involves subskills of prehension (ability to grasp an object with the fingers) and opposition (ability to oppose any of the fingers with the thumb).	Assessment usually involves criterion-based performance testing of the client in tasks requiring fine motor performance, such as checkers, cards, and art activities.
Motor planning	Ability to produce an effective motor response. Difficulty in motor planning may arise as a result of conceptual, production or motor difficulties (Roy, 1983).	Typically assessed via observation of client in activities that require the use of tools or utensils (e.g., craft activities, games).

Cardiovascular Endurance. Cardiovascular endurance involves the ability of the heart and lungs to produce enough oxygen so that an individual can engage in aerobic activities for a sustained period. This area of physical functioning is compromised whenever individuals are unable to participate in purposeful physical activity. Formal assessment of cardiovascular endurance requires advanced clinical training. Typically, recreation therapists assess cardiovascular endurance through criterion performance testing or observation (see Table 7.6, p. 110). For instance, recreation therapists will watch for signs of fatigue or shortness of breath in individuals when asking them to perform routine recreation activities.

Perceptual Motor Skills. Perceptual motor skills represent the ability to accurately perceive, integrate, and respond motorically to internal or external stimuli. Individuals with developmental disabilities such as learning disabilities, mental retardation, and cerebral palsy often have perceptual motor deficits. Impairment in this skill area is also seen in individuals with multiple sclerosis, cerebrovascular accidents, and acquired brain injury. These skills tend to diminish as a function of the aging process due to degeneration in the central and peripheral nervous systems. Table 7.7 (p. 111) defines the subskills related to perceptual motor functioning, including balance, kinesthetic awareness, fine motor skills, and motor planning and includes typical assessment procedures for these areas.

Visual and Auditory Perception. Information on a client's visual and auditory status can typically be obtained from the client's record. A client's visual and auditory status can adversely affect performance on a variety of tasks and may require you to consider adaptations in your assessment gathering procedures as well as your interventions. While not a primary target in TR assessments, recreation therapists should be attentive to client's visual fields, including field cuts, visual acuity, visual range of motion, and the ability to visually pursue a moving object. Table 7.8 explains these terms and related assessment procedures.

You will also need to gather specific information about the client's ability to hear and understand spoken language. While diagnosing auditory and receptive language difficulties are not a primary focus of TR assessments, you must understand the impact that these deficits can have on client performance. Decreased hearing can cause problems with following directions, resulting in more fatigue and difficulty with sustaining attention. Incorrect performance due to word misperception as a result of decreased acuity or receptive aphasia can complicate assessment procedures. Careful collaboration with an audiologist or a speech and language pathologist can assist recreation therapists in adapting evaluation procedures so that a client's performance is not compromised by auditory deficits. Such collaboration also allows for effective care that recognizes the implications of auditory deficits on client functioning.

Psychological Functioning

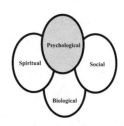

The psychological aspect in the client–system perspective is concerned with the client's

Table 7.8: Visual testing terms and sample assessment methods

Term	Definition	Assessment
Visual acuity	Ability to detect detail	Usually assessed by an optometrist. Client will have difficulty distinguishing lines, letters, or figures. Acuity problems may affect client's ability to read.
Visual range of motion	Ability to move the eyes in all directions	Visual ROM testing typically involves asking the client to follow a moving target without moving the head. Client will be unable to effectively scan the environment. Consideration of where to place materials and supplies must be made by the therapist.
Pursuit	Ability to follow a moving target with the eyes in a steady and precise way	Typically assessed during visual ROM testing by observing the control and smoothness with which the eyes can move. Can also be observed during the client's involvement in activities. Clients with visual pursuit problems will have difficulty with tasks requiring hand–eye coordination (e.g., catching a ball).

cognitive and *emotional* functioning. Record reviews can provide you with a preliminary understanding of your client's cognitive and emotional functioning. However, more specific data may be needed. The following sections explain the skills and abilities related to a client's cognitive and emotional functioning, as well as procedures or methods used for assessing functioning in these areas.

Cognitive Functioning

Assessment of cognitive functioning is a primary area in TR assessments regardless of work setting. Cognition affects the client's ability to both learn and process information. According to Haase (1997), no formal standards exist regarding how cognition should be assessed. Furthermore, the type of setting as well as other rehabilitative professionals involved in the client's care influence the methods chosen to assess cognition. Typically, recreation therapists evaluate cognitive functioning through observation or simple performance testing. More advanced evaluation of cognitive functioning is the purview of clinical psychologists and neuropsychologists.

When assessing cognition, recreation therapists must be attentive to clients' educational abilities and background. Clients will have varying reading and reasoning abilities prior to the onset of any disabling condition. Such information, which is usually found on a client's chart, is an important consideration prior to conducting an assessment. This information allows you to form a baseline with which to compare the client's current cognitive functioning. It also influences the manner in which information is presented to the client. This is especially true with clients who are not proficient at reading. The following cognitive areas should be considered as target areas for TR assessments: attention, memory, orientation, and problem solving.

Attention. Attention forms the basis for many, if not all, cognitive functions. Problems with attention affect a client's ability to be aware of important elements in the environment, process information for learning, and engage in life activities, including recreation and leisure. Attention deficits include distractibility, perseveration, decreased concentration, decreased information processing speed, confusion, impulsivity, impersistence, and persistence on irrelevant cues. Attention problems may be seen in individuals with cerebral contusions, cerebrovascular accidents, tumors, traumatic brain injury (TBI), or hypoxia (Adamovich, Henderson & Auerbach, 1985). Individuals with degenerative illnesses such as multiple sclerosis or

Alzheimer's disease may also have attention deficits, as will individuals with schizophrenia and affective disorders. There are many different types of attention skills. These skills work together to allow clients to process information. They include: arousal or alertness, the ability to attend to stimuli (selective attention), the ability to span attention (concentration), the ability to shift attention (alternating attention), and information processing. **Table 7.9** (p. 114) contains definitions and associated assessment procedures for each of these skills.

Memory. Memory is the ability to take in, store, and retrieve information (Morse, 1986). The ability to remember is crucial to a person's identity and sense of self as memories help to define who we are (Caprio-Prevette & Fry, 1996). Memory problems impair a client's ability to learn and to engage in many routine tasks. Memory deficits are often manifested in clients as difficulties with retaining new information, learning new procedures, remembering names or appointments, remembering directions, and recalling the location of items. Memory problems are seen in clients with amnesia, TBI, Alzheimer's disease, cerebrovascular accidents and progressive degenerative dementia (Haase, 1997). Clients with depression, anxiety, and psychosis may have impairments in memory, as may clients who have prolonged substance abuse (Waldinger, 1990). The information-processing perspective is the predominant approach used to understand memory (Caprio-Prevette & Fry, 1996). This model describes three levels of memory storage: sensory memory, working memory (also called short-term memory), and long-term memory. **Table 7.10** (p. 115) contains definitions for each of these skills and suggestions for assessment methods in each area.

Orientation. Orientation is a multifaceted skill that requires the integration of attention, memory, and perception (Okkema, 1993). Typically, clients are evaluated in terms of orientation to person, place, and time. Topographical orientation refers to the client's ability to navigate effectively from one place to another, to follow a familiar route, or to describe one place in relation to another. Orientation problems may be seen in individuals with a variety of disabling conditions including cerebral contusions, cerebrovascular accidents, tumors, TBI, Alzheimer's disease, progressive degenerative dementia, and some psychiatric disorders.

Most clients are oriented to self but may be disoriented to others including family or staff members or to their physical surroundings, especially if the surroundings are new. This type of disorientation can create extreme confusion and poor cooperation in clients.

Orientation to time is concerned not only with awareness of the date, but also with the season and the passage of time. Deficits in this area can result in general confusion. For instance, clients with time orientation difficulties may be unable to understand why the cafeteria is not serving breakfast foods at the dinner meal. It can also result in anxiety when clients think that anticipated visitors did not arrive when expected because the client has not correctly judged the passage of time. It may also manifest itself in poor judgment regarding appropriate clothing to wear because clients do not remember what season it is. Individuals who are not oriented to place will display many similar deficits. In addition, they may place demands on the environment or staff as a result of their disorientation (e.g., they think they are taking a vacation when they are really in a nursing home). Orientation is easily assessed in a formal or informal manner by asking clients a series of questions related to person, place, and time (e.g., "Tell me when you think five minutes have gone by."). Asking clients to locate an area within their room, home, or the nursing unit is the best method to use to assess geographical orientation.

Problem Solving. Problem solving refers to the client's ability to reason how to achieve some desired result. Problem solving is a complex task that involves cognitive and perceptual skills. Difficulty with problem solving will adversely impact a client's life, making the performance of routine and nonroutine tasks nearly impossible. Difficulty with problem solving is not limited to any one diagnostic group. Problem solving difficulties may be seen in a wide variety of clients including individuals with psychiatric disorders, TBI, cerebrovascular accidents, and individuals with degenerative disorders such as Alzheimer's disease.

Problem solving requires clients to have the ability to recognize an error when it occurs, generate possible ways to overcome the error, evaluate the feasibility of these options, and select an appropriate solution. It is important to determine which aspect of problem solving

Table 7.9: Attention component skills and sample assessment methods

Attention Skill	Definition	Assessment
Arousal	State of readiness to receive information from the environment	Structured observation in which the therapist is attentive to which type of stimuli evokes attentive response (e.g., visual, auditory, tactical, olfactory, vestibular).
Selective attention	Ability to screen out and ignore stimuli in the environment to focus on a task	Performance testing such as asking a client to perform a highly repetitive task in a highly distracting environment (e.g., playing card games in a clinic, lunch room, or day area).
Concentration	Ability to sustain attention over a long period of time. Concentration occurs automatically, but individuals can also control aspects of it. The novelty and complexity of the task as well as mental and physical fatigue often influence concentration.	Performance testing such as asking the client to perform some activity that is of interest to him or her in a quiet environment. Preferred activity selection is extremely important. Failure to select an appropriately challenging and interesting activity may result in inattention to the task as a function of boredom and not attention.
Alternating attention	Ability to shift attention from one task to another	Performance testing such as asking the client to engage in any activity that requires attention to several factors at the same time, such as cooking a multistep meal or carrying on a conversation while engaging in a game of billiards.

is difficult for a client. Such specification helps with planning interventions. **Table 7.11** (p. 116) defines each of the problem-solving stages and suggests assessment strategies to determine if clients are having difficulty in this area.

Emotional Functioning

Clients' affective or emotional functioning is of interest to all recreation therapists, regardless of their practice setting. Normal emotional functioning is challenged when individuals experience stress. Since most health crises are stress producing, the emotional functioning of most clients seen in TR can be considered at risk. Emotional functioning can also be impaired by psychiatric or physical illness or by damage to the brain. Typically, recreation therapists gain an understanding of a client's affective functioning by an initial assessment interview. Also, a record review will identify areas of concern in terms of affective functioning, such

Table 7.10: Types of memory and sample assessment methods

Type of Memory	Definition	Assessment
Sensory	First level in the information–processing model of memory. It is thought to last a few milliseconds. Large amounts of information enter the brain for further cognitive processing. The brain decides which information requires further processing, using past experiences. This information is then acted on by working memory. Other information fades from memory.	Recreation therapists are not usually involved in assessing sensory memory.
Working (Short-Term)	Portion of the cognitive system that focuses on processing information for storage and easy retrieval. The limits of working memory are reached at recall of 7 items +/– 2 (i.e., the average person can remember a 7-digit number, but remembering a 5-digit or a 9-digit number is also considered normal). More information can be stored in short-term memory if it is grouped or chunked. Individuals can recall these larger categories or chunks and the specific items within them.	Performance testing such as asking clients to recall information immediately after giving it to them (e.g., telling them 3 unrelated objects and asking them to recall them in 15 minutes). *Note*: Attention and motivation can affect immediate recall. During assessment make certain that the client has attended to the information and found it important enough to remember. Certain card games can be used to both assess and improve this component (see Parenté & Herrmann, 1996).
Long-Term	This component of the cognitive system creates the storehouse where information is coded, retained, and retrieved for use. There is no limit to the amount of information that can be stored in long-term memory; however, information does fade over time if not used.	Performance testing such as asking clients important names and dates from their earlier life. *Note*: Some texts suggest asking individuals to recall information about historical events. Care should be taken when using this approach, as such evaluation can be educationally or culturally biased.

as generalized anxiety or depressed mood. These areas may become targets for clinical TR intervention without any further assessment on your part. Usually, formal diagnosis of affective dysfunctioning is the purview of clinical psychologists and/or psychiatrists. However, recreation therapists do want to have a sense of their clients' emotional state and feelings. Areas of interest include assessing life satisfaction and hopefulness. In addition, two specific areas of affective functioning are particularly relevant to recreation. These are (a) a client's ability to experience enjoyment and (b) a client's ability to use recreation as a coping mechanism for stress.

Enjoyment is critical to recreation and leisure experiences, yet for some individuals this emotion is illusive. Anhedonia or the inability to experience pleasure is a symptom of some psychiatric disorders such as depression and schizophrenia. Other degenerative diseases, such as Alzheimer's disease, gradually rob individuals of their ability to perform activities that are rewarding and enjoyable (Teri & Logsdon, 1991). Recreation therapists must be extremely sensitized to their clients' ability in this area. Enjoyment motivates people to do things. It is often the reason people work hard, pushing themselves beyond their present abilities. For this reason, enjoyment is critical to the rehabilitation process and clinical TR practice. Reconnecting people to the things that they enjoy becomes a motivat-

ing force for the hard work of rehabilitation. No formal assessment standards exist to determine whether clients possess this ability. Typically, interviews and observational methods are used to assess a client's ability to experience pleasure. A noted exception is "The Pleasant Events Schedule-AD" (Teri & Logsdon, 1991). This is a specific rating form designed for use by caregivers to identify pleasurable and enjoyable activities for individuals who have Alzheimer's disease.

Coping is instrumental in maintaining emotional health. Coping strategies help individuals control their emotions, problem solve situations, and maintain a positive sense of self, especially during times of stress. As discussed in Chapter 3, research has indicated that recreation and leisure involvement can be a useful coping strategy. Recreation involvement has been described as a palliative coping method that can serve to "keep the mind busy" and consequently divert attention from distressing thoughts or events. It is also thought to serve as a buffer for life stress through the provision of social support and self-determination that can occur in leisure and recreation activities (Coleman & Iso-Ahola, 1993). For these reasons, you should assess the degree to which their clients can use recreation involvement as a coping strategy. **Exhibit 7.2** contains sample questions that can be used as part of an assessment interview to gather data in this area.

Table 7.11: Problem-solving stages and sample assessment methods

Problem-Solving Stage	Definition	Assessment
Problem identification	In this stage clients are unable to recognize that they have made an error. Difficulties in this stage are most frequently seen in clients who are unaware of their functional deficits.	Typically, clients are asked to follow directions given by the therapist for completing an unfamiliar task. The therapist observes the client's performance for errors and questions the client to determine if he or she is aware that an error has occurred.
Generating solutions/ Decision making	Involves the process of thinking about alternatives to solve a problem and the consequences of each alternative.	Clients may be presented with a problem or difficulty and asked to brainstorm possible ways to overcome it. The therapist observes the client's ability to generate solutions, noting whether the approach taken relies on trial and error or if the client can plan ahead and anticipate problems that the alternative solution creates. Experiential initiative activities in which clients are confronted with an unfamiliar challenge can be used for this type of assessment.

While a variety of self-report measures have been developed that examine clients' coping style, few measures examine the clients' use of recreation as a coping response. One scale that does assess the client's use of recreation as a coping strategy is the Activities as Coping Measure (Shank, 1991). It measures clients' perceptions of the usefulness of recreation for stress reduction. Sample items from the Activities as Coping Measure are described in **Exhibit 7.3** (p. 118).

Social Functioning

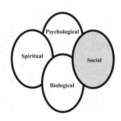

Social functioning is another primary area of interest to recreation therapists. Social functioning refers to the behaviors, language, and attitudes a person conveys during his or her interactions with one or more people. Social functioning involves both verbal and nonverbal communication. Individuals are seen as being socially competent when they are able to adapt, respond to, and balance the demands of the social situation or environment in an effective manner (Stumbo, 1994/1995). Since most recreation and leisure activities have social components, clients who have deficits in terms of social functioning may have difficulty in recreation and leisure activities.

These difficulties may arise because the client has problems with *instrumental* and/or *social–emotional* interactions. Instrumental social interactions involve those exchanges that serve "to gain tangible ends that are required for physical, material, and financial well-being" (Liberman, 1982, p. 63). Examples include: asking for information about a recreation activity, inquiring about a place to live, buying an item in a store, or informing an authority figure of something that is needed. The objective of instrumental interactions is acquiring information, or gaining something that will improve a person's physical or economic well-being. In contrast, social–emotional interactions focus on meeting an individual's affiliative needs. These interactions may involve exchanging information, opinions, and/or feelings. However, the exchange is not focused on accomplishing a tangible goal. "Social–emotional interactions deal with expressions of love, hate, ambivalence, alienation, sadness, happiness, joy, and wishes" (Liberman, 1982, p. 64). This distinction is important for both assessment and intervention planning, as clients may have difficulty with one type of interaction but not necessarily the other.

Social functioning can be impaired as a result of psychiatric or physical illness or brain injury. It may arise from inadequate learning experiences, disuse, anxiety, cognitive disturbances, or amotivational states (Liberman, 1982). However, very few people are completely competent or wholly incompetent in social and interpersonal skills (Phillips, 1978). An individual's social competence may fluctuate as a function of the environment, the other parties involved in the social exchange (e.g., authority figures vs. peers), or the emotional state of the individual (e.g., anxious, depressed). A number of competencies have been identified that need to be mastered for individuals to maintain adequate social relations. They include the ability:

- To be kind, cooperative, and appropriately compliant, as opposed to being hostile and defiant
- To show interest in people and things, to be appropriately outgoing, and to socialize actively
- To effectively use language, to comprehend the thoughts and ideas of others, and to express thoughts and ideas so they can be understood (Strayhorn & Strain, 1986)

These competencies allow individuals to successfully interact in social and intimate relationships.

Exhibit 7.2: Sample questions for assessing coping

Can you identify when you are feeling stressed or anxious? What are the warning signs for you?

Can you identify what makes you stressful or anxious? Can you elaborate on this?

What helps you deal with feelings of stress or anxiety? Is religion and prayer helpful to you?

Do you know any relaxation or meditation exercises? If so, are they helpful? Why or why not?

Has daydreaming or fantasizing helped you?

Do you share your concerns, fears, and anxieties with someone close to you? Do you find this helpful?

Are you able to find a positive aspect to most situations?

Can you use humor to deal with your situation when you are feeling anxious?

Do you find physical activity useful when you feel anxious? Why or why not?

However, deficits in social competencies may result in difficulties in any of the following areas: initiating and responding appropriately to sustained verbal exchanges, assertiveness, expression of ideas and feelings, awareness of another's needs and feelings, compromise and negotiation, and the ability to take part in cooperative and competitive activities.

Assessment techniques for social competence abound. Stumbo (1994/1995) identified and reviewed 24 different assessment tools that can be used to assess clients' social functioning. Most of these tools have been developed using psychometric procedures to ascertain that they are valid and reliable. Liberman (1982) suggests that assessments of social competence "employ multilevel and multimodal measures that tap the subjective experience of the patient (affect, cognition, imagery, sensation), the observable behavior of the patient (verbal and nonverbal response), and in some cases the physiological or biological level (electrodermal response, electromyographic response, hormone levels)." He presents four different methods, which practitioners could utilize to assess social competence. These include self-report questionnaires where clients endorse statements that reflect the social behavior being assessed, interviews, role-play tests, and naturalistic interactions.

Spiritual Functioning

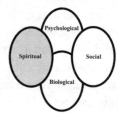

One singular definition of the word spirituality does not exist (Maher & Hunt, 1993). Spirituality has been used to describe the human need for meaning and value in life and desire for a relationship with a transcendent power (Clinebell, 1995). Spirituality is usually defined as an individual's views and behaviors that express relatedness to something greater than the self (Ziegler, 1998). While spirituality may include elements of religion, it is typically defined much more broadly. Religion implies traditional beliefs, attitudes, and practices that are part of an organization. Spirituality, in contrast, refers to "a belief system that provides a sense of meaning and purpose … and offers an ethical path to personal fulfillment which includes connectedness with self, others, and a higher power" (Hawks, 1994, p. 6). Spirituality has been defined as an important factor in an individual's perception of quality of life, in maintaining a healthy lifestyle, in the will to live, and in finding meaning in life. Typically, assessment in this area focuses on asking clients about their spiritual interests, resources, typical patterns of religious expression, and philosophical values. Questions may also

Exhibit 7.3: Activities as coping scale (Shank, 1991)

The Activities as Coping Scale is a 36-item scale determining the extent to which hospitalized clients use activities as a coping mechanism.

Response Options

1	Rarely	I rarely use activities to deal with stress in this way.
2	Once or twice	I use activities to deal with stress in this way once or twice.
3	Occasionally	I occasionally use activities to deal with stress in this way.
4	Always	I always use activities to deal with stress in this way.

Sample Items	**Response Options**			
How often do you use activities to...	1	2	3	4
Provide some fun in a serious setting?				
Have an opportunity to find spiritual comfort?				
Help you feel independent?				
Show the better side of yourself to others?				
Escape from your situation for the moment?				

focus on life goal setting and life meaning. For instance, Hopkins, Woods, Kelley, Bentley, and Murphy (1995) have a spiritual assessment comprised of 20 open-ended questions. **Exhibit 7.4** contains sample questions from this spiritual assessment. The intent of spiritual assessment is to better understand clients so that recreation therapists can create environments and opportunities that allow clients to fulfill their religious and spiritual needs.

Lifestyle

In the course of an assessment, therapists want to obtain a picture of the client's lifestyle in addition to determining the client's functional abilities. Lifestyle consists of one's way of living or the patterns of behavior in the circumstances of one's life (Breslow, 1996). Attention should be focused on the client's sleeping and eating patterns, activity patterns (including work, home, and leisure patterns), socialization patterns, and typical means of dealing with stress. An image of who the client is in terms of these patterns and what the client does in a routine day should emerge. For example, the lifestyle of a mother of three will vary greatly from the lifestyle of a college student. These circumstances will strongly affect recovery issues relating to functioning and quality of life.

In addition, recreation therapists are particularly interested in obtaining an image of the client's lifestyle as it relates to leisure and recreation behavior. Questions related to the client's satisfaction with current leisure involvement, preferred leisure activity environments, social support system for leisure, social behavior during leisure, choice making in leisure, leisure interest, leisure time management, leisure skills, leisure barriers, and typical leisure activities are areas where information should be gathered. In addition, lifestyle assessments should also focus on clients' knowledge about the role of recreation in health promotion and disease prevention. **Table 7.12** (p. 120) contains a

Exhibit 7.4: Sample questions for spiritual assessment (Hopkins, Woods, Kelley, Bentley & Murphy, 1995)

> *What is important in your life right now?*
> *What was important to you in the past?*
> *Do you expect your life to be better or worse in the future?*
> *Do you believe in a power greater than yourself? Who or what is it?*
> *Do you have a personal means for meeting your inner spiritual needs (e.g., prayer, scripture reading)?*

listing of some standardized assessment tools focused on leisure interest, skills, or attitudes. This list is not intended to be all-inclusive, rather it should alert you to some of the possible assessment instruments designed to assess this aspect of a client's lifestyle.

Developmental Perspective

When conducting an assessment, therapists must maintain a lifespan developmental perspective. A lifespan developmental perspective takes into consideration the preoccupations and challenges that are associated with an individual's chronological age. You should recall the discussion of development in the client–system perspective in Chapter 3. A developmental perspective allows you to explore clients' perceptions about how their life roles and responsibilities may be affected by their current health status (e.g., how hospitalization disrupts the everyday routine of home life and work life). In addition, you can also examine whether clients have mastered specific developmental skills and abilities associated with their chronological age. This is particularly true in pediatric settings where TR assessments are often combined with other assessment tools that examine the child's developmental level such as the Early Learning Accomplishment Profile (E-LAP) (Glover, Preminger & Sanford, 1978).

Cultural Perspective

Astute therapists know that an individual's cultural background, like development, can significantly affect the assessment process. While multiculturalism was discussed in Chapter 3, it is worth repeating that therapists must consider their clients' cultural heritage in the assessment process. In fact, accreditation standards (e.g., JCAHO) and the 1999 Surgeon General's report on mental health indicate the importance of recognizing cultural influences. While culture influences many aspects in the rehabilitation process, during the assessment process it is important that you remember that clients' actual expression of recreation and leisure is influenced by their cultural heritage.

Culture can also influence communication style. An awareness of culturally based communication differences is a priority, especially during the assessment process when clients are first acclimating to their new environment. Lack of such awareness raises the chance that you may reach erroneous conclusions despite excellent data gathering efforts. Peregoy and Dieser (1997) provide a revealing example of this issue in a review of a case report by Lane, Montgomery, and

Schmid (1995). Peregoy and Dieser question whether the recreation therapist in the case report drew accurate conclusions from the assessment data obtained from a 16-year-old American Indian male. In this case report, the recreation therapist's assessment report indicated that the adolescent was able to express why he was hospitalized, was cooperative in the interview, yet had little eye contact. Peregoy and Dieser contend that the concerns about lack of eye contact may have been ill-founded if the youth self-identified with his American Indian heritage. That is because American Indians have indirect gazes when listening or speaking as a sign of respect. If so, the lack of eye contact displayed by this 16-year-old was an appropriate behavior based on his cultural values. The therapist's concerns and any subsequent interventions that targeted this behavior

(e.g., social skills training, assertiveness training) would reflect culturally insensitive practice.

Finally, recreation therapists must be on guard for cultural bias in standardized assessment instruments. Often within the discipline of recreation therapy, the validity and reliability of an assessment instrument for use with diverse cultural or ethnic groups have not been examined, making normative comparisons inappropriate.

Physical and Social Environments

Throughout this text we have maintained that individuals cannot be understood without examining their physical and social environments. As explained in Chapter 3, this approach requires that you evaluate the environment's influence on an individual because you

Table 7.12: Sample leisure-focused assessment tools

Leisure Diagnostic Battery (LDB)
Developed by Peter Witt and Gary Ellis
Venture Publishing, Inc., State College, PA (814) 234–4561
Measures perception of competence, perceived leisure control, leisure needs, depth of involvement, and playfulness. Combined scales measure perceived freedom in leisure. Short and long versions are available.

LeisureScope
Developed by Connie Nall Schenk
Idyll Arbor, Inc., Ravensdale, WA (425) 432–3726
This pictorial tool assesses a client's leisure interests and motivation for leisure. An adapted version is also available for teens: Teen LeisureScope.

Idyll Arbor Leisure Battery
Developed by a variety of authors
Idyll Arbor, Inc., Ravensdale, WA (425) 432–3726
Combination of four assessments: leisure attitude measurement, leisure interest measurement, leisure motivation scale, and leisure satisfaction measure.

Recreation Preference Form of the OHIO Functional Assessment Battery
Developed by Roy Olsson
Therapy Skill Builders, Tuscon, AZ (602) 323–7500
The Recreation Preference Form measures leisure interests, leisure awareness, leisure barriers, motivation for leisure, and leisure strengths.

State Technical Institute's Leisure Assessment Process (STILAP)
Developed by the State Technical Institute
Idyll Arbor, Inc., Ravensdale, WA (425) 432–3726
The STILAP measures a client's interests in a variety of recreation activities. It also identifies areas the client is interested in learning about and provides a general overview of a client's leisure interests.

TRAIL Leisure Assessment Battery (T-LAB) For People with Cognitive Impairments
Developed by John Dattilo and Gail Hoge
School of Health and Human Performance, Athens, GA (706) 542–5064
This tool assesses clients' recreation history using a leisure behavior profile. It also addresses leisure choice, social preference, enjoyment, assistance needed for participation, and leisure barriers.

recognize that "A person's ability to function effectively is often as much a reflection of his environment and supports as it is a reflection of his specific skills and deficits" (Selz, Bullock & Mahon, 2000, p. 290). Referred to as "ecological assessment," this practice requires description and quantification of the physical and social environment in terms of resources and barriers. In terms of the social environment, you will want to understand the "family" constellation. Such consideration would assess whether there are people that the client can rely on for assistance, as well as whether there are people with whom the client can have fun. Conversely, consideration of whether family relationships foster dependency or create barriers for a client would also occur.

Additionally, you must be aware that changing demographics have transformed the concept of support systems, especially in terms of the traditional definition of the family unit. For instance, therapists working in pediatric settings must remember that all children do not reside with their biological parents. Many reside with grandparents, aunts, friends, stepparents or in foster care settings. In fact, many children may be members of "skipped generation" families, where children are in the custody of one or more grandparents (Sheldon & Dattilo, 1997). Recreation therapists must gently explore these differing living arrangements during data gathering. There are many reasons why clients may be hesitant to freely disclose their social and environmental supports, so you will need to exercise care, caution, and sound clinical judgment when gathering this information.

Information on barriers in the physical environment focus on clients' homes and communities in terms of obstacles that impede clients' mobility and access to life activities, including recreation and leisure activities. An *ecological assessment* strives to describe the relationships individuals have with environments and includes all life situations such as living quarters, school, social life, recreation, and any treatment agencies or legal situations occurring in clients' lives (Dowrick, 1996).

By assessing the social and physical environment, you can advocate for and develop interventions that target the environment (e.g., adaptive devices for the home). An excellent example of an ecological assessment related to client case management is contained in an analysis of the residential transitions of older adults with developmental disabilities presented by Jacobson and Wilhite (1999). These authors considered the effects of residential relocation on a 75-year-old man with a developmental disability, and drew several implications for practice and research that targeted the

environment as well as the specific client. This included involving the social network (e.g., family members and friends) in the decisions about residential relocation. The case also suggested a need for greater sensitivity to psychological attachment clients have to their present and future "home" environments. **Exhibit 7.5** (p. 123) contains areas to consider when conducting an assessment focused on physical and social environmental issues in the home including access to recreation and leisure involvement.

Thinking Trigger

What elements in your physical and social environment influence your performance as a student?

Developing Assessment Procedures

The process by which recreation therapists gather data about a client is typically guided by *assessment procedures*. Assessment procedures stipulate the type of data to be collected and the manner in which it will be collected. It is a document "that provides clear information on the standardized procedures for preparing for, administering, scoring, interpreting, and reporting assessment information" (Peterson & Stumbo, 2000, p. 226). While an agency typically develops assessment procedures during the initial conceptualization of a department, these procedures should be "evaluated and updated periodically as the agency, clients, programs, or specialists change directions" (Peterson & Stumbo, 2000, p. 214).

When developing or evaluating assessment procedures, recreation therapists should make sure that the processes used to collect data allow staff to collect *relevant information* from a *variety of sources,* using a *variety of techniques*. Furthermore, they should make certain that the procedures facilitate the collection of data on all components within the client–system perspective.

A number of structural and organizational issues will also affect an agency's assessment procedures. When designing TR assessment procedures, you must consider characteristics of the agency and TR program, such as the mission and purpose of the agency, staff resources and expertise, and types of TR services available. Client characteristics must also be considered such as length of stay and typical client needs associated with specific diagnostic groups. Other factors that will influence the assessment procedures include assessment guidelines from accrediting and regulatory bodies such as JCAHO or the Center for Medicare and Medicaid Services (CMS), formerly the Health Care Financing Agency.

Interdisciplinary Assessment

Conducting a thorough assessment of functioning in each of these areas requires an exorbitant amount of time, which is quite limited in today's work environment. Recreation therapists, therefore, are often forced to identify specific areas of functioning that are of most concern to their particular scope of practice. "Generally, the therapist focuses her effort on those areas in which the individual is likely to have the greatest need. This is determined from the therapist's general knowledge of the disability (or *health condition*) that is being addressed in treatment" (Selz, Bullock & Mahon, 1997, p. 325; emphasis added). Often you will draw on information provided by other therapists working with the client. Coordinating client care is a hallmark competency for health care practitioners in the 21st century. To accomplish this coordination, many agencies utilize an interdisciplinary assessment.

Interdisciplinary Assessment in Long-Term Care

Federal regulations require that long-term care facilities make a comprehensive assessment of a resident's needs that focuses on the resident's capability to perform daily life functions and significant impairments in functional capacity. These guidelines suggest that diverse professionals (e.g., physicians, nurses, rehabilitative therapists, activity professionals, social workers, dietitians) should contribute to this comprehensive assessment making it interdisciplinary in nature. The Minimum Data Set/Minimum Data Set Plus (MDS/MDS+) is the interdisciplinary resident assessment instrument designed by CMS to document comprehensive assessment findings. Recreation therapists are responsible for completing Section N of the MDS/MDS+ (see **Exhibit 7.6**, p. 124). This section focuses on time awake, activity involvement, activity preferences, and daily routine of the client. The "10B" and "10A" seen in this exhibit are codes used with the MDS to indicate that a client may require revisions in his or

her activity plan or care plan. A 10B trigger occurs when clients may be too active and jeopardize their health because of their failure to slow down. Trigger 10A occurs when clients have little time, low involvement, or desire a change in their daily routine. The "4, 5*" and "23" codes refer to quality indicators that facilities use to evaluate quality of care. In addition, recreation therapists may be asked to complete sections on the MDS focused on psychosocial well-being, mood, and behavior patterns. You should also contribute information that allows for accurate ratings of the client's cognitive, communication, visual, and physical functioning. More recently, recreation therapists have begun to complete Section T of the MDS/MDS+ (see **Exhibit 7.7**, p. 125) when clinical recreation therapy services, ordered by a physician, are provided.

Interdisciplinary Assessment in Physical Rehabilitation Settings

In January 2002 inpatient physical rehabilitation hospitals and units receiving reimbursement from Medicare were required to begin using the Inpatient Rehabilitation Facility-Patient Assessment Instrument (IRF-PAI). This interdisciplinary assessment instrument is used to collect patient-related data focused on functional improvement and quality of care. The IRF-PAI assesses the functional abilities of clients and assists in determining the proper reimbursement rate. It must be completed within four days of admission and at discharge for each client. The scoring and functional areas assessed using the IRF-PAI are based on the Functional Independence Measure (FIM[SM]) developed by the Uniform Data Set for Medical Rehabilitation (UDSMR). In fact, the FIM[SM] is embedded within the IRF-PAI, therefore recreation therapists need to be familiar with both the scoring and areas of functioning assessed in the FIM[SM] and the IRF-PAI. There are 18 areas assessed in both the FIM[SM] and IRF-PAI. They include self-care, sphincter management, mobility, locomotion, communication, and social cognition (see **Table 7.13**, p. 125).

For both instruments, scoring is based on a "… seven-level ordinal scale that describes the severity of disability. Disability is operationally defined in terms of the need for assistance (burden of care), the type and amount of assistance required for a disabled person to perform basic life activities effectively" (Deutsch, Braun & Granger, 1998, p. 275). **Table 7.14** (p. 126) contains the seven-level FIM[SM] scoring scale. Unlike the FIM[SM], the IRF-PAI allows clinicians to give items in the motor domain a score of zero indicating that the client has not performed the activity and a helper has not performed the activity for the client during the assessment time frame. Before such a score can be entered, other clinicians, the client's family, and the client must be consulted to confirm that the client has not performed the activity.

The FIM[SM] and the IRF-PAI were designed to be discipline-free assessment tools. Any trained clinician can complete these forms; however, the scoring should reflect the client's "typical" functioning. Therefore, clinicians often collaborate when determining a client's score in each area. Recreation therapists typically contribute information that helps determine client ratings in the areas of locomotion, communication, and

Exhibit 7.5: Assessing the home environment

The home environment contains physical, social, and organizational elements that can be targets for modification to reduce barriers and maximize functioning, social contact, and recreation involvement.

Physical Elements	**Considerations**
Physical accessibility	Are the entrances, exits, and interior doorways wheelchair accessible?
Bathroom	Are grab bars present or needed, and are the sink and cabinets accessible?
Kitchen	Is the space accessible, and are appliances, tables and countertops accessible and free of safety hazards?
Safety	Is the general living space free of clutter and trip hazards? Is furniture movable? Are electrical switches and fixtures accessible? Are smoke detectors operable?
Climate conditions	Are there apparent concerns with temperature, odors, noise, and general cleanliness?
Lighting	Is natural and artificial lighting available and accessible?
Orientation objects	Are there clocks and calendars? Are they set correctly?
Decorations	Are photographs and personal items displayed? Are there plants or other points of interest?
Outdoor areas	Is the yard or porch accessible and free of safety hazards? Is the furniture or other amenities (e.g., swimming pool) safe and accessible?
Neighborhood	How convenient is shopping, public transportation, parks and other recreation resources? How safe and accessible is the neighorhood?

Social Elements	**Considerations**
Family members and care providers	How many live in the home? What is the frequency of contact and the interaction patterns? What are the attitudes toward client needs for assistance and independence?
Family recreation	What are the shared daily and weekend recreation routines (e.g., walks, watching television, dining out)? What about vacations?
Social network	What are sources of companionship and frequency of contact (e.g., pets, neighbors, companions, community groups, faith-based groups, support groups)? How are contacts maintained (e.g., telephone, e-mail, personal visits)?

Organizational Elements	**Considerations**
Social roles in the home	How are chores and other obligations delegated and maintained?
Household schedules and interaction patterns	What are the typical daily routines (morning, day, evening, and nighttime), meal schedules, weekend schedules?
Health care	Is there any health care provided by service organizations? How are medications and health care appointments managed?
Emergency/safety	Is information about contacting doctors, police, and others easily located? Is the telephone readily available?
Recreation materials	Are tools and materials for preferred recreation activities or hobbies available? What about home entertainment resources (e.g., radio, television, VCR, CD player, newspapers, magazines)?

social cognition. Recreation therapists are also responsible for rating a client's motor and cognitive skills in naturalistic settings. Therefore, during community reintegration outings, recreation therapists collect valuable information that allows service providers to assess the degree of consistency between a client's in-center and community-based performance.

It should be noted that the FIM[SM] and the IRF-PAI do not address all basic life activities. A number of other significant areas are missing, including homemaking, ability to supervise attendants, or driving (Benson & Schell, 1997). Furthermore, recreation therapists would argue that these instruments do not assess leisure functioning, which can be viewed as a basic life activity. The Leisure Competence Measure (LCM; Kloseck & Crilly, 1997) is modeled after the FIM and is used to rate severity of disability in terms of leisure functioning. While not an interdisciplinary assessment tool, the LCM is a parallel or complementary tool that utilizes the same seven-level ordinal scale as the interdisciplinary FIM[SM] and IRF-PAI, thereby allowing recreation therapists "employed in rehabilitation facilities, a

Exhibit 7.6: Section N of the MDS/MDS+

SECTION N: ACTIVITY PURSUIT PATTERNS

1.	TIME AWAKE	(Check appropriate time periods over last 7 days) Resident awake all or most of the time (e.g., no naps more than one hour per time period) in the: a. Morning **2** *10B* **4, 5*** a. c. Evening **4, 5*** c. b. Afternoon **4, 5*** b. d. *NONE OF THE ABOVE* **4, 5** d.

(If resident is comatose, skip to Section O)

2.	AVERAGE TIME INVOLVED IN ACTIVITIES	(When awake and not receiving treatments or ADL care) 0. Most (more than 2/3 of time) **2** *10B* 2. Little (less than 1/3 of time) *10A* **23** 1. Some (from 1/3 to 2/3 of time) 3. None *10A* **23**
3.	PREFERRED ACTIVITY SETTINGS	(Check all settings in which activities are performed) a. Own room a. b. Day/activity room b. d. Outside facility d. c. Inside NH/off unit c. e. *NONE OF THE ABOVE* e.
4.	GENERAL ACTIVITY PREFERENCES (Adapted to resident's current abilities)	(Check all PREFERENCES whether or not activity is currently available to resident) a. Cards/other games a. g. Trips/shopping g. b. Crafts/arts b. h. Walking/wheeling outdoors h. c. Exercise/sports c. i. Watching TV i. d. Music d. j. Gardening or plants j. e. Reading/writing e. k. Talking k. f. Spiritual/religious activities f. l. Helping others l. m. None of the above m.
5.	PREFERS CHANGE IN DAILY ROUTINE	(Code for resident preferences in daily routines) 0. No change 1. Slight change *10A* 2. Major change *10A* a. Type of activities in which resident is currently involved a. b. Extent of resident involvement in activities b.

2 = Two items required to trigger   **23** = Quality indicator

4, 5* - N1a + N1b + N1c ≤ 1 and B1 = 0   MDS 2.0 September 2000

consistent and acceptable means of reporting at team rounds" (Kloseck, Crilly, Ellis & Lammers, 1996, p. 14). The LCM allows recreation therapists to rate the client's level of competence in leisure and report this as another basic life activity. The LCM does this by sampling representative behaviors in seven leisure domains: leisure awareness, leisure attitude, leisure skills, social appropriateness, group interaction skills, social contact, and community participation (**Table 7.15**, p. 127).

Table 7.13: Key FIM areas

Domain	Key Areas and Items
Motor	*Self-care* eating, grooming, bathing, dressing, toileting *Sphincter control* bladder and bowel management *Transfers* bed, chair, wheelchair, toilet, tub, or shower *Locomotion* walk/wheelchair, stairs
Cognitive	*Communication* comprehension, expression *Social cognition* social interaction, problem solving, memory

Exhibit 7.7: Section T of the MDS/MDS+

SECTION T: THERAPY SUPPLEMENT FOR MEDICARE PPS

1. SPECIAL TREATMENTS AND PROCEDURES	a. RECREATION—*Enter number of days and total minutes of recreation therapy administered (for at least 15 minutes a day) in the last 7 days (Enter 0 if none)*

	DAYS	MIN
	(A)	(B)
(A) # of days administered for 15 minutes or more (B) total # for minutes provided in the last 7 days		

Skip unless this is a Medicare 5 day or Medicare readmission/return assessment.

b. ORDERED THERAPIES—*Has physician ordered any of the following therapies to begin in the FIRST 14 days of stay: physical therapy, occupational therapy, or speech pathology service?*
0. No   1. Yes

If not ordered skip to item 2.

c. Through day 15 provide an estimate of the number of days when at least 1 therapy service can be expected to have been delivered.

d. Through day 15 provide an estimate of the number of therapy minutes (across the therapies) that can be expected to be delivered.

Summary

Client assessment is more than meeting an accreditation standard. It is also a systematic process of deciding what information is important to gather, how to collect the information, how to analyze the results, and what kind of actions are appropriate as a result of the data gathered. Assessment data is then the benchmark from which client progress or regression can be determined. Assessment is really an ongoing activity.

Client assessment is also the beginning of the helping relationship you will share with your client. So, in addition to providing you with information, it is also the cornerstone for establishing a therapeutic relationship, which is discussed more fully in Chapter 11.

Using the client–system as a guide in the assessment process results in a holistic image of the client as a person. This chapter provided a comprehensive overview of information that is relevant to conducting a full and complete assessment from this perspective. Although you will carefully select a few areas in which you will gather data directly using interviews, observation, or testing, it is very important that secondary data sources "round-out" your assessment picture. Such data allows you to begin meaningful intervention planning. It results in a comprehensive picture that allows you to understand the diverse skills, abilities, hopes, and desires that influence your client's functioning in the larger context of living.

Table 7.14: FIM seven-level scoring scale

Independence
The levels of assistance are:

(7) *Complete independence*: All tasks described as making up the activity are typically performed safely, without modification, assistive devices, or aids and within a reasonable amount of time.

(6) *Modified independence*: One or more of the following may be true: the activity requires an assistive device; the activity takes more than reasonable time; or there are safety (risks) considerations.

Modified Dependence
The person expends 50% or more of the effort. The levels of assistance are:

(5) *Supervision or setup*: Subject requires no more help than standby, cueing or coaxing, without physical contact, or, helper sets up needed items or applies orthoses.

(4) *Minimal contact assistance*: Subject requires no more help than touching, and expends 75% or more of the effort

(3) *Moderate assistance*: Subject requires more help than touching, or expends 50% or more (up to 75%) of the effort.

Complete Dependence
The subject expends less than half (less than 50%) or the effort. Maximal or total assistance is required, or the activity is not performed. The level of assistance required are:

(2) *Maximal assistance*: Subject expends less than 50% of the effort, but at least 25%.

(1) *Total assistance*: Subject expends less than 25% of the effort.

Table 7.15: Leisure competence measure (Kloseck & Crilly, 1997)

LCM Items	Description	Behaviors Exhibited by the Client
Leisure awareness	Client's knowledge and understanding of leisure	Personal beliefs Knowledge of leisure opportunities Awareness of strengths and weaknesses Realistic expectations
Leisure attitudes	Behaviors exhibited and/or feelings expressed by the client that suggest attitude toward leisure involvement	Initiative Self-directedness Willingness to develop new skills and hobbies Demonstration of enjoyment
Leisure skills	Skills possessed by the client that affect leisure involvement	Ability to make choices Activity skills necessary to participate in chosen activities Ability to identify and access local leisure resources
Social appropriateness	Specific social behaviors exhibited by the client that affect ability to function in leisure activities	Manners Dress Hygiene Tolerance of others
Group interaction skills	Client's ability to participate in various types of group situations	Sharing/cooperation Task as focus/minimal interaction with others 1:1 interaction Withdrawal/isolation
Social contact	Type and duration of social contact client has with others	Type, duration, and frequency of social contact
Community participation	Client's overall leisure participation pattern	Type, duration, and frequency of leisure involvement

References

Adamovich. B., Henderson, J., and Auerbach, S. (1985). *Cognitive rehabilitation of closed head injured patients: A dynamic approach.* San Diego, CA: College Hill Press.

Austin, D. (1991). *Therapeutic recreation: Processes and techniques* (2nd ed.). Champaign, IL: Sagamore Publishing.

Benson, J. and Schell, B. (1997) Measurement theory: Application to occupational and physical therapy. In J. Van Deusen and D. Brunt (Eds.), *Assessment in occupational therapy and physical therapy,* (pp. 3–23). Philadelphia, PA: W. B. Saunders.

Breslow, L. (1996). Social ecological strategies for promoting healthy lifestyles. *American Journal of Health Promotion, 10*, 253.

burlingame j. and Skalko, T. (1997). *Idyll Arbor's glossary for therapists.* Ravensdale, WA: Idyll Arbor.

Caprio-Prevette, M. and Fry, P. (1996). Memory enhancement program for older adults. A guide for practitioners. Gaithersburg, MD: Aspen.

Clinebell, H. (1995). *Counseling for spiritually empowered wholeness: A hope-centered approach.* New York, NY: Haworth Pastoral Press/Haworth Press, Inc.

Coleman, D. and Iso-Ahola, S. (1993). Leisure and health: The role of social support and self-determination. *Journal of Leisure Research, 25*(2), 111–128.

Deutsch, A, Braun, S., and Granger, C (1998). The Functional Independence Measure (FIM^SM Instrument). In Dobrzykowski, E. (Ed.), *Essential readings in rehabilitation outcomes measurement: Application, methodology, and technology* (pp. 274–278). Gaithersburg, MD: Aspen.

Dowrick, P. (1996). Psychoeducational measures: Ecological assessment. In Kurtz, L., Dowrick, P., Levy, S., and Batshaw, M. (Eds.), *Handbook of developmental disabilities: Resources for interdisciplinary care* (pp. 148–151). Gaithersburg, MD: Aspen.

Glover, M., Preminger, J., and Sanford, A. (1978). *Early learning accomplishment profile.* Chapel Hill, NC: Chapel Hill Training and Outreach Project.

Haase, B. (1997). Cognition. In Van Deusen, J. and Brunt, D. (Eds.), *Assessment in occupational therapy and physical therapy* (pp. 333–356). Philadelphia, PA: W. B. Saunders.

Hawks, S. (1994). Spiritual health: Definition and theory. *Wellness Perspective, 10*(4), 3–13.

Hopkins, E., Woods, Z., Kelley, R., Bentley, K., and Murphy, J. (1995). *Working with groups on spiritual themes: Structure exercises in healing* (Vol. 2). Duluth, MN: Whole Person Press.

Jacobson, S. and Wilhite, B. (1999). Residential transitions in the lives of older adults with developmental disabilities: An ecological perspective. *Therapeutic Recreation Journal, 33*(3), 195–208.

Kloseck, M. and Crilly, R. (1997). *Leisure Competence Measure: Adult version, professional manual and user's guide: An introduction to measuring outcomes in therapeutic recreation.* London, ON: Leisure Competence Measure Data System.

Kloseck, M., Crilly, R., Ellis, G., and Lammers, E. (1996). Leisure Competence Measure: Development and reliability testing of a scale to measure functional outcomes in therapeutic recreation. *Therapeutic Recreation Journal, 30*(1), 13–26.

Lane, S., Montgomery, D., and Schmid, W. (1995). Understanding differences to maximize treatment interventions: A case history. *Therapeutic Recreation Journal, 29*(4), 294–299.

Lasko-McCarthey, P. and Knopf, K. (1992). *Adapted physical education for adults with disabilities* (3rd ed.). Dubuque, IA: Eddie Bowers Publishing.

Liberman, R. (1982). Assessment of social skills. *Schizophrenia Bulletin, 8*(1), 62-83.

Maher, M. and Hunt, T. (1993) Spirituality reconsidered. *Counseling and Values, 38*(1), 21–28.

Morse, A. (1986). Neuropsychological tools and techniques of cognitive assessment. In P. A. Morse (Ed.), *Brain injury: Cognitive and prevocational approaches to rehabilitation* (pp. 51–88). New York, NY: Tiresias Press.

Okkema, K. (1993). *Cognition and perception in the stroke patient.* Gaithersburg, MD: Aspen.

Olsson, R. (1994). *OHIO functional assessment battery: Standardized tests for leisure and living skills.* Tucson, AZ: Therapy Skill Builders.

Parenté, R. and Herrmann, D. (1996). *Retraining cognition: Techniques and applications.* Gaithersburg, MD: Aspen.

Peregoy, J. and Dieser, R. (1997). Multicultural awareness in therapeutic recreation: Hamlet living. *Therapeutic Recreation Journal, 31*(3), 173–187.

Peterson, C. A. and Stumbo, N. (2000). *Therapeutic recreation program design: Principles and procedures* (3rd ed.). Boston, MA: Allyn & Bacon.

Phillips, E. L. (1978). *The social skills basis of psychopathology: Alternative to abnormal psychology and psychiatry.* New York, NY: Grune and Stratton.

Roy, E. (1983). Neuropsychological perspectives on apraxia and related action disorders. *Advances in Psychology,* 12, 193–320.

Selz, L., Bullock, C., and Mahon, M. (1997). Introduction to therapeutic recreation: An evolving profession. In C. Bullock and M. Mahon (Eds.), *Introduction to recreation services for people with disabilities: A person-centered approach* (pp. 299–243). Champaign, IL: Sagamore Publishing.

Selz, L., Bullock, C., and Mahon, M. (2000). Introduction to therapeutic recreation: An evolving profession. In C. Bullock, and M. Mahon *Introduction to recreation services for people with disabilities. A person-centered approach* (2nd ed., pp. 268–302). Champaign, IL: Sagamore Publishing.

Shank, J. (1991). *The activity as coping scale.* Unpublished manuscript.

Sheldon K. and Dattilo, J. (1997). Multiculturalism in therapeutic recreation: Terminology clarification and practical suggestions. *Therapeutic Recreation Journal, 31*(3), 148–158.

Shipley K. and McNulty Wood, J. (1996). *The elements of interviewing.* San Diego, CA: Singular Publishing.

Strayhorn, J. M. and Strain, P. S. (1986). Social and language skills for preventive mental health: What, how, who, and when. In P. S. Strain, M. J. Guralnick, and H. M. Walker (Eds.), *Children's social behavior: Development, assessment, and modification* (pp. 287–330). Orlando, FL: Academic Press.

Stumbo, N. (1994/1995). Assessment of social skills for therapeutic recreation intervention. *Annual in Therapeutic Recreation, 5,* 68–82.

Teri, L. and Logsdon, R. (1991). Identifying pleasant activities for Alzheimer's patients: The pleasant event schedule-AD. *The Gerontologist, 31,* 124–127.

Waldinger, R. (1990). *Psychiatry for medical students* (2nd ed.). Washington, DC: American Psychiatric Press, Inc.

Witt, P. A. and Ellis, G. D. (1989). *The Leisure Diagnostic Battery user's manual.* State College, PA: Venture Publishing, Inc.

Ziegler, J. (1998). Religion or spirituality. *Journal of the National Cancer Institute, 90,* 1256.

Chapter 8
Planning Interventions

Guided Reading Questions

After reading this chapter, you should be able to answer the following:
- After completing an assessment, what steps are taken to develop an individualized intervention plan?
- What are guidelines for writing goals and objectives in an intervention plan?
- What should be considered when selecting intervention strategies to help clients reach their goals?
- What are some strategies for motivating clients to be involved in TR interventions?
- What can interfere with planning individualized TR intervention programs?

Introduction

The preceding chapter reviewed data-gathering techniques available to recreation therapists during the assessment phase of the clinical process. The intent of data gathering is for therapists to gain a thorough understanding of clients' bio/psycho/social/spiritual needs, wants, and aspirations. This understanding allows recreation therapists to begin planning a course of action with clients. This marks the onset of the planning phase of the clinical process. The outcome of this phase is a plan of action, commonly referred to as an intervention plan. *Intervention plan* is used broadly in this text to describe plans systematically developed to assist clients with psychosocial adaptation and enhancing life quality. It is synonymous with treatment plan, service plan, habilitation plan, individualized education plan, and care plan. These plans share the common purpose of identifying the clinical services needed to achieve mutually agreed upon goals or outcomes.

This chapter describes the TR intervention planning process. This process is generic: It pertains to all clients who receive individualized clinical TR services even though the circumstances and specific format for the intervention plans will differ. Because planning is an integral step in the clinical TR process, this chapter focuses on the generic planning process that immediately follows an assessment. The chapter includes a technical explanation of writing goals and objectives and a review of several factors to consider when selecting intervention strategies. Since intervention plans are usually a formal part of a client's record, we begin this chapter with a brief explanation of comprehensive plans (developed by a team of professionals) and discipline-specific intervention plans (developed by individual recreation therapists).

Comprehensive Intervention Plans

Accreditation standards require that a team of service providers develop a comprehensive intervention plan for each client in a health care system. Comprehensive intervention plans refer to the entire scope of clinical services that will be provided to a client. Such plans incorporate the work of all disciplines into one integrated document used to direct and evaluate clinical services. These comprehensive intervention plans are typically developed and reviewed during client care conferences or treatment planning meetings. The format and structure of the comprehensive intervention plan is influenced by the agency's philosophy regarding client care, the agency's policies and procedures, and the accreditation standards to which the agency adheres (e.g., JCAHO, CARF).

Comprehensive intervention plans can differ depending on the team approach used at a particular agency. Service provider teams, also called treatment teams, are typically classified as *multidisciplinary*, *interdisciplinary*, or *transdisciplinary* (see **Table 8.1**, p. 132). Such classification reflects the agency's philosophical approach to clinical care and influences the ways the disciplines interact in providing care. In addition, some agencies use *person-centered* planning teams. These teams place the client at the center of the team and all planning is done in response to what the client wants. They focus on capacity building rather than eliminating or correcting functional deficits (Bullock & Mahon, 1997).

Regardless of the type of team approach used, it is imperative that recreation therapists participate in developing clients' comprehensive intervention plans.

This participation must include articulating to team members the manner in which clinical TR services can be used to achieve intervention goals for the client and advocating for the inclusion of clinical TR services on the client's comprehensive intervention plan.

Discipline-Specific Intervention Plans

TR standards of practice (ATRA, 2000; NTRS, 2001) require therapists to develop individualized intervention plans for clients that complement their comprehensive intervention plans. This discipline-specific intervention plan identifies goals, objectives, and interventions related to TR's scope of practice. The plan serves as the basis for evaluating client progress. In contrast to comprehensive intervention plans, discipline-specific intervention plans focus exclusively on TR clinical services. **Exhibit 8.1** contains a discipline-specific TR intervention plan that was developed for Mr. Kazigan, a 35-year-old client hospitalized for substance abuse.

TR practitioners working in community settings or in outpatient services also develop intervention plans to guide their clinical work with clients. For example, recreation therapists working with *Project PATH: Promoting Access, Transition, and Health* utilize a standard form that assists them in developing individualized goals for clients. Project PATH is a health promotion program for people with spinal cord injuries living in the community (see Exhibit 2.4, p. 23, for a complete description). Project PATH staff develop client goals related to improving wellness, fitness, functional skills, community integration, leisure skills, peer support, and resource networks. **Exhibit 8.2** (p.

134) contains excerpts from Project PATH's Individualized Treatment Planning form, which was developed by Sable, Gravink, Craig, Carr, and Lee (2001).

The Planning Process

The planning phase of the clinical TR process involves synthesizing information gathered and continuing the collaboration begun with the client during the assessment phase. This collaborative planning process involves identifying client's strengths, interests, and needs, and prioritizing problems and concerns. Planning results in a written report that includes goals, objectives, and intervention strategies. This plan, documented in the client's chart, guides all interactions with the client. The following sections explain each aspect of this planning process.

Collaborating with Clients

Planning must be approached as a collaborative process that involves the client to whatever extent possible. Collaboration is critical, as it is likely to assure that everyone—clients, families, and therapists—can work together. In some cases client collaboration may be limited or not feasible (e.g., clients with severe cognitive deficits or very young children). In these instances, family involvement must be sought. Collaboration begins with verifying assessment findings. This is done by seeking confirmation from the client and family as to the accuracy of the findings. In addition, thoughts regarding the primary targets for clinical TR services should be discussed. Sharing assessment findings and incorporating clients and their families in identifying

Table 8.1: Treatment teams in health and human service agencies

Type of Team	Definition
Multidisciplinary	Team members usually respect each other's discipline, but members work independently to assess and plan interventions according to their own perspectives, methods, and techniques. Team members independently implement the activities and approaches identified on their discipline-specific intervention plan.
Interdisciplinary	Team members value the perspective of each discipline and collaborate on identifying common client outcomes that will be targets for the entire team. Each discipline then selects and implements its own intervention strategies aimed at common outcomes.
Transdisciplinary	Team members have the highest level of collaboration. They commit to teach, learn, and work together across disciplinary boundaries. Team members develop and implement intervention plans cooperatively and often allow each other to cross disciplinary boundaries when providing care.

and prioritizing targets increases the likelihood that you, your clients, and their families are invested in the intervention plan. It also ensures that you are practicing patient-focused care (Pedlar, Hornibrook & Haasen, 2001).

Recognizing Strengths and Interests

In the planning phase (and for the duration of services) careful consideration should be given to the strengths and resources that exist within the client and his or her environment. Strengths can be used to reaffirm feelings of competence. They can also be used to deemphasize the tendency in rehabilitation to focus exclusively on client deficits, a process that can threaten feelings of competence and self-worth. Client's strengths and interests can be used in deciding on ways to achieve mutually identified goals. For instance, a supportive family can be an asset and can be used as a source of support and positive reinforcement in an intervention plan. Likewise, client interests can be used as a source of motivation to be involved and active. This is especially relevant to long-term care facilities since the MDS mandates working with resident's interests.

Recognizing client strengths also allows you to consider whether these strengths are vulnerable or at risk of being lost. In some instances you may want to design intervention strategies that allow clients to maintain existing strengths. Consider Mrs. Smith, a 75-

Exhibit 8.1: Discipline-specific intervention plan

Strengths:
Pleasant and cooperative; indicates some insight into his need for changing leisure-related behavior; has supportive family.

Areas of Concern:
Current leisure interests marked by ETOH consumption, substance use related to stress. Barriers include limited awareness of alternative activities and poor free-time management.

Goals:
1. Increase knowledge of social drinking patterns
2. Increase stress management skills through sober recreation options
3. Increase ability to structure discretionary time

Behavioral Objectives:
1.1 During leisure education group sessions, client will demonstrate increased knowledge of social drinking patterns as evidenced by (a) verbalizing how his social environment contributes to substance use, and (b) completing and discussing social drinking pattern worksheets during group with depth of insight judged acceptable by CTRS.

2.1 By discharge, client will have engaged in 3 recreation skill development activities of his choice, and will state to CTRS at least 2 ways each activity promoted relaxation.

3.1 During 3rd individual treatment session, client will identify a minimum of 3 recreational activities and include them in his personal weekend discretionary time schedule.

3.2 By end of 1st week of hospitalization, client will adhere to his weekend free time schedule w/ no more than 2 reminders (prompts) per day by CTRS or nursing staff.

3.3. During discharge planning meeting, client will submit and discuss his written stress management action plan, including a reward schedule for adhering to sober recreation activities.

Plan/Approach:
Client's schedule to include leisure education group 2x/week, stress management group 1x/week, and 30-minute sessions with CTRS 3x/week. Individual and group sessions will focus on managing stress through preferred recreation activities. CTRS will assist client in setting up a weekend free time schedule. Client's adherence to personal schedule will be verbally reinforced, and possible rewards for discharge action plan will be explored. CTRS will monitor independent use of schedule for first week and will confer with nurse-therapist about needed level of support. Also, will explore with client's spouse the necessary modifications to their weekend schedules post discharge. Evaluate progress with client at end of first weekend of hospitalization.

**Exhibit 8.2: Excerpts from Project PATH's Treatment Planning Form
(Sable, Gravink, Craig, Carr & Lee, 2001)**

Name: _____ ID#: _____ Date: _____

Date
Set/Met

Goal: Wellness Education

_____ 1.1 Participant will demonstrate an understanding of health promoting behaviors in daily activities
Objective: Participant will participate in weekly education sessions to increase knowledge
of identified risk factors /secondary conditions associated with SCI:
a. _____   b. _____   c. _____

_____ 1.2 Participant will demonstrate increased functional skill in weight shifts.
Objective: Participant will demonstrate increased functional skill in weight shifts as indicated by
increase in TR Functional Level Instrument (TRFL) score by completion of intervention.
From: _____ To: _____

Goal: Fitness

_____ 2.1 Participant will participate in a home- or community-based fitness program to address the
following areas:
___Strength   ___Flexibility   ___Pain   ___Endurance
Objectives: (to be determined by the therapist)

Goal: Functional Skill Development

_____ 3.1 Participant will demonstrate increased functional skill in transfers.
Objective: Participant will demonstrate increased functional skill in the following transfers as
indicated by increase in TRFL score by completion of intervention.
Car From:_____ To:_____   *Floor* From:_____ To:_____   *Furniture* From:_____ To:_____
Recreation Equipment From:_____ To:_____   *Other* From:_____ To:_____

_____ 3.2 Participant will demonstrate increased functional skill in wheelchair mobility.
Objective: Participant will demonstrate increased functional skill in the following wheelchair mobility
skills as indicated by increase in TRFL score by completion of intervention.
  Home
Smooth Surface From:_____ To:_____   *Rough Terrain* From:_____ To:_____
Graded Surface From:_____ To:_____   *Tight Quarters* From:_____ To:_____
  Community
Smooth Surface From:_____ To:_____   *Rough Terrain* From:_____ To:_____
Graded Surface From:_____ To:_____   *Tight Quarters* From:_____ To:_____

Goal: Leisure Skill Development

_____ 4.1 Participant will increase awareness of adapted activities.
Objectives:
1. Participant will identify 4–6 leisure activities to develop/redevelop when requested by therapist.
2. Participant will demonstrate skills in leisure activities identified when requested by therapist.

_____ 4.2 Participant will involve a family member or friend in training for adaptive activities.
Objectives:
1. Participant will involve a family member/friend in training for 1–2 activities.
2. When asked, friend/family member will explain assistive techniques required for client's
participation in activities identified in above objective.

Exhibit contains excerpts only—not entire treatment planning form.

year-old widow entering a nursing home. Mrs. Smith had volunteered for the past year at her local library as a receptionist and storyteller during the children's hour. This involvement was a source of pride and social contact for Mrs. Smith. Her relocation to the nursing home may place Mrs. Smith's "strength" at risk. As a recreation therapist, you would want to consider intervention strategies that would assist Mrs. Smith with maintaining her volunteerism or finding a satisfying substitute activity.

• • •Thinking Trigger

What are some strengths of clients that could be bypassed or lost when involved in rehabilitation? **• • •** ✫

Identifying Concerns

The next step in the planning phase is to identify any concerns related to the client's ability to engage fully in life. You will focus on those concerns most relevant to TR's scope of practice. Remember, however, that all functional concerns identified in the assessment process are not necessarily within TR's scope of practice. For instance, concerns associated with swallowing may be identified during the course of the TR assessment; however, this concern may best be addressed by a speech therapist. While recreation therapists need to be aware of swallowing precautions, they would not necessarily target this area for intervention.

It is also important to consider lifestyle issues. Clients may enter the rehabilitation process with unhealthy lifestyles. This lifestyle may be a reflection of a lack of knowledge or environmental conditions. In each instance unhealthy lifestyle behaviors related to recreation involvement should be considered appropriate targets for interventions. Consider physical activity as a lifestyle behavior, for example. If a client's lifestyle were sedentary, client education sessions focused on health promotion through physical activity would be a relevant intervention. These sessions would be aimed at providing knowledge about the health risks associated with physical inactivity. Also, any necessary environmental modifications that would promote a more active lifestyle would be addressed. By contrast, clients with eating disorders often have a lifestyle in which they exercise obsessively. In this instance a traditionally healthy lifestyle behavior is actually detrimental. Therefore, therapists would introduce alternate lifestyle behaviors that allow these clients to meet their needs.

Prioritizing

Because a comprehensive assessment will identify a range of concerns or desired changes that can be addressed during the course of service provision, you will need to make decisions regarding what areas to target for intervention. In some cases the team of service providers will determine priorities. In all cases the client's priorities ought to be foremost. Prioritizing will also be influenced by the amount of time available to work with the client, the overall mission of the agency, the resources available for clinical services (including other clinical staff), and the type of clinical TR programs available. Using this information, recreation therapists are able to focus their clinical services to most effectively meet the needs of the client and the agency.

Identifying Goals

Once the recreation therapist and the client have agreed upon the focus for TR services, the next step in the planning phase involves reframing concerns into mutually agreed upon goals or outcomes. Ethical and professional standards of practice obligate TR professionals to involve clients in determining intervention goals. When clients are encouraged to set goals they are more likely to be invested in the intervention program and motivated to make changes in their behavior. Identifying mutually agreed upon outcomes or goals, therefore, is critical to successful planning. One strategy for accessing a client's vision of recovery or end goal-state is to ask participants: *"What would it look like if life were better for you?"* This question encourages clients to focus on internal and external constraints in their life that currently hinder them. The client's response to such a question may provide excellent material for identifying client goals.

Generally, client outcomes associated with clinical TR services pertain to changes in a client's attitudes, knowledge, beliefs, and abilities that support health and well-being through recreation and leisure. Whether these goals specifically relate to physical, cognitive, or social functioning, or relate to psychosocial health and life quality, clinical TR practice is about helping clients to adapt and to achieve optimal health and well-being through recreation and leisure.

When developing goals you must integrate vast amounts of information related to the client's abilities and environmental or lifestyle issues while simultaneously imagining a future for the client. In this process attention shifts from identifying concerns to identifying what improvement would look like if the concern no longer existed. For instance, the list of concerns identified for Mr. Kazigan in Exhibit 8.1 included leisure behavior marked by alcohol consumption and lack of awareness of alternate leisure activities. In developing Mr. Kazigan's TR intervention goals, the recreation therapist and Mr. Kazigan had to identify behaviors that would be observed if these concerns no longer existed. In this case the behavior might be structuring free time with alternative leisure activities of his choice. Based on this, the therapist identified *increased ability to structure discretionary time* as a goal. The process of identifying what improvement would look like if the problem no longer existed is fundamental to developing effective goals. **Table 8.2** contains a variety of concerns that might be identified in the assessment phase and some corresponding goals that might be established in the intervention planning phase.

Some agencies require therapists to establish long-term goals (LTGs) and short-term goals (STGs). LTGs are typically described as statements predictive of the client's functioning at discharge from inpatient settings or at the subsequent annual care conference in long-term care, residential, and educational settings. In contrast STGs reflect outcomes that will be achieved in a briefer time frame (e.g., 2 weeks). As STGs are more readily achievable, they serve a dual purpose as effective markers that acknowledge progress toward LTGs and a source of motivation for both clients and therapists.

Writing Goals

Whether written as LTGs or STGs, client goals are always directional. They reflect a direction that indicates improvement in client functioning. They are statements of client change or outcomes that can be reasonably expected to result from TR interventions. LTGs and STGs use an *action verb* to illustrate the direction of change (e.g., increase interactions, enhance confidence, improve endurance). In addition, goal statements always *identify the client* as the individual performing the action. Beginning therapists often make the mistake of identifying their own actions when writing client goals (e.g., "provide client with recreation resources"); however, no therapist or member of the team should ever be mentioned or implied in goal statements. General goal writing rules are presented in **Exhibit 8.3**.

Determining the appropriateness of goals is one of the biggest challenges confronting therapists in health and human service settings. In general, goals are considered appropriate if their intended outcomes are reasonable expectations for the client and there are sufficient resources available to achieve them. "A

single activity or session is not likely to produce a desired behavioral change" (Peterson & Stumbo, 2000, p. 176). This means that therapists must consider how long and how often they or other staff will be able to work with clients when establishing goals. You must also consider whether the interventions will occur often enough—*frequency* (e.g., 2x/week for 4 weeks.)—and for a sufficient amount of time—*duration* (e.g., 45 minutes/session)—to achieve the intended result.

Writing Objectives

LTGs and STGs are further broken down into objectives. *Objectives*—sometimes called *performance measures* or *behavioral objectives*—are specific, measurable statements of client performance taken as an indicator that a goal has been achieved. In writing objectives, identify representative behaviors that reflect the outcome identified in the long-term or short-term goal. Note that representative behaviors have to be *observable and measurable* so that an objective marker can be used to assess the effectiveness of interventions. In Exhibit 8.1, the recreation therapist identified three behavioral objectives for Mr. Kazigan's goal of increased ability to structure discretionary time. These objectives had Mr. Kazigan selecting 3 recreation activities to be scheduled into his free time, adhering to his free time schedule with no more than two reminders, and submitting a written stress management action plan.

Consider another example that illustrates the interconnection between goals and objectives. Suppose you were working with a client who had a LTG of improved attention, with a STG of maintaining concentration. In developing an objective for this goal, identify behaviors that would indicate that the client has maintained concentration. *Task engagement* might be used as one such indicator. Task engagement is directly

Exhibit 8.3: Writing client goals

> **Step 1**: Identify the general condition or change that will result from the TR intervention.
>
> **Step 2**: Select an action verb to illustrate the direction of change.
>
> **Step 3**: Make the client the subject of every goal statement.
>
> **Step 4**: Diagram your goal statements, assuring that you have one sentence that contains ONLY one subject (the client), one predicate (an action verb) and one object (the condition for change).

Table 8.2: Sample concerns and possible goal statements

Type of Concern	Sample Goal Statement
Physical Functioning	
Left-side weakness	Client will increase strength for grasping in left hand.
Low endurance/fatigue	Client will increase capacity to participate in physically challenging activities. Client will articulate how the downward spiral of inactivity promotes fatigue. Client will increase knowledge of ways to use physical activity to overcome fatigue.
Lack of awareness of adaptive equipment	Client will increase ability to use adaptive recreation equipment.
Cognitive Functioning	
Disoriented	Client will navigate throughout physical environment without becoming lost, including moving along routes to/from bedroom, cafeteria, day room, and recreation room.
Disorganized	Client will identify sequential steps needed to complete a task.
Distracted by internal stimuli	Client will focus on task to completion.
Nonresponsive to person or thing	Client will purposefully interact with the physical and social environment.
Poor problem-solving skills	Client will identify ways to manage barriers to maintaining a socially active lifestyle.
Psychological Functioning	
Unable to verbalize emotions	Client will identify and recognize his or her emotional states.
Depressed	Client will use preferred leisure resources to increase pleasant experiences. Client will develop an action plan to increase the amount of physically active recreation in current lifestyle.
Social Issues	
Limited social skills	Client will engage in conversation without hostile outbreaks. Client will assert himself or herself with peers.
Limited family support	Client will identify options for peer support beyond immediate family. Client will adhere to weekly family leisure plan.
Limited awareness of social contacts	Client will identify positive outcomes associated with social support groups.
Lifestyle Issues	
Substance abuse	Client will express the relationship between recreation involvement and prior drinking patterns. Client will identify lifestyle behaviors that occur during leisure time/activities that hinder efforts to maintain health.
Sedentary lifestyle	Client will explain the role of active recreation in preventing health problems. Client will modify lifestyle through increased involvement with preferred leisure activities.
Unfamiliarity with accessible leisure resources for home	Client will demonstrate ability to use adapted computer to access Internet.

observable and measurable. You can measure the amount of time that the client remains on task (e.g., 3 minutes, 10 minutes, 60 minutes). Therefore, task engagement is a good representative behavior that would indicate that the client is achieving his or her goal of improved attention.

In addition, objectives must also identify a *criterion*. Think of a criterion as the minimum performance standard needed for satisfactory goal attainment. Consider the difference between engaging in a task for 3 minutes before becoming distracted versus engaging in a task for 30 minutes before becoming distracted. In this example, time is used as a criterion for successful performance. The criterion sets the minimum benchmark considered acceptable. Typically written as a phrase, a criterion can take a variety of formats. **Table 8.3** identifies commonly used criterion phrases.

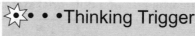

Thinking Trigger

How are criteria used in evaluating your performance in academic courses? ● ● ●

Because objectives serve as evidence that goals have been achieved, they must also identify the *condition* under which the behavior is expected to occur. "Conditions of a behavioral objective primarily set the stage by identifying necessary equipment, activities, time lines, or other events essential to the performance of the desired behavior" (Peterson & Stumbo, 2000, p. 267). Like criterion phrases, conditions are also expressed as a phrase. **Table 8.4** contains sample conditional phrases that are sometimes used by recreation therapists.

Table 8.3: Sample criterion phrases

Type of Phrase	Explanation	Sample Phrases
Amount of time	Used when the probability that the skill will occur by chance is minimal, and the speed with which the skill is performed is important	*within 5 minutes*
Degree of accuracy	Used typically with skills requiring accuracy as a criterion for success (e.g., adding numbers, estimating costs, throwing horseshoes)	*within 2 feet of the target* *within 10% of the costs*
Degree of assistance	Used when the criteria for performance is based on the amount of assistance the client needs to perform the behavior	*with minimal assistance* *with moderate assistance* *independently*
Form	Used when performance of the behavior requires specific form (e.g., swimming stroke)	*as judged by a certified aquatics instructor*
Number of trials	Used to avoid the possibility that the client performed the designated behavior by chance	*4 out of 5 times* *2 out of 5 days*
Percentages or fractions	Used when it is important that the behavior be maintained over extended periods of time	*50% of the time*
Specific subskills	Used in those circumstances when it makes sense to identify subskills representative of the target behavior, such as those associated with social conversations.	*as evidenced by:* *initiating a conversation* *responding to another's request* *speaking in cordial voice*
Therapist judgment	Used with less obvious performance, as in displaying concern for others or experiencing emotion. The behavior can only be evaluated in the context of the total intervention program and in comparsion to previous displays of attitudes and affect.	*as judged by the CTRS* *to be appropriate to the situation*

In some instances the identification of conditions increases the expectations for successful performance and, hence, goal attainment. Consider the difference between the following objectives written for a client involved in a community reintegration program for people with brain injuries:

1. *When in the TR activity room*, the client will engage in a task for 15 minutes.

2. *When in a community setting*, the client will engage in a task for 15 minutes.

In both objectives the criterion and behavior are identical. What differs is the complexity of the performance environment. The type of surroundings in which the behavior will occur has been identified by the therapist as a necessary condition associated with successful adaptation. By expecting the client to engage in the task while in a distracting community environment, the therapist is requiring that the client display higher levels of concentration and selective attention to meet his or her LTG of improved attention. **Table 8.5** (p. 140) provides useful questions and guidelines to assist you in writing behavioral objectives.

Identifying Intervention Strategies

The next task in the planning phase involves identifying specific intervention strategies that will be used to facilitate goal achievement. This includes specifying TR interventions the client will be assigned to and the type and frequency of other activity-based interventions that will be used to meet goals. In addition, intervention plans often require you to indicate when the client will again be evaluated. To a certain extent, this is evident in the behavioral objectives being used to indicate goal attainment. Recreation therapists also specify any other particular approaches they will use to help the client meet their goals—for example, collaborating with other therapists on physical functioning goals or communicating with the family about adaptive recreation resources can be important strategies for achieving desirable outcomes. Helping clients achieve community reintegration goals often requires collaboration. For example, making arrangements with video rental agents or bowling alley attendees helps pave the way for clients to practice community leisure skills. In Exhibit 8.1, the recreation therapist identified leisure education and stress management groups as interventions for Mr. Kazigan. The recreation therapist also identified specific cognitive–behavioral strategies such as positive reinforcement (e.g., verbal praise) and collaboration with nursing to monitor Mr. Kazigan's compliance and

need for support. All of these strategies were used to help Mr. Kazigan achieve his goals.

Generally intervention strategies used in clinical TR practice include a combination of activity and education-based interventions, a supportive and accommodating environment, and a therapeutic relationship. The next few chapters contain a full discussion of these aspects of practice so you can become familiar with the potential contribution each makes to the planning process, client outcomes, and overall clinical care.

Additional Planning Considerations

Several factors need to be considered when deciding on intervention strategies to use in a client's intervention plan. As explained in Chapter 3, we believe in a system perspective, which means that planning considerations include environmental or external factors as well as factors specific to the individual. Careful planning considers the influence of the following factors.

Consider the Environment

An assessment will indicate whether the client's physical and social environment helps or hinders health, leisure, and quality of life. Environmental resources can be used to support the client, while environmental problems can be targets for intervention. For example, an overprotective and anxious parent could be targeted for family education or a family support group, or a client's physical space at home could be modified to be less restrictive and more stimulating. Specific care environments should be considered as well. This means being thoughtful about the physical space and social makeup of intervention programs that clients might be assigned to, and seeking ways to sensibly collaborate with other team members to maximize client gains.

Table 8.4: Sample conditional phrases

> *Upon request...*
> *Given the necessary supplies...*
> *When asked...*
> *After 2 weeks...*
> *With visual cues...*
> *With verbal prompts...*
> *During treatment sessions...*
> *Given a list of resources...*
> *Following group discussion...*

Targeting the environment like this helps to avoid making the "fundamental attribution error" (Ross & Nisbett, 1991), which mistakenly attributes the reasons for a client's condition or behavior to the individual alone rather than recognizing the influence of external variables. Chapter 10 includes many examples of ways the physical and social environment can be used to maximize client outcomes.

Consider Culture

Cultural differences must also be considered in the planning process. In Chapter 3, we discussed the influence of cultural values, attitudes, and beliefs on health behavior and the client–provider relationship. Some cultural groups are not comfortable with being active partners in planning and monitoring their healthcare. Likewise, cultural values, beliefs and customs can influence participation in recreation and leisure activities. Thus, cultural values, customs, religious expression, or eating patterns can complicate an intervention plan unless it is culturally sensitive from the start. This important issue is addressed more fully in Chapter 11.

Table 8.5: Evaluating behavioral objectives

Part of the Behavior Objective	Question(s) to Answer	Way to Identify This Component
Behavior		
Client's performance/action representative of his or her goal	Does this sentence indicate a client behavior that I can see and measure? Is this behavior related to the goal I have set with the client?	Underline the underlined action verb used for the client's representative behavior
Condition		
Circumstances under which the client's behavior must be shown	Have I identified the circumstances that must be present for the client to do this behavior? Are there things that the client must be provided? Where or when will this behavior occur?	Place a box around the conditional phrase in your behavioral objective.
Criterion		
The minimum acceptable performance for the behavior	Have I identified how often the client must do this behavior or how long it must be present? Is there a way to distinguish between doing the behavior at an acceptable level versus doing the behavior intermittently?	Place an oval around the criterion phrase in your behavioral objective.
Example		
When sensing his hostility escalate, Mr. Kazigan will request permission from staff to use the heavy bag as a self-mediated alternative to angry outburst 100% of the time		

Consider Safety

Client safety ought to be a primary consideration when planning interventions. Many clients will have medical precautions such as ambulatory (e.g., at risk for falls), dietary, exercise, or swallowing restrictions. Safety considerations need to be made with clients who have cognitive impairments such as dementia or brain injuries. Often clients with these disorders do not recognize the risk or dangers associated with a particular activity and so appropriate supervision must be provided during TR interventions.

Consider Medication Side Effects

Medications and their side effects can affect a client's motivation, involvement, and compliance. Symptoms such as lethargy, blurred vision, constipation, dry mouth, and drowsiness, can also impair judgment and reduce enjoyment in certain activities. Recreation therapists should be knowledgeable about possible side effects associated with various medications when planning and implementing TR interventions. You can obtain this information from your place of employment or ask your clients who take medication, as they are often very well-informed.

Consider Necessary Mechanical Aids and Devices

Some clients must use mechanical aids for basic activities like mobility (e.g., wheelchairs, walkers), communication (e.g., language boards or computer-assisted speaking devices), respiration (e.g., ventilators), or bladder and bowel management (e.g., catheters and collection bags). In some instances these devices may limit the type of activities available. Most times, however, the mechanical device will merely alter the pattern of involvement or the availability of the client for involvement. Thus planning will need to include reasonable accommodations for the device.

> ✸• • •Thinking Trigger
>
> Think of a mechanical aid that a client might use (e.g., communication board). How would you accommodate this device? • • •✸

Consider Literacy

Research estimates that half of the adults in the United States have limited literacy skills and are unable to read and understand complex information (Kirsch, Jungeblut, Jenkins & Kolstad, 1993). Unfortunately, many therapists fail to consider literacy issues when planning interventions. Many mistakenly believe that literacy concerns are only an issue if clients use English as a second language or they have not completed formal schooling. However, educational attainment is not always an indication of an individual's literacy. Illiteracy can take many forms and is not limited to a specific group, education level, or socioeconomic stratum. **Table 8.6** (p. 142) lists four different types of literacy problems that therapists need to consider when planning interventions. These include prose, document, quantitative, and health literacy. Each type of literacy problem will have a different impact on the planning process. Using written materials or forms such as activity calendars to convey information about intervention schedules may be ineffective if clients have difficulty with *document literacy*. Assigning clients with limited *prose literacy* to an intervention group that uses written worksheets or journals may result in a client's refusal to attend. *Quantitative literacy* problems may be problematic on community outings that require math skills like estimating the gratuity for a restaurant check. The assumption that clients can readily understand written materials may alienate clients who are uncomfortable disclosing their literacy problems. When not recognized and compensated for during the planning process, low literacy can interfere with successful interventions.

Consider Motivation

Client motivation is a prerequisite to successful collaboration. Any efforts directed at assisting clients to make behavior changes that would result in improved functioning, adaptation, or life quality will fall short if clients are not motivated. Understanding clients well enough so that you have a sense of what motivates them is critical to successful intervention planning.

In a discussion on motivating clients, a student-led exercise had the class identify one thing that was a powerful motivator for each person, even when feeling lousy. Good food, soulful music, and being by water were high on the list. This student had captured the essence of what it takes to motivate clients. It is the ability to find something that sparks an interest so

Table 8.6: Types of literacy

Type of Literacy	Definition and Implications
Prose literacy	Needed to understand written text. Typically associated with reading skills. Lack of skills in this area results in problems with understanding and using text found in newspapers, magazines, books, pamphlets, brochures, and worksheets.
Document literacy	Required for understanding material presented in tabular formats such as applications, schedules, maps, graphs, and tables. Implications when requesting clients to read bus/train schedules, restaurant menus, checklists, activity schedules, or calendars.
Quantitative literacy	Needed for arithmetic operations, such as on bank forms, purchase orders, or restaurant receipts. Implications for basic math skills associated with exercise, medication, and nutrition information.
Health literacy	The degree to which individuals can obtain, process, and understand basic health information and services needed to make appropriate health decisions. Implications for client's understanding medical terminology and treatment protocols.

powerful that a client would act in spite of pain, boredom, fear, or poor self-esteem. Students then shared stories of dramatic moments when clients were offered something so powerful that, despite everything, they became active again. For a nursing home resident it was as simple as a daily job of delivering mail (he had been an office manager). For another person with chronic mental illness, it was pictures and music of the railroad and trains (he had been a laborer who repaired tracks). For a child, it was a cat that would curl up in his lap. Identifying a motivating force during the planning process is a very important beginning point to effective care.

Often, the source of motivation can be found by examining things that individuals value. Consider for instance Louise, who was involved in rehabilitation for a hip replacement. An important part of her therapy was improving her physical functioning and mobility skills. During treatment team meetings, the physical therapist reported that Louise did not seem invested in her physical therapy program and complained of fatigue the entire time she was working on her standing tolerance. Her recreation therapist knew how much Louise enjoyed spending time with her grandchildren. With this knowledge, the recreation therapist designed an intervention that blended the functional performance task of standing tolerance with an interest area of Louise—she had Louise bake cookies for her grandchildren. The desire to do something for her grandchildren was used as a motivator to help Louise work on her standing tolerance. Louise was motivated to engage in treatment because she was focused on something she valued.

It is also helpful to have a theoretical understanding of motivation as it relates to behavioral change. The *Stages of Change* or *Transtheortical Model* is especially useful in those instances where the focus of TR interventions is to help clients to develop healthy lifestyles through recreation involvement. Developed by Prochaska and DiClemente (1982), this theory identifies the series of stages that clients go through in making a behavioral change: *precontemplation, contemplation, preparation, action,* and *maintenance.* **Table 8.7** describes each of these stages and provides suggestions to help a client at each motivational stage.

You will need to determine where your client is in terms of these stages of change. This is not an easy task and would occur well after a therapeutic relationship is established with the client. Determining your client's readiness to make lifestyle change requires that you gently probe your client about his or her present and prior experiences with making lifestyle change. This probing may occur in the context of an activity such as asking a client to create a collage or timeline that reflects his or her efforts at making lifestyle change. It may also involve creating a poem or story about his or her efforts to change a particular behavior or make a particular decision. A client's responses to such activities may provide insight that will help you determine where he or she is in the change process so that you can tailor your interventions to support his or her efforts. Therapists may also ask questions such as those found in **Table 8.8** (p. 144) during the assessment and planning process. Of course before posing these questions with clients, therapists must feel comfortable that they

Table 8.7: Stages of change—Descriptions and intervention strategies

Stage	Description	Intervention Strategies
Precontemplation	Individuals have no intention of changing their behavior. They may not have even considered the need for change, or they may have tried to change a behavior before and given up. Because they have no intention of taking action, people in this stage are difficult to engage in rehabilitation.	Interventions must be targeted at increasing the client's awareness of the need to make a lifestyle change. Tactful suggestion, peer mentors, or recommended readings may help clients at this stage become more aware of their need to make a change.
Contemplation	At this stage individuals have acknowledged that a problem exists and have begun to think about making a change. People can remain in this stage for some time—knowing that they have a problem but never finding the time or energy to do anything about it.	Intervention strategies useful for clients in this stage include encouragement, additional information, and assistance with developing the skills needed to take action or with developing a change plan.
Preparation	At this stage people are close to taking action. They have moved from thinking about the reasons why they can't change their behavior to thinking about how they could begin to take action. Most people in this stage have thought about several things that they might do to change a behavior and may have even developed a plan.	Intervention strategies useful at this stage include helping clients to set realistic goals, focusing on changing only one behavior, identifying rewards that can be used for acknowledging small gains in behavior change, and finding supports to help clients maintain their new behavior. In addition, discussions that focus on identifying those things that have served as barriers to maintaining change need to occur with a focus on modifying or changing these barriers.
Action	At this stage the individual begins to follow the plan they have developed.	Strategies effective in helping the client follow through during the action stage include having clients publicly state their desire to change and eliciting support to engage in the plan. Stimulus control strategies in which reminders or cues are used to assist the client with engaging in the desired behavior are also appropriate.
Maintenance	Individuals at this stage have made a behavioral change in their lifestyle; however, to continue it and not slip back into old patterns, vigilance and attention to detail is needed.	In this stage therapists can help clients by discussing the potential for relapse and developing strategies to overcome these setbacks.
Termination	At this stage the behavior has become so ingrained that it is a routine part of the individual's lifestyle.	Vigilance is no longer needed as the person has incorporated the behavior into his or her daily life.

have established a therapeutic relationship with the client and that they have the needed facilitation and communication skills so that clients experience the exchange as helpful and not threatening.

Often when planning interventions, therapists inadvertently assume that clients are at the action stage in the change process and will eagerly follow through with all intervention plans; however, this is not always the case. For instance, clients may decline to be involved in TR because they are unsure about its role in overall treatment and may question how TR services will help them achieve their desired goals. These clients may be in the contemplation stage of behavioral change—they recognize that they want their lives to be different but are unsure what to do about it. During the planning phase you can begin to foster motivation by helping clients understand why they are being asked to engage in particular activities and how such involvement would benefit them. These benefits should reflect what the client wants and values.

Summary

This chapter focused on the second phase of the TR clinical process: the planning phase. The ability to develop client-specific intervention plans is fundamental to clinical practice. Therapists must carefully weigh a number of issues to plan effective interventions, including clients' wants, needs, and aspirations. Cowger (1994) provides practice guidelines that can be used when working with clients in the intervention planning process (and throughout your services). While some focus exclusively on the assessment process, others reflect a general approach toward planning and service delivery. These include:

- Give priority to the client's understanding of the facts
- Believe the client
- Discover what the client wants
- Move the focus toward personal and environmental strengths
- Use language the client can understand
- Make goal setting a joint activity between you and your clients

Table 8.8: Questions for determining client's readiness for change

Stage of Change	Questions to Assess Stage
Precontemplation	What are your thoughts about *(identified behavior)*? What effect has *(identified behavior)* had on your life? Is this *(identified behavior)* something you have thought about changing?
Contemplation	Why do you think *(identified behavior)* is problematic? Why do you think you should consider changing *(identified behavior)*?
Preparation	Have you thought about what you need to do change *(identified behavior)*? Do you have a plan for changing *(identified behavior)*? Have you considered other ways to change *(identified behavior)*? Who would support you with changing *(identified behavior)*?
Action	Have you told anyone that you are intending to change *(identified behavior)*? Have you identified rewards for yourself that will keep you motivated as you try to change *(identified behavior)*?
Maintenance	What will you do if you fall back into *(identified behavior)*? Have you thought about how you will handle setbacks? Who will you use to help motivate you to maintain the changes you've made in *(identified behavior)*?
Termination	Have you ever been able to change a lifestyle behavior? How did you manage to change this behavior? Are there any new behaviors that you want to change?

- Reach a mutual understanding based on the assessment
- Avoid blame and blaming
- Avoid labeling

As Cowger conveys in his practice guidelines, the planning phase determines the course and style of all subsequent interactions with a client. Ultimately, it results in a systematic written plan of action that identifies goals, objectives, and intervention strategies that utilize a client's strengths.

In some cases it is difficult to plan as systematically as we discussed in this chapter. For instance, short-term, acute care settings leave little time for thorough assessments, and contact time is often unpredictable. Even so, you will be expected to address relevant client outcomes whenever you can. In pediatric care settings for example, a primary goal for all clients is that they are able to use play and recreation to manage stress associated with illness and hospitalization. Even a chance encounter in the playroom is an opportunity to use medical play to address this goal. Likewise, short stays in a psychiatric or alcohol treatment program makes planning very difficult. Often clients end up in an intervention group prior to being assessed. In some settings, they are free to select what intervention groups they will attend, and how often. Thus, a recreation therapist must be prepared to do a quick assessment on the spot, and adjust his or her group interventions to those who attend. Just as there are "teachable moments" there are "therapeutic encounters" that are planned and implemented simultaneously.

Even when planning can be systematic, it is important to understand that any intervention plan is merely a starting point. Even though you have been very careful to think about appropriate goals and suitable strategies to reach these goals, you must stay flexible. Goals sometimes have to be modified or abandoned altogether and different strategies have to be used. An effective recreation therapist is adaptable. The technical knowledge and skills needed to write goals and behavioral objectives must always be complimented by your clinical judgment about when and how to use intervention strategies and why these strategies can be helpful. The following four chapters focus on the art of implementing intervention strategies. These include chapters on using activity and education-based interventions, the environment, therapeutic relationships, and group work in clinical TR practice.

References

American Therapeutic Recreation Association. (2000). *Standards of practice for therapeutic recreation* (rev. ed.). Alexandria, VA: ATRA.

Bullock, C. and Mahon, M. (1997). *Introduction to recreation services for people with disabilities: A person-centered approach*. Champaign, IL: Sagamore Publishing.

Cowger, C. (1994). Assessing client strengths: Clinical assessment for client empowerment. *Social Work, 39*(3), 262–268.

Kirsch, I., Jungeblut, A., Jenkins, L., and Kolstad, A. (1993). *Adult literacy in America: A first look at the results of the National Adult Literacy Survey* (2nd ed.). Washington, DC: Office of Educational Research and Improvement.

National Therapeutic Recreation Association. (2001). *NTRS Standards of practice for TR services and annotated bibliography*. Ashburn, VA: NTRS.

Pedlar, A., Hornibrook, T., and Haasen, B. (2001). Patient-focused care: Theory and practice. *Therapeutic Recreation Journal, 35*(1), 15–30.

Peterson, C. and Stumbo, N. (2000). *Therapeutic recreation program design: Principles and procedures* (3rd ed). Needham Heights, MA: Allyn & Bacon.

Prochaska, J. and DiClemente, C. (1982). Transtheoretical therapy: Toward a more integrative model of change. *Psychotherapy: Theory, Research and Practice, 19*(3), 276–288.

Ross, L and Nisbett, R. (1991). *The person and the situation: Perspectives of social psychology*. New York, NY: McGraw-Hill.

Sable, J., Gravink, J., Craig, P., Carr, T., and Lee, D. (2001). *Project PATH treatment planning form*. Unpublished manuscript.

Chapter 9
Using Activity-Based Interventions

Guided Reading Questions

After reading this chapter, you should be able to answer the following:
- What inherent characteristics exist in activities that allow them to be used therapeutically?
- What is experiential learning?
- How do recreation therapists facilitate experiential learning?
- What are some activity or education-based interventions commonly used by recreation therapists?
- What is a program protocol?
- How can health promotion be incorporated into education-based interventions?
- What should recreation therapists consider when selecting activities for clinical practice?

Introduction

Activities are the core of TR practice and used by recreation therapists for two primary purposes. First, TR specialists provide activities to clients so they can use them at their own discretion to *re-create* themselves physically, psychologically, socially, and spiritually. Providing recreation opportunities allows clients to be self-determining in their pursuit of health, leisure, and life quality. Second, activities, games, and other learn-ing exercises are used in clinical practice as planned interventions to help people learn about themselves, cope with and adapt to change, and gain knowledge, skills, and abilities necessary to maintain health and live meaningful lives. In this sense activities are used as a means to achieving health and rehabilitation goals. Sylvester, Voelkl, and Ellis (2001) describe this as *activity therapy*. While both uses of activities are important, we will focus our discussion primarily on the use of activities in clinical interventions as it coincides with the focus of this text.

This chapter provides a brief overview of activities used in clinical practice, often referred to as TR *modali-ties* and *facilitation techniques*. We begin with a discus-sion of the therapeutic potential inherent in activities. Next we describe various categories of activities and offer guidelines for their selection.

Before we begin with these topics, we must offer a clarification. We purposely use the term "activities" to represent both recreation and other action-oriented processes used in clinical TR practice. We recognize that this risks blurring the differences between recre-ation activities and activities used as purposeful inter-vention. We acknowledge (as discussed in Chapter 1)

that recreation is a category of human activity that is unobligated and expected by the participant to bring about feelings of renewal and revitalization. In this culture recreation implies the antithesis of work, whereas therapy consists of an obligated effort that is sometimes unpleasant and nonnegotiable. In fact, clients often equate therapy with work. Thus clients may appear confused or are resistant when they learn that recreation is a part of their intervention or therapy services.

While these terms may seem incompatible, we believe that in TR clinical practice the same activity can be used for therapy *and* can be recreation for a client. It depends on how the decision is made to do the activity and for *what* purposes. Consider the following example.

Tom, a 22-year-old male with a brain injury resulting from a car accident, attends a day program. Tina, a recreation therapist, works with clients in this day program. Like many other college students, computers were a large part of Tom's life prior to his accident. He used the computer to play games, chat online, and send and receive e-mails from family and friends. He is currently unable to operate a computer because of functional losses associ-ated with his injury and tells Tina he wants this "lifeline" back again. Tina and Tom together decide to use computer activities as an interven-tion. For Tina, the use of computer activities can help Tom improve his cognitive skills, such as sequencing, as well as his recreation skills. This is important since without some functional improvement Tom will not be able to use the computer satisfactorily during his free time. For

Tom, the computer was a hobby that brought him pleasure. He is excited about learning how to resume this part of his life. As Tom and Tina work together using this intervention, Tom's cognitive abilities improve. This renewed feeling of competence motivates Tom to use the computer in his free time.

An important factor in this scenario is that Tina facilitated changes for Tom by thoughtfully and carefully using computer activities appropriate to Tom's clinical as well as recreational needs. We recognize that this is not always the case. Sometimes activities, like writing exercises and discussions in a stress management program are used in clinical TR practice. These would probably not be considered recreation. In these examples, however, activities are integral parts of clinical interventions. Therefore, rather than clarifying these subtle but important distinctions throughout the chapter, we have chosen to use the generic term "activities."

The Value of Activity as a Means

Using activities in clinical practice depends on your understanding of the therapeutic potential inherent in them. The structure of an activity and the process of doing an activity create therapeutic opportunities that can be used to help clients reach necessary and desirable goals. A critical factor in facilitating clients' learning, adaptation, and growth is being able to evaluate the potential therapeutic value of activities and then being able to match therapeutic potential with client needs. This matching is one of the primary clinical skills of a TR professional. Generally, activities used in TR practice provide the potential for acquiring and improving functional skills, psychosocial learning, diversion, creative expression, and symbolic meaning in one's life.

Acquiring and Improving Functional Skills

Any activity requires a variety of physical skills (e.g., strength, mobility, coordination), cognitive skills (e.g., memory, planning, comprehension), affective skills (e.g., emotional control and expression), and social skills (e.g., conversation, cooperation). Participation in activities enables clients to develop, improve, or adapt skills needed to function in most life domains. An *activity analysis* is the most useful way to identify the functional skills required by particular activities (see **Exhibit 9.1**). With the information gained from conducting activity analyses, therapists can select and adapt activities that facilitate or improve clients' functional skills.

Sometimes the structure or actual behaviors inherent in activities facilitate skill development. For example, children playing on an obstacle course are developing gross motor skills as well as language skills. Likewise, playing a table game can help children with developmental disabilities acquire basic social skills such as turn-taking.

Skill development can also be aimed at a client's capacity or competence to use recreation as a contribu-

Exhibit 9.1: Activity analysis

Activity analysis identifies the inherent characteristics of an activity and the physical, social, cognitive, and emotional requirements needed for successful participation. While analysis occurs independent of specific clients, it produces information that allows therapists to modify or adapt the activity to accommodate wide-ranging functional abilities. Thus, activity analysis helps with matching activities to particular client needs and intended intervention outcomes. Beginning with an activity as it is traditionally performed, therapists ask questions related to the skills needed for each domain of functioning. For example:

- What specific fine and gross motor movements/skills are needed in this activity?
- Are there specific motor patterns required for the successful participation in this activity (e.g., throwing, jumping, bending)?
- What types of social interaction skills are needed for successful participation? Does this activity require academic skills related to reading and writing?
- What feelings get provoked in this activity?
- Additional analyses pertain to activity facilitation matters such as required equipment, space, and time duration.

See Peterson & Stumbo (2000) and Sylvester, Voelkl & Ellis (2001) for specific activity analysis forms

tion to health and well-being. This is often the case with fitness activities. Beyond this activities can be relevant for reinforcing interventions of other disciplines, thereby maximizing functional gains within the overall treatment context. For example, activities that require or stimulate conversation can be used to reinforce a speech therapist's effort to help a client use compensatory communication skills (see **Exhibit 9.2**).

Exhibit 9.2: Case in point—Facilitating the acquisition and improvement of functional skills

> Rhonda, the recreation therapist on a CVA (stroke) unit, conducts a "high tea" twice a week for clients with impaired communication skills. Clients are encouraged to practice their communication skills in the relaxed atmosphere of this social gathering.

Skills developed and used in recreation are easily transferable to other tasks and situations. In this sense recreation serves as a threshold experience, where functional competence gained in recreation can be the bridge to functioning in other life domains. Each successful experience leads to greater confidence and thus a willingness to meet more challenging demands in daily life. For instance, clients with developmental disabilities may learn or develop skills such as turn-taking, counting, and matching by playing card games. Clients can also use these skills in their prevocational work training program.

TR activities are also a valuable mechanism for functional improvement and adaptation because of the process inherent in them. Engaging in an activity involves a cognitive and affective process as well as the actual behavior itself. This *process* involves the sequence of planning the activity, taking action to follow through with the plans, making adjustments as needed in response to one's action, and completing the activity with appropriate ending and closure. This sequence involves the task skills Mosey (1973) considered to be essential to all human action. *Task skills* include the ability to organize materials needed for an activity; the ability to follow oral, written, or demonstrated directions; and the ability to solve problems as they arise (see **Exhibit 9.3**). The sequential process inherent in recreation activities has also been highlighted by Bullock and Mahon (1997) as containing instrumental skills that can be generalized to many other tasks and situations.

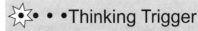

Thinking Trigger

In Exhibits 9.2 and 9.3 recreation therapists Rhonda and Dan chose recreation activities because their inherent therapeutic potentials matched the functional needs of their clients. Can you identify the match? What other activities could Rhonda or Dan use?

Psychosocial Learning

Activities are an excellent catalyst for clients to address a variety of psychological and social issues related to learning, adaptation, and growth. The structure and process of activities provide a means for clients to experience and confront thoughts, perceptions, and beliefs related to themselves and their relationships with others. Professions other than TR have also recognized the therapeutic value in using activities with clients. Nurses, psychologists, and educators sometimes use activities to help clients cope, express themselves, and develop greater self-efficacy. Nurses, for example, reportedly use guided imagery, storytelling, humor, bibliotherapy, and journal writing to help clients cope with chronic illness (Miller, 1992).

Psychologists Nickerson and O'Laughlin (1982) found activities to be an excellent alternative to verbal, insight-oriented counseling interventions. They believe the nonverbal nature of activity interventions minimizes the biasing effects of language, which helps when working with diverse cultures. Activities also could bypass the defensive, censoring functions of language and expose a client's typical pattern of behaving. In either instance activities allow opportunities for clients to try out new, more effective ways of behaving.

Exhibit 9.3: Case in point—Facilitating the acquisition and improvement of functional skills

> Ralph, a 38-year-old man with a brain injury, has difficulty with sequencing. Ralph and Dan, his recreation therapist, decide to work on making a birdhouse from a kit. This activity involves following a number of sequential steps diagramed in written instructions. Because Ralph wants to make this same kit with his 11-year-old son and because of the task skills associated with successfully completing the project, Dan decided it was a good intervention activity to use with Ralph.

Board games, for example, are a particularly useful intervention with children and adolescents. Games can be used to confront and manage feelings associated with winning and losing and to learn through analogy how to live within the rules. An example of how Joyce, a recreation therapist, uses games as an intervention is explained in **Exhibit 9.4**. Game play has also been successfully used as *kinetic psychotherapy*, a form of group therapy with school-age children to teach prosocial skills and conflict resolution (Schachter, 1982). Recreation therapists have also developed board games to use with clients.

Exhibit 9.4: Case in point—Facilitating psychosocial learning

> Joyce, a recreation therapist, uses the "Anger Solution Game" with a group of preadolescent boys hospitalized for conduct disorder problems. Through the game they talk about situations that provoke anger and behaviors that are positive solutions. They also talk about rules and why one needs to follow them.

Psychosocial learning also occurs through activities because of the opportunity to learn through doing. This is known as *experiential learning*. Engaging in activities and reflecting on one's entire experience (e.g., thoughts and feelings) can result in new levels of awareness and insight. This understanding can be used to change perceptions and influence future behavior. Experiential learning activities are usually conducted with a group of clients so that social interactions within the group can be used to facilitate learning and growth.

According to Luckner and Nadler (1997) experiential learning occurs when carefully chosen activities are supported by reflection, critical analysis, and synthesis

(see **Figure 9.1**). It follows a cycle that involves *experiencing* the structured activity, *reflecting* on the new experience in comparison to past experiences, *generalizing* by making inferences from this experience to everyday life, and *applying* this learning to their life.

Experiential learning affects clients in three ways: It alters cognitive structures, modifies attitudes, and expands the repertoire of behavior skills (Johnson & Johnson, 1982). Activities can provide learners with concrete and tangible feedback about the consequences of their actions, which clients reflect on and incorporate into their thoughts and beliefs. Also, within group activities a person's behaviors are immediately evident to others who can provide feedback about what the person said or did in the activity. Based on this feedback, and with the support of others, clients can experiment with new behaviors and evaluate their effectiveness. For instance, if a child's need to be first in everything is bothersome to peers, this child can try to behave with more patience and restraint during recreation activities.

Finally, experiential learning typically involves using activities as metaphors to explore issues in clients' lives (Gass, 1993). Activities that require group participation and cooperation can be used as a metaphor for exploring similar relational issues. Physically challenging activities can be used to examine thoughts and feelings clients have about confidence, decision-making, and tendencies to seek and use the support of others. Sometimes, the challenge inherent in an activity is a metaphor for life challenges. In **Exhibit 9.5**, Jim, a recreation therapist, uses experiential learning activities and metaphors with clients.

Exhibit 9.5: Case in point—Facilitating psychosocial learning

> Jim, a recreation therapist, uses an adventure-based counseling program with middle-school boys who have attention deficit hyperactivity disorder (ADHD). Program activities help the boys learn about themselves and how to get along with peers. Twice a week the group engages in trust activities and other team-building activities. At the end of each session the boys talk about their behavior in the group. The program culminates in a weekend camping trip that requires the group to apply what they have learned about respect, cooperation, and teamwork. Their group challenge is to build a bridge over a stream. Jim facilitates discussions with the boys about their experiences throughout the weekend. They use the bridge as a metaphor during the discussions.

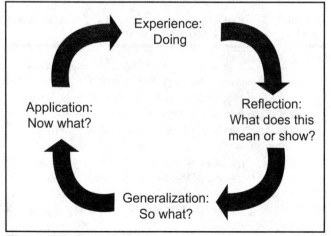

Figure 9.1: Experiential learning cycle

Thinking Trigger

In exhibits 9.4 and 9.5 recreation therapists Joyce and Jim chose activities that promote psychosocial learning. Why? What metaphors might Joyce or Jim use with their clients? If you were the recreation therapist, how would you encourage the clients in either example to make connections between the activity experience and their everyday life? How would you use the bridge as a metaphor in Exhibit 9.5?

Diversion

Diversion is another valuable yet often disregarded therapeutic potential inherent in activities. It is understandable that recreation therapists are sometimes offended when other professionals consider their work with clients frivolous and unnecessary, and dismiss it as merely diversion. However, this may simply reflect a lack of understanding about the healing properties of diversion, especially as a mechanism for coping and adapting. This may also result from our failure to communicate to others the therapeutic intentions of activities we offer or use with clients. Getting distance from problems, worries, or concerns is a classic function of recreation and a major coping skill for managing stress. In this regard diversion through recreation and other activities needs to be promoted and protected. **Exhibit 9.6** illustrates one of the ways that recreation therapists can promote the diversional use of recreation as a coping mechanism.

Furthermore, enjoyment and the sense of renewal that comes from pleasant diversion can also leave clients open to addressing other goals. Recreation therapists will frequently report that an asset they have

Exhibit 9.6: Case in point—Facilitating coping and adaptation through diversion

During the day the hospital's greenhouse is used by Jean, the recreation therapist, as a place for improving functional skills. During the evening Jean invites clients to use it as a haven for retreat and renewal. Soft music, pleasant smells, and a comfortable sitting area create a pleasant environment where clients can briefly escape from their worries.

over other professionals is the nonthreatening nature of their interventions. Consequently, the casual and often enjoyable nature of TR activities actually motivates clients to be more active. Clients will often report that TR represents opportunities for fun, which can be a primary motivator for many individuals.

Creative Expression

Certain activities can be liberating and energizing opportunities for spontaneous self-expression—they contain neither predetermined boundaries nor fixed processes. The participant is free to create without constraints of logic or orderliness. These activities give expression to one's inner self, such as art, music, and movement. Nathan and Mirviss (1998) provide an excellent resource on creative activities. Their informative explanation of creativity includes characteristics such as curiosity, imagination, novelty, discovery, spontaneity, and risk. When used as interventions, the creative arts "can be a means of both reconciling emotional conflicts and fostering self-awareness and personal growth" (p. 7). **Exhibit 9.7** displays one of the ways creative activities can be used in clinical practice.

Exhibit 9.7: Case in point—Facilitating self-expression

Yvonne, a recreation therapist working with adolescent girls struggling with eating disorders, has the girls use creative arts activities including making facial masks and writing poetry to portray their images of health and happiness.

Symbolic Meaning

Finding meaning in one's life is an ultimate existential challenge for every human being. "Seeking and finding meaning in ourselves, our activities, and the broader world of people and things around us is a remarkable, but often undervalued, gift that permits adaptation and growth for both the individual and society" (Fidler & Velde, 1999, p. 12). According to Richter and Kaschalk (1996) recreation therapists have the opportunity to promote meaning and identity in clients' lives through recreation activities; however, a therapist cannot give meaning to a client. Authentic meaning "only declares itself in the life context of a given individual or a particular social group" (Fidler & Velde, 1999, p. 12). Each individual's perspective influences what is valued and ultimately meaningful. Thus it takes special effort to understand each client and find ways to create opportunities for "meaning-making." For many clients, meaning is synonymous with spiritual fulfillment (O'Keefe, 2000). **Exhibit 9.8** contains an example of an activity facilitated by a recreation therapist that holds the potential to promote meaning and identity in clients.

Exhibit 9.8: Case in point—Facilitating opportunities for "meaning-making"

> Jody, a recreation therapist, works on a specialized Alzheimer's unit. As part of her family education program, she arranges for married couples whose relationships have been ravaged by Alzheimer's disease to dance to the songs of their past, including their wedding song.

Activity-Based Interventions Commonly Used in TR Practice

Austin (2001) maintains that virtually any activity considered recreation could be used in TR clinical practice. This creates enormous possibilities when you consider that recreation is socioculturally defined and therefore can include many activity forms unfamiliar to recreation therapists. Likewise, there are many "nontraditional" forms of recreation (Peterson & Stumbo, 2000, p. 47) that clients use for relaxation, diversion, and self-expression. Although the range of possibilities is enormous, a definable scope of activities used as interventions exists in TR practice. These activities are referred to as modalities and/or facilitation techniques. According to burlingame and Skalko (1997), a *modality* is "the type of activity used to deliver treatment" (p. 179), whereas a *facilitation technique* is a method or procedure used to intervene with client problems or needs (Kinney & Witman, 1997). Facilitation techniques involve a combination of activity and a therapist's interaction skills to facilitate change. Dattilo (2000) defines facilitation techniques as "a systematic procedure by which individuals are empowered to overcome difficulties or obstacles" (p. 6).

Table 9.1 contains a listing of modalities and facilitation techniques identified by various authors as used in TR practice. Austin (1999) and Dattilo (2000) provide thorough explanations of many of these modalities/facilitation techniques, and you are encouraged to consult their work directly.

Additional activity resources are available through vendors such as Venture Publishing, Inc., Idyll Arbor, Wellness Reproductions, S & S Crafts, and Childwork/Child Play. Finally, many recreation therapists use the Internet for activity-based intervention ideas, especially the recreation therapy website developed by Charlie Dixon (http://www.recreationtherapy.com). The diversity of activity-based interventions available for use with clients is one of the unique advantages of the profession; however, it can also be overwhelming. For ease of discussion, we have created eight broad categories of TR interventions, incorporating many from Table 9.1.

The grouping of activity-based interventions in **Table 9.2** (p. 154) attempts to link similar activities under broad, conceptual categories. The categories within Table 9.2 are not mutually exclusive—some of the activity-based interventions could be listed in more than one category. Likewise, the listing of interventions is not all-inclusive. Activity variations occur often in practice as a result of the creativity of therapists (e.g., tape art, intergenerational programs, service learning projects). The types of activities utilized in practice are quite diverse and continually changing.

Table 9.2 illustrates similarities among the most common activities used by recreation therapists. Sometimes the categories reflect the primary outcome associated with particular interventions (e.g., Mind–Body Health Interventions, Fitness Interventions, Social Skills Interventions, Self-Discovery/Self-Expression Interventions). Other times, the intervention categories reflect types of activities (e.g., Games, Creative–Expressive, Nature-Based), as these activities are not primarily associated with one particular outcome. In addition, a few TR interventions mix education with skill development, most notably leisure education. This category is addressed separately as Education-Based Interventions.

Many interventions listed in Table 9.2 require specialized or advanced training in addition to a TR degree. Recreation therapists are professionally and ethically bound to obtain appropriate training as needed before you attempt to use such activity-based/education-based interventions in your clinical practice. The following sections describe each category of activities and their associated interventions.

Interventions Primarily Focused on Mind–Body Health

This category reflects interventions based on an understanding of the interconnectedness of mind and body. Their use is growing in popularity, in part due to the current emphasis on health promotion and because research has demonstrated their effectiveness with a variety of disabling conditions. Several of these interventions are considered *complementary and alternative medicine* (see Chapter 2). They intend to decrease stress and promote relaxation. They are sometimes used for pain management and improved immune functioning. The Mind–Body Health Interventions are described in **Table 9.3** at the end of this chapter.

Interventions Primarily Focused on Physical Activity and Fitness

The interventions in this category share a common characteristic: each requires the use of large muscle groups, resulting in caloric expenditures and increased cardiac output. Activities within this category typically aim at improvements in physical health (e.g., cardiorespiratory functioning, muscle strength, endurance, flexibility) and psychological health (e.g., reduced anxiety, depression). When used as clinical interventions, recreation therapists need to remember that participants must engage in these activities often enough (frequency), long enough (duration) and at a level appropriate to their current level of fitness and age (intensity) to achieve health benefits. Therefore, using

Table 9.1: TR modalities and facilitation techniques

Carter, Van Andel & Robb (1995)	Austin (1999)	Dattilo (2000)	Kinney, Witman & Kinney (2002)	
			Modalities	**Facilitation Techniques**
Adventure/challenge education	Adventure/ challenge	Adventure therapy	Activities of daily living	Behavior management
Aerobic exercise	Animal-assisted	Anger management	Adventure/initiative	Cognitive retraining
Assertiveness training	therapy	Aquatic therapy	Animal-assisted treatment	Family interventions
Attitude therapy	Aquatic therapy	Assistive	Aquatics	Group interventions
Behavior modification/ management	Aromatherapy	technology	Arts and crafts	Guided imagery
Cognitive retraining	Assertiveness therapy	Exercise	Assertiveness training	Humor therapy
Humor	Bibliotherapy	Expressive arts	Athletics/sports	Leisure education
Leisure education	Cognitive rehabilitation	Humor	Bibliotherapy/ storytelling	Leisure counseling
Reality orientation	Creative arts	Leisure education	Camping/outdoor activities	Play therapy/skills
Reminiscence therapy	Horticulture therapy	Moral development discussion	Community reintegration	Pre/postoperative play
Remotivation	Humor	Play	Dance/movement	Reality orientation
Resocialization	Leisure education	Reminiscence	Drama	Reminiscence
Sensory training	Reality orientation	Sports	Empowerment/ self-esteem	Remotivation
Social skills training	Relaxation techniques	Stress management	Exercise/fitness/ aerobics	Resocialization
Stress management	Reminiscence	Tai chi	Games	Sensory stimulation
	Remotivation	Therapeutic horseback riding	Horseback riding	Social skills training
	Resocialization	Therapeutic use of animals	Horticulture	Stress management
	Sensory training	Values clarification	Meditation	Values clarification
	Social skills training		Music/singing	
	Tai chi		Parties/special events	
	Technology		Problem solving	
	Therapeutic community		Project/service activities	
	Therapeutic touch		Weight training	
	Validation therapy			
	Values clarification			

these interventions clinically requires specialized training in safety precautions, CPR, contraindications to participation, instructional techniques, adaptive devices, and activity modifications. Additional information about the three major categories of fitness related activities—aquatics, exercise, and sport—can be found in **Table 9.4** at the end of this chapter.

Creative–Expressive Interventions

Creative–expressive activities include the visual arts, music, drama, dance, storytelling, and arts and crafts. When used therapeutically, these activities promote changes in cognitive, physical, emotional, or social functioning (Uhler, 1979). They can also promote self-expression and enhance leisure experiences for persons with disabilities (Ludins-Katz & Katz, 1990). Nathan and Mirviss (1998) provide an excellent resource on the use of the creative arts in therapy. They describe activities that address issues of self-worth and esteem, communicating thoughts and feelings, and experiencing relaxation and escape. Note that art therapists, music therapists, and dance/movement therapists differ from recreation therapists in their use of the creative arts. Art, music, and dance/movement therapists have specialized training often rooted in psychology. They have advanced study in the use of one art medium, especially in terms of the inherent therapeutic characteristics of the medium. Thus, recreation therapists should not misrepresent their use of art, music, dance or movement activities. The use of music by a recreation therapist, for example, does not constitute music therapy and should not be labeled or promoted as such. **Table 9.5** at the end of this chapter contains descriptions of activities typically included in this category.

Self-Discovery/Self-Expression Activities

Closely related to the creative–expressive activities are those interventions primarily used to facilitate self-discovery. These interventions vary but all focus on helping clients achieve insights into their values, attitudes, beliefs, and behaviors. Research suggests that these interventions can affect common outcomes including improved self-concept, self-worth, and self-esteem (Groff & Dattilo, 2000; McKenney & Dattilo, 2000; Sheldon & Dattilo, 2000). Therapists can receive specialized training for interventions in this category. Most adventure therapy programs, in particular, require advanced training. Descriptions of some of the more common self-discovery/self-expression interventions used in clinical TR practice are listed in **Table 9.6** at the end of this chapter.

Social Skills Interventions

Some clients with whom recreation therapists work display deficits in social functioning. As discussed in Chapter 7, social functioning refers to the behaviors, language, and attitudes a person conveys during his or her interactions with one or more people and involves both verbal and nonverbal communication. Individuals

Table 9.2: Activity-based and education-based interventions

Mind–Body Health	Physical Activity for Fitness	Creative Expression	Self-Discovery/Self-Expression
Aromatherapy	Aquatics	Arts and crafts	Adventure challenge
Breathing	Exercise	Dance/movement	Bibliotherapy
Guided imagery	Sports	Drama	Journaling/writing
Humor		Music	Reminiscence
Massage		Storytelling	Values clarification
Medical play		Visual arts	
Meditation			
Relaxation			
Sensory stimulation			
Tai chi			
Yoga			
Social Skills	**Nature-Based Interventions**	**Games**	**Education-Based Interventions**
Assertiveness training	Animal-assisted therapy	Cards	Assistive technology training
Anger management	Horticulture	Computer/video	Family/caregiver education
Resocialization		Puzzles	Community reintegration
Remotivation		Table/board	Leisure education
Reality orientation			

are seen as being socially competent when they are able to respond to and balance the demands of the social situation or environment in an effective manner (Stumbo, 1994/1995). Interventions designed to develop social skills typically employ a cognitive–behavioral approach and use modeling, skill rehearsal, and homework assignments where clients practice social skills in natural settings. Social skills interventions typically used by recreation therapists are described in **Table 9.7** at the end of this chapter.

Nature-Based Interventions

Nature-based interventions use plants, animals, and other living things to address a variety of clients' needs and goals. For many clients, plants and animals are or were an integral part of their lives, so the motivation to be involved in these activities is usually high. In addition, nature-based activities provide opportunities for clients to care for and nurture, which can be a welcomed change from being the one cared for by others. Outcomes associated with nature-based activities range from improved physical, cognitive, social, and emotional functioning to increased satisfaction with leisure and life. **Table 9.8** at the end of this chapter describes common nature-based activities used in TR practice.

Games

A wide variety of games are available for use by recreation therapists. Games adapt to all ages and ability levels and often have rules that may be modified to facilitate involvement. Games involve clients in tests of strategy, choice, and chance and may be engaged in alone (e.g., solitaire) or with other participants (e.g., chess). They may be cooperative or competitive in nature and may or may not require specialized equipment. Games may be commercially purchased or staff and participants may create them. Cards, puzzles, board/table games, and computer/video games are popular activities often found in clients' homes. The activities in this category are diverse and allow recreation therapists to address a variety of functional, psychosocial, and recreational needs.

Education-Based Interventions

In many instances recreation therapists combine a sequence of activities and other learning exercises into education-based interventions. These interventions

focus on an active process of information exchange and instruction aimed at changing clients' knowledge, attitudes, behaviors, and skills. They can involve activities and facilitation techniques discussed previously. For example, a stress management education intervention can incorporate several activities from various categories in Table 9.2 (e.g., guided imagery, deep breathing, journaling) with discussions about stress and coping behavior. There are at least four primary education-based interventions used in clinical practice: assistive technology training and education, community reintegration, family/caregiver education, and leisure education (see **Table 9.9** at the end of this chapter).

Program Protocols and Practice Guidelines

Sometimes activities and education-based interventions are developed into programs with several distinct and interrelated sessions. When this is done, recreation therapists write a protocol or program description. A *protocol* refers to "systematic intervention descriptions designed and delivered to attain predetermined client outcomes" (Hood, 2001, p. 191). *Program protocols* include statements of purpose and intended outcomes for the program as well as descriptive explanations of who will take part, what specific interventions will be provided, and how these interventions will be implemented. A variation on these program descriptions is *clinical practice guidelines*, which assist practitioners in making decisions about how to use certain activities as clinical intervention. The guidelines are established based on research and other evidence of best practice. Rather than dictating a step-by-step delivery, they support the clinical decision-making of a practitioner (Hood, 2001).

Frequently TR intervention programs are implemented with groups of clients. Chapter 12 describes in detail how group interventions are facilitated. For now, we want to show how education-based interventions and protocols interface. To do that, **Exhibit 9.9** (p. 156) presents a schematic model—*Healthy Living through Leisure*—that integrates concepts of health, wellness, and leisure and can be used to create health promotion and leisure education programs that assist clients with behavior change.

Each of the four parts to this model represents an important dimension of the behavior change process. The first part, *becoming informed,* focuses on raising awareness about health and wellness and the role of leisure in a person's life currently. This exploration includes environmental factors as well as personal information, and culminates in a lifestyle self-assessment. The next part examines a client's *motivation and readiness* to make lifestyle changes. At this point, clients establish meaningful and realistic goals or outcomes. The third part begins the activation stage, which focuses on *decision making* and *skill development*. Clients rework their goals by creating action plans for behavior change. These action plans focus on lifestyle changes that promote health through recreation involvement. The final part of this model focuses on *ensuring behavioral change*. Support is rendered for implementing the action plan, problem-solving setbacks, and using rewards regularly.

The Healthy Living through Leisure model is simply a framework. Therapists must select the specific activities that will be used in each of the four stages to promote the outcomes identified. In this way the framework can be individualized to help create specialized programs for specific groups of clients based on

their needs. An example of how the model was used to design a specific program protocol for women with physical disabilities appears in **Exhibit 9.10** (pp. 158–159).

Selecting Activities for Clinical Practice

Given the range of options available for activity-based interventions, how do you decide which to use? General agreement exists within the TR literature about the basis for selecting activities for use in clinical practice. Bullock, Mahon, and Selz (1997) believe that *client needs and preferences* and the *professional judgment of the therapist* drive the decisions. Peterson and Stumbo (2000) urge selection based on *client characteristics, resource factors, and activity content and delivery processes*. Austin and Crawford (2001) recommend selecting activities based on their *therapeutic potential* (e.g., chance for gaining mastery).

Exhibit 9.9: Healthy living through leisure

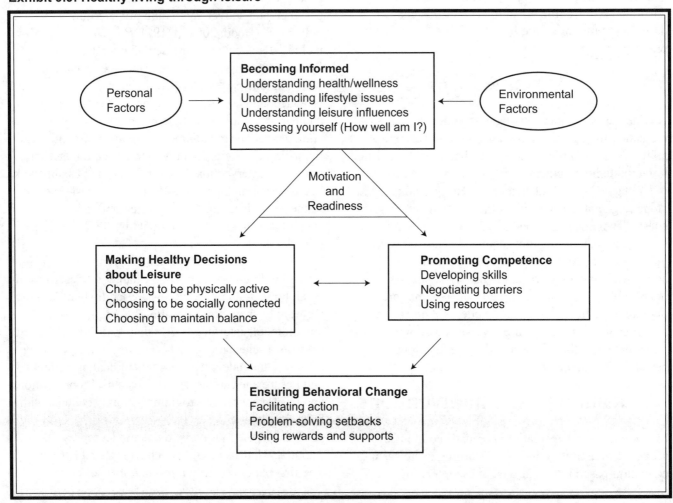

To make thoughtful selection decisions, you will need knowledge and understanding of three primary things: *clients*, *activity-based interventions*, and *yourself*. To help you with selecting activities for use as clinical interventions, we have highlighted several key issues within these three areas. **Exhibit 9.11** (p. 160) contains a 12-point checklist to use when selecting activity-based TR interventions. While this checklist is not all-inclusive, it is an helpful starting point for preparing to use an intervention for the first time. You should also periodically revisit this checklist since clients constantly change.

Summary

This chapter provided an overview of activities and discussed the inherent therapeutic potential that exists within activities. It also provided information to assist you in selecting activities for clinical interventions and grouping activities into intervention programs via a program protocol. Activities are the bedrock of TR practice (Kinney, Warren, Kinney & Witman, 1999). Inherent within the structure and process of activities are opportunities for clients to learn, adapt, and grow. When used as clinical interventions intended to assist clients with learning, adaptation, and growth, they must be selected and implemented thoughtfully. Merely assigning clients to an activity or making activities available for their discretionary use does not equate with clinical practice, as there are no assurances that necessary and desirable outcomes will result. Clinical practice involves the systematic and purposeful use of recreation and other activity-based interventions with the intent of *effecting change* in clients' attitudes, beliefs, behaviors and/or skills necessary for health and well-being. Use of activities, therefore, must be thoughtful and planned. While many professions recognize activities as useful, consideration of this final Thinking Trigger will enable you to discover the uniqueness of therapeutic recreation.

 • • •Thinking Trigger

If activities are used by many other helping professionals (e.g., nursing, psychology, occupational therapy, art therapy, music therapy), how would you explain the differences when activities are used by recreation therapists?

Here are a few more questions to consider as you formulate your response to this thinking trigger, as sometimes answers lie within questions.

- If activities have the potential to be helpful to clients in meeting their needs and goals, might more opportunities to benefit from carefully facilitated activities be better?

- Who benefits and who loses when you get into "turf" or "practice" battles around who can or should use activities to help clients?

- Do all helping professions have an equal commitment to activities as both a means to improving functioning and as a source of recreation and leisure fulfillment?

- Of all the helping professions, including TR, which is committed to helping clients improve through activities and then using these same changes in knowledge, attitudes, and skills in ways that promote health through recreation and leisure involvement?

Exhibit 9.10: Women and Wellness program protocol

Background and Rationale

Women who have chronic illness and physical disabilities (e.g., multiple sclerosis, spinal cord injury, cerebral palsy, Parkinson's) are at risk for many secondary health problems. Research indicates that these women have sedentary lifestyles, yet would like to become more physically and socially active. Major barriers appear to be lack of knowledge about resources and a lack of awareness of behavioral strategies to maintain health. Many of these women also lack social support.

Specific Health Promotion/Leisure Education Targets

Awareness and understanding of wellness

Understanding of leisure's connection to holistic health and wellness

Knowledge of current lifestyle's contribution to health status

Ability to develop action plans that promote physically and socially active lifestyles

Ability to follow an individualized exercise plan

Statement of Purpose

The purpose of this program is to provide women with physical disabilities opportunities to examine their current lifestyles in terms of holistic health and wellness, and to develop knowledge, attitudes, and skills related to creating and maintaining physically and socially active lifestyles.

Goals

At the conclusion of this program, participants will be able to demonstrate:

    Knowledge and understanding of wellness

    Knowledge and understanding of secondary health risks associated with their primary illnesses and disabilities

    Ability to develop and maintain behavioral action plans for healthy, active lifestyles

    Ability to contribute to peer support groups related to health maintenance

Referral Criteria

Program is seeking women with chronic illnesses and physical disabilities and living in the greater Philadelphia community.* Self-referrals are accepted. Must have a physician's clearance for exercise component of workshops and must provide own transportation.

__Note__: Program is advertised in newspapers, disability organization newsletters, as well as through flyers sent to local MS Society and Independent Living Centers in Delaware Valley. All inquiries and self-referrals were contacted for a preprogram interview. This helps to ensure participants are fully informed and understand the program's expected level of commitment.

Exhibit 9.10: Women and Wellness program protocol (continued)

Content	Process
Workshop I Overview of program Exploring wellness Wellness in women's lives Physically and socially active leisure Personal lifestyle assessment	Discuss three characteristics of wellness and six dimensions of a healthy lifestyle. Illustrate with a diagram attached to a large felt board for visual display Review lifestyle assessment and answer questions about completing it Distribute workbook: "*Charting Your Course*"
Workshop II Review completed lifestyle assessment Set personal priorities for change Develop action plans Review strategies for success	Direct a discussion on thoughts or issues that carried over from last workshop Record priorities on flipchart to show commonalities within group Use large posterboard featuring specific steps in developing action plans Distribute and review personal journal Distribute workbooks on stress management, leisure, relationships, and nutrition
Workshop III Options for being physically and socially active Benefits of exercise Physically active leisure Thera-Bands Exercise action plan Peer support group	Direct a discussion on thoughts or issues that carried over from last workshop Discussion on current and possible forms of physical and social activity Handout guidelines and precautions for exercise Distribute and demonstrate Thera-Bands and provide individual guidance while participants practice various exercises Give out *Active Living Magazine* and program materials Discuss peer support follow-up meetings and come to consensus on first get-together

This program is copyrighted.
Developed in part through a grant from the National Institutes of Health Grant #HD35059-01.

Exhibit 9.11: 12-point checklist for selecting activity-based interventions

☐ What are my clients' interests, strengths, needs, and priorities? How can my clients relate their involvement in this intervention to their goals? Can this intervention be a source of motivation for my clients?

☐ What religious, ethnic, or cultural values, beliefs, and customs of my clients warrant sensitivity? Is there any aspect of this intervention that could be offensive?

☐ What has an activity analysis revealed about the functional demands inherent in the activity that I am using as an intervention?

☐ What are ways to modify or adapt the intervention to clients' specific needs or limitations?

☐ How much contact time is needed for clients to benefit from this intervention? Is there a timing issue related to when these interventions are best used with clients?

☐ Have I involved my clients in selecting the activities that will be used as part of my intervention?

☐ How would I explain the structure, process, and outcomes of the intervention to my clients or their family members? Could I explain it in a manner that makes sense to them and their needs?

☐ What carry-over value exists for this intervention? Can my clients use this intervention in their home or community? Will any carry-over knowledge and skills contribute positively to helping my clients maintain their health through recreation and leisure involvement?

☐ What procedural guidelines, if any, specify ways to use this intervention?

☐ Am I competent to conduct this intervention with my clients? What have I done or should I do to make myself more competent with this intervention?

☐ What specialized training is required or recommended before using this intervention?

☐ What kind of supervision will I need when I use this intervention?

References

Allsop, J. and Dattilo, J. (2000). Therapeutic use of tai chi chuan. In J. Dattilo (Ed.), *Facilitation techniques in therapeutic recreation* (pp. 245–272). State College, PA: Venture Publishing, Inc.

Austin, D. (1999). *Therapeutic recreation: Processes and techniques* (4th ed.). Champaign, IL: Sagamore Publishing.

Austin, D. (2001). Therapeutic recreation process. In D. Austin and M. Crawford (Eds.), *Therapeutic recreation: An introduction* (3rd ed., pp. 45–56). Needham Heights, MA: Allyn & Bacon.

Austin, D. and Crawford, M. (2001). *Therapeutic recreation: An introduction* (2nd ed.). Needham Heights, MA: Allyn & Bacon.

Barr, J. and Taslitz, N. (1970). The influence of back massage on autonomic functions. *Journal of Physical Therapy, 50*, 1679–1689.

Becker, B. and Cole, A. (1997). *Comprehensive aquatic therapy*. Boston, MA: Butterworth-Heinemann.

Berrisford, J. (1995). Implications of pet-facilitated therapy in palliative nursing. *International Journal of Nursing, 1*(2), 86–89.

Broach, E. and Dattilo, J. (2000). Aquatic therapy. In J. Dattilo (Ed.), *Facilitation techniques in therapeutic recreation* (pp. 65–98). State College, PA: Venture Publishing, Inc.

Broach, E., Dattilo, J., and Deavors, M. (2000). Assistive technology. In J. Dattilo (Ed.), *Facilitation techniques in therapeutic recreation* (pp. 99–132). State College, PA: Venture Publishing, Inc.

Broach, E., Dattilo, J., and Loy, D. (2000). Therapeutic use of exercise. In J. Dattilo (Ed.), *Facilitation techniques in therapeutic recreation* (pp. 355–383). State College, PA: Venture Publishing, Inc.

Bullock, C. and Mahon, M. (1997). *Introduction to recreation services for people with disabilities: A person-centered approach*. Champaign, IL: Sagamore Publishing.

Bullock, C., Mahon, M., and Selz, L. (1997). Introduction to therapeutic recreation: An evolving profession. In C. Bullock and M. Mahon (Eds.), *Introduction to recreation services for people with disabilities: A person-centered approach* (pp. 299–344). Champaign, IL: Sagamore Publishing.

burlingame, j. and Skalko, T. (1997). *Glossary for recreation therapists*. Ravensdale, WA: Idyll Arbor.

Carter, M., Van Andel, G., and Robb, G. (1995). *Therapeutic recreation: A practical approach* (2nd ed.). Prospect Heights, IL: Waveland Press.

Coyle, C. and Santiago, M. (1995). Aerobic exercise training and depressive symptomology in adults with physical disabilities. *Archives of Physical Medicine and Rehabilitation, 76*, 647–652.

Dattilo, J. (1999). *Leisure education program planning: A systematic approach* (2nd ed.). State College, PA: Venture Publishing, Inc.

Dattilo, J. (2000). *Facilitation techniques in therapeutic recreation*. State College, PA: Venture Publishing, Inc.

Dattilo, J., Loy, D., and Keeney, R. (2000). Therapeutic use of sports. In J. Dattilo (Ed.), *Facilitation techniques in therapeutic recreation* (pp. 439–475). State College, PA: Venture Publishing, Inc.

Ellmo, W. and Graser, J. (1995). *Adapted adventure activities*. Dubuque, IA: Kendall/Hunt.

Fidler, G. and Velde, B. (1999). *Activities: Reality and symbol*. Thorofare, NJ: Slack.

Gass, M. (1993). The evolution of processing adventure therapy experiences. In M. Gass (Ed.), *Adventure therapy: Therapeutic applications of adventure programming.* (pp. 219–229). Dubuque, IA: Kendall/Hunt.

Groff, D. and Dattilo, J. (2000). Adventure therapy. In J. Dattilo (Ed.), *Facilitation techniques in therapeutic recreation* (pp. 13–40). State College, PA: Venture Publishing, Inc.

Haight, B. and Burnside, I. (1993). Reminiscence and life review: Explaining the differences. *Archives of Psychiatric Nursing, 7*(2), 91–98.

Hesley, J. and Hesley, J. (1998). *Rent two films and let's talk in the morning: Using popular movies in psychotherapy*. New York, NY: John Wiley & Sons.

Hood, C. (2001) Clinical practice guidelines. In N. Stumbo (Ed.), *Professional issues in therapeutic recreation: On competence and outcomes* (pp.189–213). Champaign, IL: Sagamore Publishing.

Johnson, D. and Johnson, F. (1982). *Joining together: Group theory and group skills*. Englewood Cliffs, NJ: Prentice Hall.

Kinney, J., Warren, L., Kinney, T., and Witman, J. (1999). Use of therapeutic modalities and facilitation techniques by therapeutic recreation specialists in the northeastern United States. *Annual in Therapeutic Recreation, 8*, 1–11.

Kinney, T. and Witman, J. (1997). *Guidelines for competency assessment and curriculum in therapeutic recreation: A tool for self-evaluation.* Hattiesburg, MS: American Therapeutic Recreation Association.

Kinney, J., Witman, J., and Kinney, W. (2002). *Therapeutic activities and facilitation techniques: A national study.* Unpublished manuscript.

Kreitzer, M. (1998). Meditation. In M. Snyder and R. Lindquist (Eds.), *Complementary/alternative therapies in nursing* (3rd ed., pp. 123–138). New York, NY: Springer.

Landy, R. (1994). *Drama therapy: Concepts, theories and practices* (2nd ed.). Springfield, IL: Charles C. Thomas.

Luckner, J. and Nadler, R. (1997). *Processing the experience: Strategies to enhance and generalize learning* (2nd ed.). Dubuque, IA: Kendall/Hunt.

Ludins-Katz, F. and Katz, E. (1990). *Art and disabilities: Establishing the creative art center for people with disabilities.* New York, NY: Brookline Books.

Malley, S. and Dattilo, J. (2000). Stress management. In J. Dattilo (Ed.), *Facilitation techniques in therapeutic recreation* (pp. 215–244). State College, PA: Venture Publishing, Inc.

Mason, L. (1985). *Guide to stress reduction.* Berkeley, CA: Celestial Arts.

McCue, K. (1988). Medical play: An expanded perspective. *Children's Health Care, 16*(3), 157–161.

McKenney, A. and Dattilo, J. (2000). Values clarification. In J. Dattilo (Ed.), *Facilitation techniques in therapeutic recreation* (pp. 477–495). State College, PA: Venture Publishing, Inc.

Miller, J. (1992). *Coping with chronic illness: Overcoming powerlessness* (2nd ed.). Philadelphia, PA: F. A. Davis.

Mobily, K. and Verburg, M. (2001). Aquatic therapy in community-based therapeutic recreation: Pain management in a case of fibromyalgia. *Therapeutic Recreation Journal, 35*(1), 57–69.

Mosey, A. (1973). *Activities therapy.* New York, NY: Raven Press.

Murray, S. (1997). *Patient's lived experience of acute physical rehabilitation and recovery contained in a creative journal.* Unpublished doctoral dissertation, Temple University, Philadelphia, PA.

Murray, S. (in press). Finding a friend at the end of your pen: What makes journaling therapeutic for patients and professional growth for students. In C. LeNavenec and L. Bridges (Eds.), *Creating connections between nursing care and the creative art therapies: Expanding the concept of holistic care.* Springfield, IL: Charles C. Thomas.

Nathan, A. and Mirviss, S. (1998). *Therapy techniques using the creative arts.* Ravensdale, WA: Idyll Arbor.

Nickerson, E. and O'Laughlin, K. (1982). *Helping through action: Action-oriented therapies.* Amherst, MA: Human Resource Press.

Nickerson, E. and O'Laughlin, K. (1982). It's fun—but will it work? The use of games as a therapeutic medium for children and adolescents. In E. Nickerson and K. O'Laughlin (Eds.), *Helping through action: Action-oriented therapies* (pp. 117–123). Amherst, MA: Human Resource Press.

O'Keefe, C. (1997). *The role of legacy building in chronic illness.* Paper presented at the NTRS Institute, Salt Lake City, UT.

O'Keefe, C. (2000). *Spirituality and the ethics of caring.* Paper presented at the NTRS Institute, Phoenix, AZ.

Peterson, C. and Stumbo, N. (2000). *Therapeutic recreation program design: Principles and practices* (3rd ed.). Needham Heights, MA: Allyn & Bacon.

Richter, K. and Kaschalk (1996). The future of therapeutic recreation: An existential outcome. In C. Sylvester (Ed.), *Philosophy of therapeutic recreation: Ideas and issues* (Vol. 2, pp. 86–91), Arlington, VA: National Recreation and Park Association.

Sausser, C. and Dattilo, J. (2000). Therapeutic horseback riding. In J. Dattilo (Ed.), *Facilitation techniques in therapeutic recreation* (pp. 273–301). State College, PA: Venture Publishing, Inc.

Schachter, R. (1982). Kinetic psychotherapy in the treatment of families. In E. Nickerson, and K. O'Laughlin (Eds.), *Helping through action: Action-oriented therapies* (pp. 243–250). Amherst, MA: Human Resource Press.

Sheldon, K. and Dattilo, J. (2000). Therapeutic reminiscence. In J. Dattilo (Ed.), *Facilitation techniques in therapeutic recreation* (pp. 303–326). State College, PA: Venture Publishing, Inc.

Smith, K. (1998). Humor. In M. Snyder and R. Lindquist (Eds.), *Complementary/alternative therapies in nursing* (3rd ed., pp. 269–284). New York, NY: Springer.

Snyder, M. (1998). Journal writing. In M. Snyder and R. Lindquist (Eds.), *Complementary/alternative therapies in nursing* (3rd ed., pp. 203–210). New York, NY: Springer.

Snyder, M. and Cheng, W. (1998). Massage. In M. Snyder and R. Lindquist (Eds.), *Complementary/ alternative therapies in nursing* (3rd ed., pp. 63– 74). New York, NY: Springer.

Stumbo, N. (1994/1995). Assessment of social skills for therapeutic recreation intervention. *Annual in Therapeutic Recreation, 5,* 68–82.

Sylvester, C., Voelkl, J., and Ellis, G. (2001). *Therapeutic recreation programming: Theory and practice*. State College, PA: Venture Publishing, Inc.

Uhler, E. (1979). The arts as learning and socialization experiences for the severely handicapped. In C. Sherril (Ed.), *Creative arts for the severely handicapped* (pp. 183–190). Springfield, IL: Charles C. Thomas.

Vickers, A. (1996). *Massage and aromatherapy: A guide for health professionals*. London, UK: Chapman Hall.

Waller, D. and Gilroy, A. (1992). *Art therapy: A handbook*. Philadelphia, PA: Open University Press.

Wang, J. and Snyder, M. (1998). Breathing. In M. Snyder and R. Lindquist (Eds.), *Complementary/ alternative therapies in nursing* (3rd ed., pp. 15– 22). New York, NY: Springer.

West, O. (1990). *The magic of massage: A new and holistic approach*. Mamaroneck, NY: Hastings House Publishers.

Williams, R. and Dattilo, J. (2000). Therapeutic use of humor. In J. Dattilo (Ed.), *Facilitation techniques in therapeutic recreation* (pp. 385–408). State College, PA: Venture Publishing, Inc.

Table 9.3: Mind–body health interventions

Intervention	Description
Aromatherapy	Aromatic essential oils derived from plants may have therapeutic use (Vickers, 1996). Essential oils are applied through massage, used in a warm bath, or inhaled when released in the air through a diffuser or vaporizer. Most oils need to be diluted in a base or carrier oil before use, especially when being applied to the skin. Whether inhaled or absorbed through the skin, aromatherapy works by triggering a biochemical reaction that alters mood and action. For example, lavender encourages stillness, soothes tired muscles and aids sleep, while lime and rosemary restore vitality and invigorate. Aromatherapy requires special knowledge about essential oils and related safety precautions.
Breathing	Proper breathing helps to improve one's mood by improving circulation, normalizing muscle tone, and enhancing respiration (Wang & Snyder, 1998). Breathing instruction is often combined with other interventions such as yoga or relaxation training. For example, breathing techniques can be taught to children and adolescents for use in managing anxiety due to medical procedures. There are a variety of different breathing techniques such as deep breathing, three-part breathing (Mason, 1985), and integrative breathing.
Guided Imagery	Guided imagery uses "positive suggestions to create mental representations of things clients know or fantasize about" (Austin, 1999, p. 75). Imagery employs all six senses—visual, aural, tactile, olfactory, gustatory, and kinesthetic. Guided imagery has been used to help clients plan and initiate problem-solving strategies by redefining their situation and visualizing a desirable future. Imagery is also often used to assist clients with managing stress. In both cases, clients are empowered to control their situations. For example, learning to induce a state of relaxation in the face of stress can be enhanced by visualizing one's most pleasant environment (e.g., the beach), "hearing" the sounds of the ocean, "feeling" the warm grains of sand, and "tasting" a cool drink that refreshes thirst. Imagery has proven effective in controlling nausea among cancer patients. Children with leukemia increased cancer fighting T cells by imagining "Pac Man" racing through their bodies gobbling up cancer cells (Miller, 1992). However, imagery can occasionally cause anxiety or guilt feelings, especially when relaxation cannot be attained. Training and supervision is very important before attempting to use guided imagery to alter a physiological condition.
Humor	Humor can be used therapeutically to achieve specific outcomes such as reductions in anxiety, pain management, and improved immune system functioning (Williams & Dattilo, 2000). Humor often induces laughter, which stimulates the release of endorphins, which are the body's natural pain killers and mood elevators. Humor can also promote social interaction, thereby reducing feelings of isolation. Humor can be classified as spontaneous or formal (Smith, 1998). Spontaneous humor is the type of humor we use daily in our interactions with colleagues, family, and friends. It can involve making fun of situational absurdities in our daily life. Formal humor involves a premeditated act and includes activities such as sharing a joke, cartoon, or humorous story. Purposeful humor interventions can range from a specific humor room containing videos, books, and other resources, to portable humor carts and bulletin boards, or joke-telling hours.
Medical Play	Structured and unstructured play activities may be centered on medical issues, procedures, or equipment. There are a variety of different forms of medical play (McCue, 1988); however, all allow children to explore and express fears and anxieties related to their health condition and medical care, to manage the stress of illness and medical care, and to increase familiarity with and receive accurate information about pending medical procedures. Fantasy medical play involves dolls and other props that allow children to play out events related to their condition (e.g., car accidents, ambulances). Medical art allows children to be creative with medical supplies such as tongue depressors and gauze bandages. Indirect medical play typically involves children using medical equipment for a nonmedical function (e.g., using a syringe as a water pistol, an IV tube as a straw). Finally, there is preprocedural play, which

Table 9.3: Mind–body health interventions (continued)

Intervention	Description
Medical Play (continued)	involves children in role rehearsal/reversal. This form of medical play allows a child to pretend to be a doctor or nurse and to carry out medical procedures on a doll or a puppet using real medical supplies and equipment.
Meditation	Meditation is the self-directed practice for relaxing the body and calming the mind. By helping the client feel "centered," meditation reenergizes the individual physically, mentally, emotionally, and spiritually. During meditation clients systematically and continually focus their attention on a single target—a meaningful word or phrase repeated in rhythm with one's breathing. Some of the more common meditation techniques include Transcendental Meditation, centering prayer, Benson's relaxation response, mindful meditation, and Carrington's clinically standardized meditation (Austin, 1999; Kreitzer, 1998).
Massage	Massage is the manipulation of soft tissue using touch and pressure to relax and heal the body and mind (Barr & Taslitz, 1970). Soothing strokes and gentle rubbing can release tension and heighten physical and psychological comfort. Various techniques include Swedish massage, Esalen massage, neuromuscular massage, Shiatsu, and reflexology (Snyder & Cheng, 1998). Many massage therapists follow an eclectic approach and borrow techniques from different types of massage (West, 1990). Use of therapeutic message requires specialized training.
Relaxation Training	Relaxation techniques focus on helping clients learn to identify and control excess bodily tension that results from stress. Two techniques include progressive relaxation and autogenic training. In progressive relaxation, clients are taught a systematic process of alternating tension and relaxation in a progressive order of muscle groups. By focusing on each isolated muscle group and the sensations associated with muscle tension and relaxation, one can learn, with practice, to induce a sense of relaxation. Autogenic training is similar to progressive relaxation; however, clients are taught to focus on physiological sensations normally regulated by the autonomic nervous system. Thus, they focus on muscle groups and body parts and sensations like weight (e.g., heavy, light), temperature (e.g., warm, cool), and heart rate (e.g., fast, slow). Simple "biofeedback" techniques are sometimes taught such as taking one's pulse prior to and following an autogenic training session. Relaxation training often includes music, imagery, and deep breathing.
Sensory Stimulation	Sensory stimulation interventions involve both sensory training and sensory stimulation (Austin, 1999). Sensory training is used with regressed and confused clients to maintain awareness and optimal functioning. Activities normally involve all six senses (taste, touch, sight, smell, hearing, and bodily movement). Sensory training is often combined with reminiscence and remotivation activities. Sensory stimulation interventions are used with clients who have advanced dementia or with severely brain injured clients in a coma to increase arousal and responsiveness. Intervention sessions can either focus on multiple senses or one in particular. Stimulants can include familiar music, touch, or meaningful objects.
Tai Chi	This traditional Chinese martial art emphasizes body relaxation, mental concentration, and movement coordination. Tai chi involves slow, graceful, learned movement sequences. There are a variety of different styles of tai chi, but all emphasize coordinated, rhythmical movements, relaxed muscles, weight shifting, and deep breathing techniques (Allsop & Dattilo, 2000).
Yoga	Yoga integrates physical posturing, focused breathing, and meditation to promote physical and mental well-being and to integrate mind, body, and spirit. Yoga is also believed to be the union between one's physical being and the "Cosmic Being" (Malley & Dattilo, 2000). When used as a therapeutic intervention, yoga has been shown to reduce anxiety and hypertension and to improve mood, body awareness, and social adaptation.

Table 9.4: Physical activity interventions

Intervention	Description
Aquatics	Aquatic interventions involve active or passive exercise done in water, ranging from swimming and water aerobics to gentle stretching. Aquatic interventions target physical and psychosocial outcomes, including strength, endurance, flexibility and balance, as well as improvements in managing pain, mood disorders, and chronic fatigue. Aquatic activities are particularly beneficial to individuals with disabilities because the buoyancy, increased resistance, and warmth of the water creates a more favorable environment for achieving health benefits than land-based exercise (Becker & Cole, 1997). Various aquatic approaches have been developed for individuals with disabilities. These include swimming, which can be taught using techniques like the Halliwick or Dolan methods, and exercise using Watsu or tai chi methods (see Broach & Dattilo, 2000 for further information). Mobily and Verburg (2001) provide an explanation for aquatic exercise as a method for pain management. Using aquatic activities as interventions requires formal instruction. Specialized training leads to certification in adapted aquatics or aquatics therapy.
Exercise	Exercise includes physical activity that involves planned, structured, and repetitive bodily movements done for the purpose of improving or maintaining one or more components of physical fitness, such as cardiovascular endurance, muscular strength, muscular endurance, or flexibility. Exercise also contributes to psychological outcomes. As such, exercise is a primary component of health promotion programs, and a significant influence on reducing the chances of secondary health problems (e.g., pressure sores, depression) among people with disabilities. *Aerobic exercise* involves activities that require clients to move their muscles in a repetitive, rhythmic, and continuous manner over a period of time (usually at least 5 minutes) and results in increased breathing and heart rate. Popular aerobic exercises include brisk propelling or walking, jogging, and cycling. Specialized programs involving a sequence of exercises have been developed for individuals who use wheelchairs. These are typically called "chair aerobics." *Anaerobic exercise* involves activities that require clients to use their muscles to either work against a resistant object (e.g., pushing their arm against a table top) or move a resistant object (e.g., lifting a weight or stretching a Thera-Band). Anaerobic exercises increase muscle strength and size and improve muscle endurance, balance, coordination, and joint stability. They also improve bone strength and reduce the risks of falling and/or injury to muscles and joints. To achieve these benefits, the resistance or weight must be greater than what the muscles would encounter in their daily tasks. Weight training is the most popular form of anaerobic activity. Other types include isometric and manual resistive exercise. (See Broach, Dattilo & Loy, 2000 and Coyle & Santiago, 1995 for a more complete discussion on the therapeutic use and benefits of exercise.)
Sports	Sports encompass a wide variety of competitive activities that can be engaged in on an individual or team basis. Sport involvement by individuals with disabilities has been associated with a variety of physical and psychological benefits (see Dattilo, Loy & Keeney, 2000). Some sports require modification of equipment and rules; however, in most cases the modifications are limited to those required by a specific functional limitation. Recreation therapists will need to be knowledgeable about adaptive equipment, classification procedures, rules, and modifications associated with different sport activities to introduce, teach, and support their clients' sport involvement. A variety of organizations support and promote sport for individuals with disabilities, including Special Olympics International, Paralympics, the American Association of Adapted Sports Program, and Disability Sports, USA.

Table 9.5: Creative–expressive interventions

Intervention	Description
Arts and Crafts	This intervention involves art produced for utilitarian purposes—the end product serves a pleasant and useful purpose in peoples' homes or lives (Nathan & Mirviss, 1998). These activities may use a combination of art and/or natural mediums. Flower arranging, holiday crafts, macramé, wood carving, metal enameling, rubber stamping, knitting, or weaving are some of the many arts and crafts activities available for use with clients. Arts and crafts are used as clinical interventions to achieve physical, cognitive, social, and emotional outcomes along with facilitating creative expression.
Music	Music interventions involve listening to or creating music, singing, or playing a musical instrument. Music is an effective medium for improving and maintaining sensory motor and perceptual motor skills, as well as social interaction. For example, rhythm instruments can stimulate cognitive and physical functioning for persons with dementia, while drumming can be a creative outlet for adolescents. Whether used individually or with groups, music is often combined with other interventions to enhance effectiveness, including the visual arts, guided imagery, relaxation, reminiscence, and exercise. All genres of music ought to be considered (e.g., folk, jazz, classical, hip-hop, new age), as well as music associated with clients' culture and generation.
Dance/Movement	Dance/movement interventions stimulate physical, social, and emotional expression. Interventions can range from learning or relearning how to dance. Movement activities can help clients with body awareness and self-image, as well as be a source of social interaction. Interpretive dance/movement activities can be used with children who have developmental disabilities to learn concepts like up and down or in and out, as well as provide opportunities to express imagination triggered by a story, poem, or nursery rhyme.
Drama	Acting allows clients to communicate images, messages, characters, or mood that may or may not be a part of their everyday reality (Landy, 1994). Examples include play and character acting (including role-plays), puppetry, mime, and theater games. In play and character acting, clients assume "roles" allowing them to portray fictional characters or themselves. Mime activities are quite similar to play and character acting; however, clients must express their character using only nonverbal means. Puppetry activities include finger puppets, hand puppets, and shadow puppets. Puppetry allows children to disguise themselves, thus it is less threatening than direct self-expression. Theater games encourage spontaneity and experimentation. For example, an object or prop can be passed around a circle of clients and each person acts out an unusual use of the object or tells a creative story about its origins (see Nathan & Mirviss, 1998).
Storytelling	Storytelling is the oral narration of fact or fiction. Stories may be personal tales, folk tales, fairy tales, or religious, moral, or historical stories. They may be read from written literature or they may be created by a group of clients as part of the intervention. When used therapeutically stories can stimulate meaningful conversation and shared recollections. Personal narratives can be the beginning of oral histories and life review.
Visual Arts	This is the formation of products using various art material and artistic technical knowledge (Waller & Gilroy, 1992). Visual arts can focus on aesthetics—the beauty of one's creation. An added therapeutic value is the process involved in creative expression. Using a variety of mediums clients explore their creative impulses and examine their spontaneous expression without regard for the end product. Painting, sculpting, pottery, and drawing are some of the activities that comprise the visual arts.

Table 9.6: Self-discovery/self-expression interventions

Intervention	Description
Adventure Therapy	Also called adventure challenge and adventure-based counseling, these interventions involve physically, socially, and psychologically challenging activities. The challenge comes from real or perceived risks inherent in unfamiliar and novel activities that encourage effort and problem solving. Adventure therapy activities include individual and group games and initiative activities, or outdoor/wilderness experiences. Popular adventure therapy activities include "trust activities (e.g., trust walks, falls), cooperative activities (e.g., lap sit), group problem-solving tasks (e.g., human knot), initiative games (e.g., electric fence and wall), low rope courses (involving maintaining balance while moving across a course made of rope, wire, and wooden beams constructed a few feet off the ground), and high adventure activities (e.g., rappelling, caving high ropes courses, zip lines, tree climbs, kayaking, wilderness camping)" (Austin, 1999, p. 93). The essence of adventure/challenge has been adapted for clients with physical and neurological limitations (Ellmo & Graser, 1995). Specialized training in adventure-based counseling techniques is important, especially since effective interventions require competence in the technical and safety aspects of the activities, and skills in processing clients' experiences. Training is available from several organizations. Most notably, Project Adventure, Inc. provides a full range of training, educational and technical materials and supplies, and consultations.
Bibliotherapy	Intervention that uses reading materials such as short stories, novels, plays, poems, and other written accounts of human experiences. These materials allow clients to identify with and relate to the events or underlying messages and to appreciate that others share similar experiences. For example, adolescents may read poetry and discuss their interpretations or use a story as a metaphor for their own life circumstances. Likewise, persons dealing with chronic illnesses can read the accounts of others who also struggled with managing their illness. A related procedure is the use of videos or films to provoke thoughts, feelings, and discussion (Hesley & Hesley, 1998). Therapists select readings or videos based on client needs or issues. These materials and subsequent reactions are used to help clients find comfort, support and insight into their own problems and emotional responses.
Journaling	Creative intervention process where clients record their thoughts, feelings, and reflections in a journal. "The very process of writing may lead a writer to discoveries about him/herself that lie hidden from conscious thought" (Nathan & Mirviss, 1998, p. 235). The intentional and purposeful use of reflective writing contributes to physical, emotional, and spiritual outcomes. Journaling is used with a wide variety of clients to promote self-reflection, self-discovery, and personal growth. For instance, clients can use reflective writing and pictures to chronicle and find meaning in their rehabilitation experience (Murray, 1997, in press). It is also sometimes used as an adjunct to cognitive–behavioral interventions to promote insight into antecedents or triggers for problematic behaviors. Various writing activities are used in journaling interventions, including free writing, poetry, structured or formatted journaling (often involving sentence completion activities), or intensive journaling (Snyder, 1998). For further information contact the Center for Journal Therapy, Arada, CO.
Reminiscence/ Life Review	Used primarily with older adults, therapeutic reminiscence facilitates an integrative reflection and valuing of one's life. In therapeutic reminiscence memories are evoked and reconstructed in an effort to stimulate cognition and reaffirm the client's dignity and self-worth. Reminiscence activities typically include props or visual aids to stimulate memories, such as pictures, old songs, films, and news accounts of historical events of the past. A particular type of reminiscence activity is life review, which is a critical analysis of one's past (particularly unresolved conflicts) with the purpose of integrating them and achieving a sense of worth, coherence, and reconciliation (Haight & Burnside, 1993). A variation on life review is "legacy building" whereby individuals who are terminally ill narrate stories of their past onto audiotapes and videotapes (O'Keefe, 1997). Meaning is made of one's memories and tangibly shared with family and others through the audio or videotape.
Values Clarification	Process of clarifying values and attitudes pertinent to choices and actions associated with various parts of a person's life, such as health and leisure. As such, values clarification is an important part of leisure education interventions. Clients are encouraged to explore what is important to them and to develop their own value system that will guide their behavior. Typical values clarification activities include structured individual and group exercises involving writing, value sheets containing statements and clarifying questions, and group discussions (McKenney & Dattilo, 2000).

Table 9.7: Social skills interventions

Intervention	Description
Assertiveness Training	Assertiveness training assists clients with distinguishing between aggressive, passive, passive-aggressive, and assertive behaviors. Clients are encouraged to explore beliefs that stop them from being assertive and are taught a variety of techniques (e.g., making "I statements") that they can use to be more assertive in their social relationships. Typically conducted with groups of clients, assertiveness training involves structured activities, including board games, card games, and role-playing.
Anger Management	Anger management interventions assist clients with learning how to cope with and express anger in socially acceptable ways. Using cognitive–behavioral approaches, clients are encouraged to explore components of anger, including thoughts, bodily responses, and attack responses aroused when they are feeling threatened (McKenney & Dattilo, 2000). By understanding their reactions when threatened, clients are better able to explore alternative behavioral approaches for managing their anger. Interventions aim at learning to channel anger, thereby increasing self-esteem and respect for the rights of others. Anger management interventions use structured activities such as board games, role-plays, and systematic thinking strategies that are learned, rehearsed, and applied in social situations.
Resocialization	Resocialization interventions "increase awareness of self and others by helping clients to form relationships, establish friendships, and discover new interests" (Austin, 1999, p. 119). Used primarily with isolated geriatric clients, resocialization involves group discussions facilitated by the group leader, which focus on building relationships and living together in their social community. Simple, undemanding activities are used to counteract social isolation.
Remotivation	Remotivation activities are used with isolated, somewhat confused clients (including those with brain injuries) who need encouragement and support to rediscover interests and reengage with the world around them. Remotivation activities use a group structure, oriented around a theme or topic, and pass through five sequential phases, including setting a climate of acceptance, using a story to introduce the theme as a bridge to reality, using questions or props to stimulate sharing the world we live in, further exploration of clients' appreciation of the work of the world based on their experiences, and supportive and encouraging comments from the leader to end the session in a climate of appreciation.
Reality Orientation	Reality orientation is used with clients who are confused or disoriented. This intervention involves social interactions with orientation to basic facts such as time, place, names, daily events, and places/things in the client's environment. When conducted as a group intervention, therapists record basic reality orientation information on a reality orientation board. These boards may also contain information such as the weather, upcoming meals, events, or holidays. This information is reviewed with clients through social conversation, and if clients are confused they are cued to use the board to assist them with responding correctly. During reality orientation, therapists use a variety of activities designed to help diminish confusion in clients such as identifying staff, familiar objects, and/or places related to activities of daily living (e.g., restrooms, cooking utensils, recreation activity areas).

Table 9.8: Nature-based interventions

Intervention	Description
Animal-assisted Therapy	Animal-assisted therapy encompasses interventions that utilize animals and includes animal visitations, pets, and the use of animals as an active participant in therapy sessions, commonly referred to as pet therapy or pet-facilitated therapy (Berrisford, 1995). Interactions with animals can promote feelings of acceptance and can be reliable sources of enjoyment and pleasure. A wide variety of animals, including dogs, rabbits, birds, cats, and dolphins are used to help clients benefit physically, cognitively, socially, and emotionally. Animal use ranges from friendly visits at nursing homes to specific functional improvement programs where animal, client, and therapist interact to stimulate communication, motor, and cognitive performance. A related but specialized variation of animal-assisted therapy is *therapeutic horseback riding*. A passive form of riding called *hippotherapy* has been shown to improve vestibular, proprioceptive, tactile, communication, and cognitive functioning. Additionally, horseback riding has been an effective medium for developing social skills, self-esteem, and various academic skills (Sausser & Dattilo, 2000). More specific information about pet-facilitated therapy and therapeutic horseback riding can be obtained from the Delta Society and the North American Riding for the Handicapped Association (NARHA). Both organizations provide information and support for program development and specialized training.
Horticulture	Horitculture interventions use plant material and indoor and outdoor gardens to achieve therapeutic outcomes associated with cognitive and physical functioning and emotional well-being. Horticulture activities have the added benefit of humanizing sterile institutional settings, and the flowers and vegetables that result from horticultural activities can be used in other activities like cooking and crafts. Horticulture interventions can be as simple as watering potted plants to more complex interventions that involve planting and caring for indoor and outdoor gardens. Adapted horticulture tools and other gardening aids are available, such as long handled tools and raised garden beds. Therapists interested in using horticulture activities as part of their intervention options need to be knowledgeable about plants and plant care. Additional training in the therapeutic use of horticulture is available from the American Horticulture Therapy Association.

Table 9.9: Education-based interventions

Intervention	Description
Assistive Technology Training	Assistive technology training and education involves activities ranging from exposure to and awareness of assistive devices to actual training programs for clients in the use of assistive devices to support play and recreation. While assistive devices can be used as needed in all TR interventions to accommodate clients, assistive technology and training programs are specifically designed to help clients acquire or improve functional skills through the use of assistive devices and be self-determining in their play and recreation. Assistive technology devices that support these outcomes include switches, computers, virtual reality, augmentative and alternative communication systems, and video games (Broach, Dattilo & Deavors, 2000).
Community Reintegration	Community reintegration interventions assist clients with returning to the community following treatment for a medical or behavioral health issue. These interventions typically include learning functional skills needed to interact with one's physical and social environment and activities that allow clients to apply these functional behaviors in natural community settings. An important component of these programs is environmental resources (e.g., agencies, facilities, and people) that support recreation and leisure pursuits. As such, community reintegration intervention programs often incorporate leisure education.
Family/caregiver Education	Family/caregiver education programs are used as part of comprehensive client care, particularly in facilities caring for children and elderly persons. These TR interventions use a variety of materials (e.g., print, video) to inform caregivers about illnesses and disabilities and ways to promote play, recreation, and leisure in the lives of their loved one. These education programs also focus on the role of recreation and leisure in the lives of caregivers since this issue has a direct bearing on their capacities to care.
Leisure Education	Leisure education has been defined as "an individualized and contextualized process through which a person develops an understanding of self and leisure and identifies and learns the cluster of skills necessary to participate in freely chosen activities that lead to an optimally satisfying life" (Bullock and Mahon, 1997, p. 381). Several models of leisure education describe a process of exploring leisure attitudes and values, and teaching recreation and leisure skills (e.g., Dattilo, 1999, Peterson & Stumbo, 2000). All models share the following key elements: leisure awareness and appreciation, knowledge of leisure resources, development of leisure participation skills including activity skills, decision-making skills, and social skills.

Chapter 10
Incorporating the Environment

Guided Reading Questions

After reading this chapter, you should be able to answer the following:

- How does a person's environment affect his or her behavior?
- What is meant by the physical, social, and organizational components of the environment?
- What is dehumanizing about hospitals, institutions, nursing homes, and other so-called "care" environments?
- How can a TR professional humanize a care environment?
- What does contextual training mean, and how does this occur in TR clinical practice?
- What are some developmental needs of clients that can be supported or impeded by their environments?

Introduction

Health and human services ought to be designed with a holistic view of individuals as part and product of their environment. Any attempt to help clients learn, adapt, and grow is incomplete without fully understanding the environment in which the individual functions. Likewise, quality of life cannot be understood, improved, or maintained without consideration of the physical and social elements of the environment. This is known as an "ecological perspective" of human behavior. In Chapter 3 we asserted that an ecological perspective ought to guide TR practice. We presented several examples of TR professionals working with clients, their families, and other community service providers to ensure that home and community environments supported clients' recreation and leisure involvement. In this chapter we continue with an application of the ecological perspective in clinical practice as it occurs in specific health and human service settings.

The theories described in Chapter 5 and the TR clinical process described in Chapter 4 and Chapter 6 underscore the importance of the environment in shaping people's attitudes and behavior. If TR interventions are going to help clients improve their physical, cognitive, emotional, social, and spiritual health, then environmental influences must be addressed. Thus, an essential function of practice is to combine activities with environments that have been designed to help clients learn, adapt, and grow. This principle pertains to all environments where clinical practice occurs. This includes group homes, psychiatric day programs and social clubs, adult day centers, nursing homes, hospitals, clients' homes, and the community at large. We begin this chapter with an overview of the environment's impact on human behavior and then present a variety of ways in which the physical and social environment can be incorporated into clinical practice. Although our examples primarily represent hospitals and nursing homes, the four conclusions or propositions identified in this chapter can be applied to any environment where clients are served through TR.

The Environment and Human Behavior

The environment is a composite of seven elements, each having the potential to be a positive or negative force on human emotion, comfort, and behavior (Compton, 1992). These include *natural* (e.g., air, water), *built* (e.g., objects and structures created by people and technology), *ambient* (e.g., temperature, humidity), *temporal* (e.g., mechanical, psychological or physiological references to time), *regulatory* (e.g., laws, rules, regulations), *communicative* (e.g., oral and written exchange of information), and *sociocultural* (e.g., people, mores, traditions, rituals) components. These components interact to create a total context for providing care. Each service delivery environment has a *physical* dimension comprised of natural, built and ambient components, a *social* dimension involving communicative and sociocultural components, and an *organizational* dimension focused on the regulatory component.

All care environments can be described in terms of their physical attributes, the level and complexity of social interaction, and the overall care philosophy, policies and procedures that regulate what, when, and how things occur. Likewise, when home health care is provided, the client's home becomes the care environment. This environment could be described in terms of its physical properties (e.g., size, number of rooms, location of bathroom, clutter and trip hazards, access to community services), the number and types of people and pets who reside there (e.g., relatives, interaction patterns), communication resources like telephone, television, and Internet, and the structure that regulates what goes on in this home (e.g., division of chores, meal schedule, day and evening routines).

Environmental influences on thought, feelings, and behavior are quite apparent in health and human service settings. The intuitive notion that a room with a view would be more pleasing for hospitalized patients was actually tested in research. Ulrich (1984) examined the medical records of 23 matched pairs of patients and found that those who had a hospital room with a window recovered more quickly and required less medication than those who did not. Coping with any stressful situation involves effort to find a sense of balance with one's surroundings, so that a reasonable degree of stimulation, relaxation, comfort, and belonging is experienced. Being able to regulate transactions with the environment provides a sense of control and competence, which is important to life quality as well as coping with stress.

The environment–behavior relationship can be explained theoretically. It begins with Kurt Lewin's concept of "life space." His explanation of person–environment transaction was represented in the formula, B = f(PE). According to Lewin (1951), behavior (B) is a function (f) of an interaction between personality (P) and the environment (E). As we interact with the environment, we make judgments or interpretations about the demands on us and our abilities to respond. A person's capability to respond to the environment is termed "fit." Nahemov and Lawton (1973) explained environmental fit in terms of a balance between an individual's capabilities and the "press" or demands of the environment. Kahana (1975) contended that individuals seek to find a sense of "congruence" between characteristics of their environment and their needs and preferences. When there is a mismatch between environmental demands and individual competency, either boredom or stress results. In contrast, psychosocial adaptation and improved quality of life are more likely to occur when there is a fit between needs, wants, and expectations and the resources in the environment.

Environmental congruence, or fit, is a judgment made by individuals according to their needs and their expectations. For instance, Parmelee and Lawton (1990) (as cited in McGuire, Boyd & Tedrick, 1996) contend that the dichotomous issues of autonomy and

security are at the core of person–environment relations, especially for older adults. Adults in nursing homes, for example, simultaneously need to exercise some control in their daily living and yet feel secure that others (i.e., staff) will take care of them. When there is no sense of fit, an individual who feels competent and in control may exert effort to change environmental conditions; others who feel less competent and thus less control will accept the situation as unchangeable and adjust their self-perceptions.

An additional option is for the individual to accept the support of others. According to Steinfeld and Danford (1997), the environment can be considered a prosthetic support for functional independence. "In contemporary rehabilitation practice, with its emphasis on independent living, a common intervention would be to provide environmental support to achieve or maintain competence in the face of stress" (p. 39). Examples of environmental supports include barrier-free access to the outdoors, remote control devices for lights, stereo, and television, and energy-efficient sport wheelchairs. Each supports independent functioning.

☆• • •Thinking Trigger

What experiences have you had in which the environment influenced your behavior, feelings of competence, and sense of belonging?   • • •☆

Based on a review of the literature about environmental influences on human behavior, four basic conclusions can be drawn. Together, they provide direction for examining the relative quality of environments where clients live, work, play, and receive care. Also, these conclusions can be used as a guide for creating and modifying environments so that they will be conducive to learning, adaptation, and growth. The remainder of this chapter reflects these four conclusions and contains examples of ways recreation therapists use the environment as an integral element in their clinical interventions, care, and support of clients. The four conclusions drawn from the literature regarding environmental influences are:

Design features of built environments influence a sense of mastery and competence (efficacy). The physical and social environment either inhibits or enhances autonomous action. Opportunities to make choices and exercise control, and the existence of adaptive equipment suitable for varied functional abilities are the mark of environments that promote feelings of mastery and competence.

Individuals process information from the environment and modify their behavior to find congruence and a sense of "fit." Care environments can unwittingly reinforce stigmatizing messages of illness and disability by emphasizing what clients cannot do, as opposed to strengths and capabilities. In contrast, environments that share responsibility with clients and provide numerous and varied opportunities for clients to be active, engaged, and vital reinforce messages of health and personal dignity.

Design features of built environments affect communication and social contact. Environments either encourage or discourage human contact. Defined places to interact, printed materials, and signage are critical environmental elements that influence human interactions. Environments help people to regulate the amount of social contact they have by offering spaces for privacy and social retreat.

Environments provide models for social learning. All environments have a social dimension that provides opportunities for individuals to support one another and learn from one another. Healthy, growth-promoting environments celebrate client abilities and structure opportunities for them to contribute to the greater good of the whole.

To be effective in TR clinical practice, you need to be prepared to modify the physical, social, and organizational dimensions of existing environments, and advocate for environmental qualities that support clients' health, leisure, and quality of life.

Humanizing Care Environments

In practice TR professionals try to *humanize* care environments to maximize therapeutic gains for clients; however, this challenge can be daunting. Upon walking into a hospital, a psychiatric unit, a nursing home, or any other place where people receive health or human services, one immediately forms an impression of the type of care that can be expected. While it is possible that caring compassion and a commitment to the well-being of clients can transcend the most impoverished environment, there is little question that environmental features have a great deal of influence on the individuals being served.

Generally, design standards for health care facilities reflect the primary orientation of Western medicine—to treat and correct medical conditions. Facilities are typically designed for efficient and effective medical care and for the convenience of the care providers (staff) rather than the care recipients (clients). Traditionally, the client's biomedical needs were the only thing considered in planning these facilities. Fortunately, the design of care environments is improving, and there is greater awareness of environmental influences on healing, health, and quality of life. Consider the Crozer-Keystone Health System's advertisement in **Exhibit 10.1**. Providing patients with lush greenery and soothing sounds of falling water is impressive, yet even simple environmental enhancements can be effective. A greenhouse and a fully equipped horticulture center can be found in some facilities; most other places can still use simpler yet effective modifications like portable gardening carts, posters of nature scenes, or small potted plants for each room.

☆• • •Thinking Trigger

When a family member or visitor walks into the facility where you have interned or worked, what impressions might they form about the quality of care? How can therapeutic recreation practice influence these impressions? • • •☆

Similarly, nursing homes were traditionally designed with an image of the resident as a person "at the end of the line," frail, and near death. The primary intention of nursing home environments was custodial care of the elderly. Many newer facilities are now being designed with greater attention to the full range of client care needs. Nevertheless, even with better design features, health care and human service agencies need professionals who know how to incorporate the social and organizational dimensions of the environment

Exhibit 10.1 Advertisement about health care environment

Can the sound of water help cure cancer?

At Crozer-Chester Medical Center we believe in the power of medical technology, research, and equipment in the fight against cancer. But we also believe in the healing properties of nature and the human spirit. So we have designed the new 40,000-square-foot Crozer Regional Cancer Center as a place that recognizes the power of both mind and body in treating cancer. The latest technology will coexist with an environment of waterfalls, green plants, and serene spaces that allows patients to receive treatment in one calm and quiet place.

along with improved physical designs. The responsibility to make sure that environments benefit clients holistically mostly falls in the domain of therapeutic recreation. You must be willing to help administrators recognize how the environment can help rather than hinder psychosocial well-being, thereby complimenting biomedical care. Administrators of long-term care environments have counted on recreation therapists to structure the facility in ways that promote residents' dignity and self-worth. In essence then, your work involves a deliberate and purposeful use of health and human service environments in ways that embrace the humanity of the clients.

What does it mean *to humanize* care environments? Basically, it means seeing the *person* in the *patient* or *client*. No one is sick all of the time, in all aspects of self. Despite the most serious of illnesses, every individual has something of value, a worthiness that deserves dignifying. Before individuals became ill, or were placed in long-term care, they came from somewhere else that gave them a sense of identify and meaning. Those past environments represent their "psychoenvironmental history" (Howell, 1998), and this history will influence their responses to the care environment. Keller (1997) encouraged recreation therapists to request newly admitted clients in nursing homes and adult day centers to bring a cherished possession with them. Most clients will readily identify an item such as a photograph, religious items, or symbolic jewelry. Keller reported that researchers found "cherished possessions may serve as 'anchor points' that facilitate adaptation to new environments and provide historical continuity, comfort, and a sense of belonging" (p. 88). Indeed, each client has a story to tell, and it is a story that never begins and ends with his or her medical diagnosis. Cherished possessions can be creatively incorporated into reminiscence and life-review activities, and they can be used in intergenerational programs. Likewise, familiar, meaningful possessions can be a source of comfort for other clients as well, such as a child's special blanket or an adult's bathrobe. These items reveal the person's humanity in spite of their temporary role as client.

To humanize care also means to appreciate the strengths and capabilities of the person and to allow an expression of these assets in order to balance the obvious limitations that care environments magnify. It means creating opportunities for individuals to meet their basic human needs for affection, recognition, and social affiliation. *Humanizing care* means to honor one's "personhood" by truly respecting the person's right to self-determination, informed consent, privacy,

and confidentiality. This means making sure that organizational procedures allow clients to be partners in their own care. Finally, *humanizing* care means recognizing and respecting the individual's developmental needs and preoccupations, as well as their cultural background. Fidler and Velde (1999) identified 10 human needs that can be met by the physical, social, and organizational characteristics of one's environment. These needs (see **Table 10.1**) can be addressed through a wide range of activities potentially available in the environment.

Environmental Modification

Humanizing care environments occurs through environmental modification. Caring environments ought to be designed to maximize comfort and healing. Yet, a major criticism of care environments, as seen *Through the Patients' Eyes*, is that they can be far from this ideal (Gerteis, Edgman-Levitan, Daley & Delbanco, 1993). Quite often, environments that are intended to give quality care are overly medicalized and impersonal, or they are stark, institutional, and uninviting. Either way, they can be a major deterrent to the healing process and to being physically and socially active. As mentioned earlier, even though some newer facilities are designed in a more "client-friendly" manner, recreation therapists are in a position to modify or manipulate environments in ways that improve the chances for healing and recovery. Recreation therapists can use creativity in transforming overly medicalized or institutionalized settings by simple modifications and clever "re-engineering." This includes modifications to the physical, social, and organizational dimensions of the environment.

Modifying Physical and Organizational Components

As a beginning point for you to consider, we present six common approaches to using physical and organizational features of the environment so that clients' bio/psycho/social/spiritual needs are supported. These approaches can be modified or adapted to various care settings, and these approaches and their examples are not all-inclusive.

Provide Useful Information in Printed and Electronic Formats

An obvious example would be calendars informing clients of daily, weekly, and monthly events. While posting a calendar in the nursing home unit is a regulatory mandate, to humanize the environment recreation therapists ought to make sure these calendars are visually attractive and that clients and family members can easily locate and read them. Newsletters keep the community of staff and clients informed, and can be planned, prepared, and distributed by clients. Clients and their families can benefit from informational brochures that describe resources in the agency and nearby community for their independent use (e.g., gift shops, VCR and video rental opportunities, park benches, places of worship for quiet and solace). Coloring books that include illustrated information about hospitalization and medical procedures are helpful to children and parents alike. The facility's closed-circuit television can be used to inform, guide, and encourage attention to play, recreation, and leisure needs of the client and family. As a final example, the Patient Activities Department at the National Institutes of Health (NIH) developed a brochure for people who sat idly in outpatient clinics. The *Creative Approaches to Waiting* brochure was filled with lots of developmentally appropriate suggestions for managing boredom and anxiety while waiting for appointments. Similar informational brochures can also be used to help clients and families plan ways to control the environmental impact of long hospital stays, recuperative periods at home, or relocation to nursing homes or assistive living facilities.

Creatively Display Recreation-Related Products and Materials

Clients sometimes make beautiful art projects that deserve to be displayed. A display case containing a variety of completed projects can call attention to clients' creativity and skills, and how these abilities and talents can be expressed through recreation. Also, attractively displayed materials can be a motivator for active involvement. Linda Simeca of the Clinical Center, NIH, arranged to display prints of various artists in hallways and included placards that gave information about the life and times of the artist (e.g., Monet, Van Gogh, Wyeth) and the school of art represented (e.g., impressionist). Linda worked with cardiac rehabilitation patients who were expected to walk progressively further distances each day. Linda developed a guidebook for clients so they could keep a log of their "art appreciation" project and the distance they

Table 10.1: Human needs that can be supported by the environment (Fidler & Velde, 1999)

Autonomy	To be self-determining and as self-dependent as personal needs and capacities define
Volition	To have alternatives and opportunities to act on one's choice
Individuality	To know one's uniqueness, to distinguish self from others, and to confirm one's interests and skills
Affiliation	To have a sense of belonging and to experience interdependence
Consensual validation	To receive feedback from one's actions (with objects and people) that clarify and acknowledge one's contributions
Predictability	To have a sense of order in one's life and the opportunity to limit ambiguity and uncertainty
Self-efficacy	To be able to make things happen and have a sense of competence
Adventure	To have opportunities to explore, to discover, to experiment, and to risk
Accommodation	To be free from physical and mental harm and to live in an environment that tolerates and supports limitations as well as capabilities
Reflection	To have respite from activity and a chance to review, reflect, and contemplate

walked each day. The art transformed a hospital floor by creating an on-site gallery of attractive artwork, and clients had an incentive and aesthetically pleasing diversion as they walked each day.

Humor Rooms and Displays

The healing power of humor is being recognized by a wide range of health professionals, including doctors, nurses, and psychologists. Ham (2000) offers numerous suggestions for recreation therapists to incorporate humor into the entire environments. For example, humor bulletin boards can feature cartoons, jokes, and other brief humorous stories for clients and their families. "Laughter wagons" can be moved from room to room offering clients humorous videotapes, audiotapes, and magazines for their personal use and enjoyment. In some settings dedicated "humor rooms" are available where clients can spend some recovery time enjoying videotapes and other humorous materials. Props, like clown noses or make-up, hand puppets, balloons, and other "mirth makers" can be used by clients and families (Hafen, Karren, Frandsen & Smith, 1996).

Self-Expression ("Graffiti") Stations

Everyone involved in a care environment is loaded with thoughts and feelings that deserve opportunities for expression. Graffiti stations offer a place for spontaneous (and anonymous) expression. Large blackboards with chalk or white boards with dry erase markers (or even large rolls of butcher paper) can be placed in a central location for clients to express themselves, whether to vent feelings or try their hand in poetry. This can be an interesting repository for thoughts and feeling that might not be known otherwise, and a barometer for issues that might be going on for clients on a psychiatric unit, in a day treatment program, or in a group home. Of course, encouraging free expression does open the possibilities for angry, hurtful, and profane comments. Usually there are rules restricting such comments.

Personalized Space

As mentioned earlier, photographs and other items of personal significance, and things brought from home provide a sense of continuity. Children can personalize their space with "cherished" objects (e.g., special blanket, stuffed animal) to add a sense of comfort and security. A favorite chair or afghan can create a home-like ambience for older adults. Public displays of such items help tell the person's "story" and often stimulate conversation. Personalizing space also helps to reduce the psychologically damaging "placelessness" characteristic of long-term care environments (Howell, 1998). Even short hospital stays can be more personal when clients have shelves and bulletin boards in their rooms to display cards and other items from home that lend familiarity and comfort (Walker, 1993). Similarly, MedCare Designs started a program that allowed children to "borrow" different posters for their hospital rooms, thereby decorating according to their interests (Iwanicki, 1999).

Nurturing through Nature

The healing and comforting qualities of nature contributes to the "care" in care environments. The outdoors can be brought indoors by arranging birdfeeders and birdbaths in clear view from windows, as well as flowers in window boxes. Horticulture rooms provide opportunities for intervention, socialization, and pleasure. Simple things like seasonal murals, videotapes on nature, and small potted plants for each client can be sources of enjoyment and comfort. Aquariums offer pleasant diversion, while domestic animals and birds, whether periodic visitors or permanent residents of the environment, offer a chance to give and receive nurturing care. Additionally, being outdoors in natural settings that surround facilities can be one of the pleasures clients find in many TR programs. Outdoor gardens and walking paths can lend comforting familiarity for some, while makeshift putting greens can be a motivator for others. On a larger scale, adventure-based counseling programs that involve ropes courses and group initiative activities rely on the natural setting as an essential dimension of therapeutic challenge for clients.

These six commonly recommended approaches to modifying physical and organizational components can help create a humanized care environment conducive to health. These same environmental modifications can be extended to home environments in order to improve continued recovery after discharge or to maintain independence. Indeed, recreation therapists are increasingly involved in helping clients prepare for discharge by evaluating the home environment and making recommendations for changes. Chapter 7 provided a sample of issues for consideration when evaluating clients' homes. The ultimate intention is to reduce the chances of "excess disability" (as discussed in Chapter 3) and to maximize opportunities for recreation and leisure involvement.

Modifying the Social Component

All care environments have an array of people with distinct contributions to make to the life of the environment. This includes clients, family, friends, acquaintances, service providers, or others. In the 1970s inpatient psychiatric care was delivered in a *therapeutic milieu*. These therapeutic communities recognized the potential value in *all* human interactions. Often it was the role of the recreation therapist to learn of some special interests of a staff member and arrange to incorporate these abilities into the overall milieu. For instance, a psychiatric nurse knew a lot about hair care and make-up, and believed that personal appearance and presentation had much to do with self-esteem issues. Together with the recreation therapist, a self-image program was developed for female clients to learn ways to present themselves with confidence through attentive grooming. While the average length of stay in psychiatric hospitals today is around 5–7 days, the importance of the social milieu continues to be recognized, and all care providers have an obligation to collaborate on meaningful environmental interventions and modifications that promote effective care.

Recreation therapists also create opportunities for clients to be helpful and supportive of each other. This ranges from informal opportunities for clients to socialize and form a temporary support network, to more structured therapeutic intervention groups where client interaction actually becomes a central part of the change process. Within this range, clients have opportunities to gain from relationships they form with others. They can serve as models, coaches, and confidants. Some rehabilitation programs train former clients to be volunteers and to offer peer counseling. Recall the discussion of peer modeling as a way to increase a client's self-efficacy beliefs. That is, when clients have exposure to others like them doing things they also want to do, they can increase their beliefs that it is possible. At the Community Hospital of Los Gatos Rehabilitation Center in California, former clients serve as volunteers in recreational therapy groups.

> While the volunteer does not assist in hands-on clinical duties, he/she may participate in inpatient recreational therapy groups. Having a volunteer sit in on such a group in which patients perform therapist-led upper extremity exercises and tabletop activities motivates patients; they are working with someone who

has successfully gone through the rehab process. (Tomczyk, 1998, p. 28)

In some cases, recreation therapists work with the client's natural support network to modify the environment so that clients have the necessary accommodations and supports to live fully and function optimally. Members of the support network are often pivotal factors in helping clients change and grow. Very often, people in the client's life must change in order to support the client and ensure continued gains. Working with members of a client's natural support network (i.e., family, friends) ought to begin during hospitalization. With the client's permission and as time permits, family and friends can be incorporated into the care program so that their familiarity with, for example, physical transfers, cognitive cueing, adaptive equipment, and the like will be an added support for the client. Chapter 3 contained other examples of how recreation therapists worked in clients' homes with spouses and other caregivers. Also, recreation therapists serve as life skills coaches, helping clients adjust to the physical, social, and organizational demands inherent in home and work environments and the larger community. In all of these cases, the aim is to modify elements of the social environment so that clients get the best support possible.

Care environments can offer a supportive social component to family members as well as clients. This primarily comes in the form of social support programs, designed to facilitate four types of *social support* (Cohen & Willis, 1985).

- Informational support (advice and guidance)
- Emotional support (comfort care and security)
- Esteem support (feedback that increases feelings of competence)
- Social integration or belongingness (shared identity and commonalties)

Family support groups can use recreation as an enjoyable supplement. For example, families involved in pediatric oncology treatment can have their social support enhanced by sharing relaxing diversions from their stress. It is important to note, however, that incorporating "family" may mean more than the nuclear family. For many, family includes extended family members as well as the immediate family. Also, grandparents may be the primary care providers and guardians of children. Obviously, organizational policies and regulations need to be sensitive to such cultural differences (Ma & Henderson, 1999). Recreation therapists will have to be culturally competent in addressing organizational responses to clients and families of diverse cultural backgrounds.

Finally, creating activity space that clients can freely access and use facilitates healthy social interactions in health and human service environments. In addition to having designated activity areas that are supervised, care environments can be enlivened with other spaces that promote creative and adaptive behaviors. With some simple "environmental re-engineering," recreation therapists can create *social nooks* by rearranging chairs around a coffee table with magazines, photo albums, and the like. These social nooks can be spontaneous rest stops for clients and their visitors. They can also be comfortable areas for clients to use for semiprivate conversations, as an alternative to larger, more public spaces or the isolation of their rooms.

• • •Thinking Trigger

> Many suggestions and examples have been provided about modifying care environments. What other ideas came to mind as you read this section? • • •

Using Care Environments for "Contextual Training"

Environments can also be used as part of TR interventions when they involve "*contextual training.*" Contextual training can occur in health and human service facilities as well as in the natural community. Essentially, contextual training involves placing clients in situations (context) that approximates the real physical and social situations that will constitute their daily living. Contextual training intends to evoke a response in clients such that they must use their physical, cognitive, or social skills, thereby reinforcing skill training that has occurred elsewhere. The more the practice situations approximate reality, the greater the chance for skill transfer and generalization. Contextual training, however, involves more than functional skill development. With encouragement and support from therapists and each other, clients can use the concrete and tangible feedback they get to explore the accuracy of their environmental perceptions and their emotional responses to these experiences. Contextual training directly reflects self-efficacy theory in that clients

experience changes in their sense of competence through *performance accomplishments*—the most effective way to change efficacy beliefs.

Contextual Training in the Facility

Two facility-based contextual training examples involving TR come from physical rehabilitation programs. The first program is known as "Easy Street," which has been used extensively throughout the country. For example, Magee Rehabilitation Hospital, a regional spinal cord injury treatment center located in Philadelphia, PA has a rooftop training environment complete with a car that clients use to practice transferring, sidewalk curbs (with and without curb cuts), and an automated-teller machine. A variation of Easy Street is located at Shriner's Hospital for Children and is managed by the recreation therapy department. This training environment includes rows of theatre style seats for wheelchair transfer practice, and simulated fruit and vegetable bins found in grocery stores (the angled ones where it seems once you select some fruit, the whole stack starts tumbling). These facilities, and others like them around the country, offer clients opportunities to learn real skills that will be transferred to community and home situations. Independence Square "is designed and built to provide clinical staff, patients, and their care givers opportunities to experience aspects of everyday living on the journey to regain personal autonomy" (Shriner's Hospital for Children, Philadelphia, 1998).

Contextual Training in the Community

Community-based training offers clients an effective way to confront and alter their personal beliefs on personal control. In particular, community-based contextual training provides opportunities to improve a sense of competence and self-efficacy through performance accomplishments in *real* rather then contrived situations.

Another expression for contextual training is *in-vivo training*. Basically, the term "in-vivo" implies training in real-life situations. While this term is originally associated with psychologist's treatment of phobias and anxiety disorders through desensitization, community integration/reintegration is TR's equivalent of in-vivo training. This involves taking clients into a natural community setting (e.g., a shopping mall, the dressing room in a store) to experience and contend with realistic, everyday challenges that will require varied skills and abilities. Encountering architectural and attitudinal barriers provides opportunities to confront fears and insecurities, testing the degree to which one has the physical skills to maneuver, cognitive skills to problem solve, and social skills to negotiate. Thus, the intervention environment extends well beyond the confines of the facility, and offers unmatched opportunity to learn, adapt, and grow.

Cognitive rehabilitation programs incorporate contextualized training to help improve functioning, including attention, planning, judgment, perception, processing, problem solving, communication, and social skills. Cronin (1997) described a TR community reentry program for clients that addressed problems associated with head injury (e.g., poor judgment), role adjustments (e.g., relationship with significant other), and problems associated with premorbid status (e.g., high-risk recreation pursuits). First, clients are taught a variety of independent living skills in the clinic. These include money management, time management, social awareness, community mobility including transportation system, and healthy lifestyle behaviors related to exercise and nutrition. Next, training is moved into an environment where greater risk and complexity increases the instructional challenge for clients. Restaurants, shopping malls, movie theaters, dressing rooms, fitness facilities, banks, and subways become the training ground for client's cognitive and safety skills. Eventually, training incorporates the home environment, as well.

Similarly, community behavioral health care agencies incorporate community skills training as a major component of overall psychiatric rehabilitation. Rather than using traditional insight-oriented interventions, clients are helped through behavior management interventions focused on promoting functional skills needed to live in the community. Techniques, such as modeling and coaching, are used to support clients as they involve themselves with community agencies like banks, bowling alleys, and YMCAs. The tangible consequences of their actions provide the most realistic feedback about their behavior, which can be used to confront faulty perceptions and insufficient planning or reward adaptive behaviors.

Contextualized training should target environments that *the client wants* for living, working, and playing, and teach behaviors and skills that *the client values* and believes to be necessary to function in these environments. This is what "client empowerment" is all about. The extent to which clients value the outcomes associated with certain behaviors has a direct bearing on the extent to which they are motivated to learn the behavioral skills.

Humanizing Pediatric Care Environments

Recreation therapists working in pediatric facilities must contend with the impact of medical environments on children and families. Hospitals can be overwhelming, intimidating, and frightening places for children and their families, adding to the stress already experienced from medical problems. This issue was a major impetus for founding the Association for the Care of Children's Health (ACCH) in 1977. A cross-section of pediatric health care workers, including physicians, nurses, social workers, and "play leaders" began to coalesce around the issues of caring for children in hospitals that were really designed for adults. The physical environment, coupled with organizational policies and procedures designed for treating adults were potentially harmful for children. The creation of ACCH provided the organizational structure for harnessing these concerns, and a strong, multidisciplinary voice for advocating change in pediatric health care environments.

Historically, inpatient and outpatient pediatric facilities tended to be designed only with children's medical needs in mind. The designers of newer facilities, however, have realized that environmental design is critical to quality care. Dedicated children's hospitals are now designed to reflect total care, and are creating physical environments that are responsive to the child's *developmental needs* as well as medical needs. Newer facilities also reflect a greater commitment to "family-centered care." Both of these factors have resulted in innovative design elements for pediatric facilities. Laura Poltronieri, director of health care architecture at an architectural and interior design firm, reported that many children's hospitals are converting to private rooms that feature sleep space for parents and caregivers. Special family resource and respite rooms offer support and "decompression zones." Teen rooms and play spaces are being integrated into units. Lobby areas are more "client-friendly," and support a variety of visiting, educational, and entertainment activities. These spaces "will serve as 'safe havens' from painful procedures. They will provide privacy for families and allow children to personalize and control their spaces" (Poltronieri, 1999, p. 12).

Recreation therapists must be vigilant about protecting the importance of play and recreation in addressing developmental needs of children and adolescents in care settings. Playrooms need to be constructed and equipped with resources that stimulate and challenge cognitive, physical, and social skills as well as offer children outlets for coping. Children with severe cognitive and motor impairments are especially in need of play environments that stimulate all levels of development.

Specially designed sensory stimulation rooms that contain swing baskets, air mats, and light machines allow children with severe physical disabilities to play with an exceptional sense of freedom and control. Similarly, Shriner's Hospital offers pediatric rehabilitation clients "Rehab 1,2,3," a multilevel area containing slides, a drawbridge, a tunnel and maze, and a keyboard system. These elements invite children to interact with the environment by using their cognitive and physical skills. According to Dickason and London (2001), "This environment is an example of a trend to create motivational designs that foster self-initiated skill building and training" (p. 265). For adolescents, lounges or teen rooms are important places to find some privacy and independence from adults and authority. So, while space is always limited and at a premium, recreation therapists need to be persuasive in their justification for space, and creative in their use of available space. In fact, recreation therapists have been giving valuable input to architects who are redesigning many pediatric rehabilitation units to incorporate social, psychological, and developmental needs of children, adolescents and parents (Iwanicki, 1999).

Pediatric facilities are also paying more attention to social environmental features that address social needs of children and their families. Various creative approaches are used to increase contact children and adolescents have with other clients their age. For example, the Starlight Project, funded by movie producer Steven Spielberg, utilizes computer technology and the Internet to allow children in one hospital to interact with peers in other hospitals across the country. Recreation therapists are primarily responsible for helping children use the technology. The Internet is also being used for clients to create web pages that keep family and friends in touch, and e-mail accounts are being provided as a means for communication and support (see **Exhibit 10.2**).

Family-centered care, a well-established care philosophy in pediatrics, is a primary way to meet a child's developmental needs. Parents are invited to be equal care partners, and are offered services that will help the family system function as well as improve the medical health of the child. For example, it is quite common for recreation therapists in pediatric settings to offer support groups for parents and siblings. These groups may provide information and education about the medical condition and the immediate and long-term impact this condition may have on the child's friendships, family relationships, play needs, and behavior. Recreation therapists can also offer important support to parents and siblings by providing opportunities for them to use recreation as their own means for coping with the stress that is created on the family unit when one member is ill.

Humanizing Geriatric Care Environments

Research during the last quarter of the 20th century established that long-term care environments can contribute to the physical, psychological, and social decline of elderly persons. In response to this pervasive threat to life quality for nursing home residents, the federal government issued mandates for better care environments. The 1987 Omnibus Budget Reconciliation Act mandated that nursing home facilities provide a full and complete range of activities as an essential

Exhibit 10.2: World Wide Web resources for social contact

Examples of Web programs that have emerged recently include:

> http://www.visitingOurs.com
> http://www.thestatus.com
> http://www.caringbridge.com

Each website is being used in medical settings to allow patients to post updates on their condition or to communicate on any other matter with family and friends. The same electronic message can be sent to many people simultaneously, saving the patient the hassle of repeating the same story. In turn, patients receive support continuously from people no matter how far away they may be. For some this is better than keeping a journal because they had no one responding to their thoughts and feelings. The creator of CaringBridge.com, Sona Hunter, reported that the webpages are a perfect way for friends to check in without intruding. This has also served as a "support network" for families battling similar health crises.

component to meeting quality of life standards. Furthermore, these facilities were mandated to provide "care for residents in a manner and in an environment that maintains or enhances each resident's dignity and respect in full recognition of his or her individuality" (*Federal Register,* 1991, p. 48871). Consequently, it is up to TR specialists to transform nursing homes into therapeutic environments that are designed and used in ways that evoke the vitality of clients, despite functional decline due to medical problems and normal aging.

Howe-Murphy and Charboneau (1987) talked about converting impoverished environments into enriching ones. Enriched environments for elderly persons contain physical, social, and organizational characteristics that promote the resident's dignity. This includes opportunities for residents to share in planning and decision making about activities, decorations, and rules through resident councils. Additionally, physical spaces are redesigned to maximize independent movement, and social arrangements are structured to give residents the chance to share their interests, abilities, stories, and support with each other.

McGuire, Boyd, and Tedrick (1996) maintain that the place where older individuals live ought to provide opportunity for mastery, competence, interaction, privacy, and stimulation. They have presented several general programming goals that have implications for designing the physical and social dimensions of long-term care environments, including increased independence, contact with reality, increased control, involvement of the family, and continued involvement in life.

McGuire and his colleagues summarized three essential areas to consider for environmental modification:

1. Environmental cues (e.g., cues to identify spaces and distinguish personal from public spaces, cues to assist in locating individual areas)

2. Environmental stimulation (e.g., enhancing new learning, promoting use of all senses, appropriate uses of challenge)

3. Environmental support (e.g., providing opportunities for choice and control, increased sense of competence)

Note that these recommendations imply environmental modification in all three dimensions of the environment—physical, social, and organizational. Providing TR services in geriatric care facilities involves so much more than planning and running activities. A total environmental context needs to be created and maintained so that older adults will be motivated to be as independent as possible, doing activities that they prefer and find meaningful, in a variety of settings, with others they want to be with. This also means working with administrators to examine policies that govern the facility, and instituting change as needed.

An excellent example of a total environmental modification involving physical, social, and organizational changes is described by Buettner and Martin (1995). They modified a nursing home environment significantly by creating a "leisure empowerment" environment. A major component of this leisure empowerment environment was designating a large room as a *leisure lounge* replete with diverse age-appropriate recreation materials, including art materials, music and exercise resources, simple sporting equipment, and a wide variety of table games and puzzles. Residents had input on the initial selection of materials, and were encouraged to make suggestions for additional materials once they became accustomed to using the leisure lounge. According to Buettner and Martin, these rooms should be colorful, well-lit, and large enough to permit wheelchairs to be maneuvered between tables and chairs. Shelves should be low enough that residents can easily view activity materials and supplies, and there should be baskets to easily transport materials to and from tables. Above all, leisure empowerment environments must use age-appropriate materials and foster a maximum level of choice, control, and independent behavior.

Special Considerations for the Physical Component of Geriatric Care Environments

There is increasing attention to the importance of designing environments that are physically safe and accommodating for geriatric clients who have a wide variety of needs and abilities. Common features of a supportive physical environment include:

- Good lighting (e.g., natural lighting, task focused lighting, reduced glare)

- Visual presentation (e.g., large print, color contrasts for changes in elevation, designated perimeters)

- Stable surfaces (no slippery surfaces or loose rugs)

- Modulated auditory stimulation (e.g., minimal background noise, minimal high decibel sounds)

- Adaptive sensory aids (e.g., magnifying glasses, reading stands, communication boards)
- Spaces designed for privacy as well as social congregating

An obvious goal of environmental modification is to accommodate the cognitive and physical limitations of the residents. Injuries resulting from falls is a major risk associated with long-term care environments, and one that recreation therapists need to help prevent. Environmental conditions that contribute to falling include inadequate lighting, sun glare, slick floors, unstable furniture, unlocked wheelchairs, excessive clutter, and lack of adaptive equipment (Buettner & Martin, 1995).

Buettner and Waitkavicz (1997) reported on a model recreation therapy program designed to prevent falls for older adults in long-term care. An interdisciplinary team comprised of an occupational therapist, nurse, and recreation therapist developed and used an environmental evaluation to assess the risks found in areas where falls had occurred, including recreation areas. Modifications were made to the environment and a program was then designed to improve the abilities of residents to avoid falls. The program consisted of a graded walking program in the morning, sensory integration and balance activities in the afternoon, and exercising to music in the evening to improve strength, balance, and flexibility. In addition, this program had a cognitive element comprised of group sessions where clients were educated about fall prevention and discussed their fears of falling and other misconceptions that limited their involvement in activities.

Of course, safety and security can be overdone and can be counterproductive, limiting the chance for clients to learn, adapt, and grow. Planned environments, such as rehabilitation hospitals, nursing homes, and adult day centers need to ensure that they do not become so uniform and predictable that they evoke a sense of boredom. According to McGuire, Boyd, and Tedrick (1996), "the goal of environmental design is to provide a setting that allows an individual to be as independent as possible while retaining excitement and challenge" (p. 212).

Special Considerations for the Social Component of Geriatric Care Environments

McGuire, Boyd, and Tedrick (1996) suggest that family members be included in programs within nursing homes for residents to maintain as much continuity with life as possible. According to these authors, the Philadelphia Geriatric Center in Pennsylvania encourages family members to make their visits more meaningful and enjoyable by helping their relatives decorate their rooms, helping with personal grooming, assisting with writing letters, making telephone calls, or sending greeting cards. They are also encouraged to bring grandchildren and family pets, and to take their relative out into the community for meals, shopping, and attendance at special family affairs. When the family cannot come to the nursing home, residents can feel connected to family and friends through "video visits." Family members can make videotapes of "interviews" with children and grandchildren and various special events like birthdays and graduation ceremonies. These videotapes can be tremendous sources of comfort and support when residents feel lonely and agitated.

Sometimes, especially in the case of persons with Alzheimer's disease, visiting family members can experience disappointment, frustration, guilt, and sadness. These feelings can be deterrents to continued visits, which is the exact opposite of what their family member needs. Caregiving for a relative in an institution produces stress that is different from that experienced by caregivers in the community. "Many of the stresses in caregiving within the institutional care setting are of an emotional nature and are experienced *in visits* with an older adult relative" (Dupuis & Pedlar, 1995, p. 186). While there are increasing caregiver support programs in the community, including those designed around recreation and leisure interventions, the need for institution-based caregiver support programs is becoming more apparent.

Dupuis and Pedlar (1995) designed and evaluated a structured music program for family members and their loved-ones who resided in a geriatric care facility. The program consisted of twice weekly sessions over a six-week period, combining singing, listening to songs, and reminiscence. Evaluation of the program, using interviews and observations, indicated that the program produced numerous benefits for family members and loved ones (i.e., clients). Specifically, the quality of visits was enhanced due to the sense of relaxation experienced by family members and residents. Family members reported positive feelings related to being able to share enjoyable activities, which for some were similar to past interests and activities. The program also revealed a side of their loved one that family members had forgotten or overlooked. A sense of reciprocity was also experienced during visits. That is, family members were able to receive a level of attentiveness and responsiveness from their loved one as well as being able to give attention and care. Family members reported that the program served as a coping mechanism, helping them accept the disease and feel better about the situation. Of equal importance was the social support that was generated among the families involved in the program. They reportedly felt less alone and were able to exchange informational and emotional support with each other.

Environmental Issues in Dementia Care

In response to the increasing numbers of older adults with Alzheimer's disease and related dementias, and the complexity of this illness, specialized care environments have been opening rapidly. In 1992, the federal government's Office of Technology Assessment issued a report containing several principles that shape thinking and action related to special care. One principle, in particular, recognized the importance of person–environment transactions, and concluded that appropriate environmental interventions could enhance function and quality of life (Kovach, Weisman, Chaudhury & Calkins, 1997). Kovach and her colleagues compared a traditional nursing home unit having a majority of residents with Alzheimer's, and a new dementia care unit that was specially designed to enhance the independence of persons with Alzheimer's disease. These researchers found that the environmental features of the dementia care unit contributed to greater use of activity space and significantly greater social interaction. The special care unit had six key design principles:

1. Noninstitutional image
2. Smaller groups of residents (two clusters of 12)
3. Variety of small activity spaces
4. Meaningful wandering path (allowing for continuous movement) overlooking activity spaces
5. Positive and secure outdoor space
6. Special glass cases containing personal memorabilia

Environmental stressors can provoke certain behaviors in dementia residents that have little to do with the disease and much to do with their surroundings. Special care units can positively impact resident's well-being by reducing environmental stress. "The distinction between reducing stress-related behavior and curing disease is an important one for caregivers of residents with dementia. It helps them develop an attitude towards residents as normal yet disabled people whose quality of life needs to be maintained rather than as sick people who need to be cured" (Zeisel, Hyde & Levkoff, 1994, p. 9). Cohen and Weisman (1997) have suggested that care environments should be considered in terms of therapeutic goals. Looking back at the human needs displayed on Table 10.1 (p. 177), recreation therapists can plan activity programs to meet these human needs of residents.

Increasingly, recreation therapists work on special care units, and this trend will continue. They will be expected to help with modifying traditional nursing care units and to create environments that are conducive to quality care and quality of life for older adults with Alzheimer's and related dementia. Beyond the human needs presented on Table 10.1 (p. 171), their work on special care units can be oriented toward therapeutic outcomes identified by Mace (1991), including decreased agitation and restlessness, reduced use of psychotropic drugs, improved orientation, increased awareness of self in relation to others, and a regained sense of humor.

Zeisel, Hyde, and Levkoff (1994) developed an excellent model that organizes and describes the influences that the physical environment of special care units has on residents and caregivers. The components of this model help to achieve the therapeutic outcomes identified by Mace (1991). The eight primary environmental concepts include:

1. Wandering paths that are continuous and have understandable cues for wayfinding
2. Interesting events that encourage walking
3. Immediate and unobtrusive exit controls
4. Private and personalized bedrooms
5. Common and varied activity areas
6. Accessible and interesting outdoor areas
7. Interiors that safely maximize autonomy
8. Sights, sounds, and smells that residents can understand
9. Building design components that have home-like features (e.g., furniture, décor)

Any environmental modification of special care units can be guided by a close examiniation of this model.

Environmental Modifications Using the Eden Alternative

Perhaps the most comprehensive environmental reengineering effort within nursing homes has been through a bold, innovative approach called the *Eden Alternative*. The brainchild of Dr. William Thomas, the Eden Alternative is dedicated to transforming nursing homes from places that are, in essence, "living mortuaries" to complex, biologically diverse "human habitats." Thomas (1994) considered nursing homes to be highly regimented institutions breeding three "plagues" of loneliness, helplessness, and boredom. Activity personnel and their programs do not escape Thomas' sweeping condemnation.

> And what contemporary nursing home would be complete without the endless round of "activities programs" which often have more to do with meeting the expectations of the regulators than serving the true needs of the residents? As the therapeutic mentality extends its reach, more and more pieces of a life well lived are taken over and remade into treatments rendered by certified therapists. The pleasure of animal companionship and the enjoyment of children, music, art, movement and touch are increasingly the focus of professional therapists and their treatment plans. (pp. 18–19)

Thomas argues that nursing home personnel confuse treatment with "care." True caring, contends Thomas, is helping another to grow by removing barriers to growth and enlarging one's ability to grow. Caring is guided by three fundamental principles: a recognition and appreciation of every resident's capacity for growth; defining the work of nursing home personnel by the needs and capacities of the residents, not that of the staff; and an understanding that care is continuous and long lasting. These principles would be embodied in a human habitat characterized by a harmonious blend of biological and social diversity.

An "Edenized" nursing home is a complex interdependent community that integrates people, plants, and animals. Animals including dogs, cats, birds, and rabbits reside in this community where they offer companionship and a reciprocal exchange of care. Indoor and outdoor plants are an added dimension to the life cycle and also offer opportunities for elderly persons to be responsible and nurturing. Gardens are a source of food as well as beauty. Finally, children provide social diversity in this human habitat. Children are woven into the fabric of life in an Edenized nursing home through on-site childcare centers, after-school programs, and summer day camps. Thus, the Eden Alternative goes well beyond intergenerational, horticulture, and pet visitation programs. The Eden Alternative is a living community that integrates biological and social diversity that defines the community, as opposed to scheduled programs that are determined and highly regulated by staff. An Edenized nursing home is a living environment based on the principles of ecology and anthropology rather than medical science and bureaucracy.

The Eden Alternative is spreading throughout the country. It is also controversial, primarily because it rejects the assumed value of professional caregivers, including recreation therapists. Its tenets can be appealing, yet it requires that nursing home personnel fully embrace its philosophy. While that may be difficult for some, especially in these times of tightening regulations and severely constricted reimbursement, the Eden Alternative can serve as a beacon for everyone who is committed to truly caring for older persons. It is obvious that Edenizing most closely reflects the intent of therapeutic recreation to help people learn, adapt, and grow. It is difficult to conceive of any nursing home that could not benefit from more companionship, more opportunities for residents to give as well as receive care, and more spontaneity. Some will resist these ideas because of assumed risk for injury and other problems for residents, yet part of what gives the real world substance is the inherent risk in living as opposed to merely existing. Others will resist because job descriptions are blurred and the top-down management style has contributed to institutionalizing staff. This is the largest impediment to the Eden Alternative. Management and staff must risk giving up control and instead share responsibility and accountability.

Summary

The purpose of this chapter was to review the role and function of the environment in the care and treatment of clients. Therapeutic recreation practice involves using the physical and social dimensions of the environment to support the health and life quality of people who are hospitalized or living in nursing homes or other care environments. Practice also involves challenging the organizational dimension of the care environment so that it too contributes to the clients potential for health and life quality. Examples pertaining to children and older adults were used to illustrate ways in which the physical and social environment can be an asset to quality care. As a recreation therapist, you can lead the way in humanizing environments that are overly medicalized and impersonal, or that diminish the dignity of clients. The essence of humanizing care environments is captured quite poignantly by Benson (1996), a landscape architect and recovering alcoholic. He contended that recovery environments ought to be spaces that divert, relax, and amuse. These "therapeutic landscapes" ought to draw power to individuals by providing opportunities for introspection as well as interaction. Recovery-oriented spaces "can, at their best, *impel*, not compel patients to discover for themselves a pathway to health" (p. 91).

References

Benson, R. (1996). What's a nice guy like me doing in a place like this? A landscape architect and recovering alcoholic's thoughts on designing therapeutic landscapes. *Journal of Therapeutic Horticulture, VIII,* 88–91.

Buettner, L. and Martin, S. (1995). *Therapeutic recreation in the nursing home.* State College, PA: Venture Publishing, Inc.

Buettner, L. and Waitkavicz, B. (1997). Preventing falls in long-term care: A model recreation therapy program. Available online: http//www.recreationtherapy.com/articles/falls.htm

Can the sound of water help cure cancer? (2000, March 17). *The Philadelphia Inquirer,* p. H7.

Cohen, S. and Willis, T. (1985). Stress, social support, and the buffering hypothesis. *Psychological Bulletin, 98*(2), 310–357.

Cohen, V. and Weisman, G. (1997). Long-term care design: National Alzheimer's design assistance project—Promoting innovation through exemplary settings. *Journal of Healthcare Design, 9,* 125–128.

Compton, D. (1992, April). *Environmental influence on leisure behavior.* Paper presented at the Midwest Therapeutic Recreation Symposium, Missouri.

Cronin, T. (1997). *Cognitive rehabilitation: Application in the community reintegration process.* Paper presented at the ATRA National Conference, Nashville, TN.

Dickason, J. and London, P. (2001). Pediatric play. In D. Austin and M. Crawford (Eds.), *Therapeutic recreation* (3rd ed., pp. 255–268). Needham Heights, MA: Allyn & Bacon.

Dupuis, S. and Pedlar, A. (1995). Family leisure programs in institutional care settings: Buffering the stress of caregivers. *Therapeutic Recreation Journal, 39*(3), 184–205.

Fidler, G. and Velde, B. (1999). *Activities: Reality and symbol.* Thorofare, NJ: Slack.

Gerteis, M., Edgman-Levitan, S., Daley, J., and Delbanco, T. (1993). *Through the patient's eyes: Understanding and promoting patient-centered care.* San Francisco, CA: Jossey-Bass.

Hafen, B., Karren, K., Frandsen, K., and Smith, L. (1996). The healing power of humor and laughter. In *Mind/body health: The effects of attitudes, emotions and relationships*. Boston, MA: Allyn & Bacon. 541–583.

Ham, G. (2000, November/December). Long-term care—does laughing matter? *ATRA Treatment Networks, 1*(5), 3.

Howe-Murphy, R. and Charboneau, B. (1987). *Therapeutic recreation intervention: An ecological perspective*. Englewood Cliffs, NJ: Prentice-Hall.

Howell, S. (1998). Integrative environments for the older adult. *Journal of geriatric psychiatry 31*(1), 55–64.

Iwanicki, H. (1999 April/May). The making over of a rehab unit. *REHAB management*, 58–63.

Kahana, E. (1975). A congruence model of person–environment interaction. In P. Windley, T. Byerts, and F. Ernst (Eds.), *Theory development in environment and aging*. Washington, DC: The Gerontological Society.

Keller, J. (1997). Cherished possessions: Being an effective helper with older adults. *Parks & Recreation, 32*(5), 86–89.

Kovach, C., Weisman, G., Chaudhury, H., and Calkins, M. (1997 May/June). Impacts of a therapeutic environment for dementia care. *American Journal of Alzheimer's disease*, 99–110.

Lewin, K. (1951). *Field theory in social science*. New York, NY: Harper & Row.

Ma, G. and Henderson, G. (1999). *Rethinking ethnicity and health care*. Springfield, IL: Charles C. Thomas.

Mace, N. (1991). Dementia care units in nursing homes. In D. Coon (Ed.), *Specialized dementia care units*. Baltimore, MD: Johns Hopkins University Press.

McGuire, F., Boyd, R., and Tedrick, R. (1996). *Leisure and aging: Ulyssean living in later life*. Champaign, IL: Sagamore Publishing.

Nahemov, L. and Lawton, M. (1973). Toward an ecological theory of adaptation and aging. In W. Preiser (Ed.), *Environmental design research, 1,* 24–32. Stroudsburg, PA: Dowden, Hutchinson & Ross.

Poltronieri, L. (1999, March 12). New design trends prepare pediatric facilities for future. *Hospital & Healthcare News*.

Shriner's Hospital for Children, Philadelphia (1998). New Philadelphia Shriner's Hospital offers unique approach to pediatric rehabilitation. *Connections, 9*(2), 3.

Steinfeld, E. and Danford, G. (1997). Environment as a mediating factor in functional assessment. In *Functional assessment and outcome measures for the rehabilitation health professional*. Gaithersburg, MD: Aspen, 37–56.

Thomas, W. (1994). *The Eden Alternative: Nature, hope and nursing homes*. Columbia, MO: University of Missouri.

Tomczyk, C. (1998, April/May). The value of volunteers. *REHAB management*, 26–28.

Ulrich, R. (1984). View through a window may influence recovery from surgery. *Science, 224,* 420–421.

U. S. Department of Health and Human Services, Health Care Financing Administration. (1991, September 26). Medicare and medicaid regulations for long-term care facilities. *Federal Register, 56*(187), 48867–48880.

U. S. Office of Technology Assessment (1992). *Special care units for people with Alzheimer's and other dementias: Consumer education, research, regulatory, and reimbursement issues* (OTA-H-543). Washington, DC: U. S. Government Printing Office.

Walker, J. (1993). Enhancing physical comfort. In M. Gerteis, S. Edgman-Levitan, J. Daley, and T. Delbanco (Eds.), *Through the patient's eyes: Understanding and promoting patient-centered care*. San Francisco, CA: Jossey-Bass, 119–153.

Zeisel, J., Hyde, J., and Levkoff, S. (1994, March/April). Best practices: An environment–behavior (E–B) model for Alzheimer special care units. *The American Journal of Alzheimer's Care and Related Disorders & Research*, 4–21.

Chapter 11
Developing Therapeutic Relationships

Guided Reading Questions

After reading this chapter, you should be able to answer the following:

- What are some personal attributes of helping professionals? How might these attributes affect your relationships with clients?
- What is a *therapeutic relationship* and how does it differ from relationships you have with friends and family?
- What factors must be considered to establish a therapeutic alliance or partnership with clients?
- What skills and abilities combine to produce multicultural and communication competencies?
- How do timing, emotional closeness, and self-disclosures impact therapeutic relationships?
- What ought to happen between a recreation therapist and a client when they terminate a therapeutic relationship?

Introduction

Every aspect of TR clinical practice pivots on the relationships that therapists have with their clients. An effective therapeutic relationship is one of the primary elements of TR clinical practice, along with activity-based interventions, and a supportive and accommodating environment. Of these three, the relationship between a client and a recreation therapist is most essential. The importance of the client–therapist relationship has been implied throughout earlier chapters. For instance, viewing clients as active *partners* in their care and respecting their developmental and cultural backgrounds is an essential part of the client–system perspective. Furthermore, the clinical change process presented in Chapter 6 places significant emphasis on communication between clients and TR professionals. Thus, we believe a therapeutic relationship is the central element for facilitating client learning, adaptation, and growth.

It can be very gratifying to help clients improve their functioning, feel more hopeful, or live more effectively as a result of your actions. Yet helpful client–therapist relationships are not automatic. While therapeutic relationships are based on the therapist's desire and intention to help, that alone is never enough, especially when the relationship is central to helping clients make lifestyle change. Therapeutic relationships depend on skills and abilities that you acquire and maintain in your clinical practice. They also depend on your possession of a core set of personal attributes consistently associated with effective helping relationships.

While the client–therapist relationship is unique to each client, several ingredients are fundamental to all relationships. This is illustrated in **Figure 11.1** (p. 190). Specifically, attributes and characteristics of a client and a recreation therapist come together in a service delivery setting. The service setting usually determines general expectations for TR services and the amount of time available to work together. Ideally, the therapeutic relationship reflects a partnership of shared responsibility for the client's learning, adaptation, and growth. The most critical aspect of the relationship is communication, which is influenced by the recreation therapist's sensitivity to the client's unique developmental, cultural, and situational factors. Cormier and Hackney (1999) describe the helping relationship as occurring in a context that appreciates "individual differences along such dimensions as race, ethnicity, socioeconomic level, gender, religious and spiritual affiliation, sexual orientation, age, developmental stage of life and so on" (p. 2). These factors, along with the client's values, attitudes, and beliefs about health, leisure, and disability influence what they want and expect from TR interventions. The outcomes of therapeutic relationships are focused on necessary and desired changes for clients, although recreation therapists often derive benefits as well.

Although therapeutic relationships involve two people, this chapter concentrates on factors associated with the recreation therapist. We assume an understanding of the potential range of issues that clients bring to the relationship, based on reading earlier chapters. We begin this chapter by describing fundamental attributes and characteristics of helping professionals. These attributes and characteristics are critical as they affect your response to clients. To be an effective helper, recreation therapists must understand what aspects of themselves influence client change and growth. Next, three competencies that are essential to therapeutic relationships are discussed. These include an ability to create partnerships, an ability to practice from a multi-cultural perspective, and an ability to communicate effectively. The chapter concludes by presenting several challenging issues that often arise in client–therapist relationships.

Personal Attributes of Helping Professionals

Most individuals who are drawn to helping professions like therapeutic recreation have basic personal attributes that provide a foundation for professional learning and growth. Brammer and MacDonald (1999) contend that personal attributes are ultimately used by helping professionals to produce growth-facilitating conditions, such as trust and encouragement, which are instrumen-

tal in assisting clients. The following section presents an overview of these attributes. Arguably, there may be others. Those presented here are synthesized from the work of several notable authors (e.g., Brammer & MacDonald, 1999; Corey & Corey, 2002; Egan, 1994). As you read consider the extent to which each attribute has motivated you to become a helping professional.

Altruism and Compassion

Therapeutic recreation students are frequently asked, "Why are you in this field?" A common response is "I enjoy helping others." Altruism, the desire to serve others and to advance their best interests, is one of the main reasons for entering a helping profession such as TR. Similarly, when TR students are asked what motivated them to select their major they often point to the fact that they have or had a relative with a disability or chronic illness. Their love, concern, and compassion for this individual inspired them to pursue a helping profession. This same motivation is found among students in other disciplines as well. For many, the pain and suffering of others, social injustices, and poor life

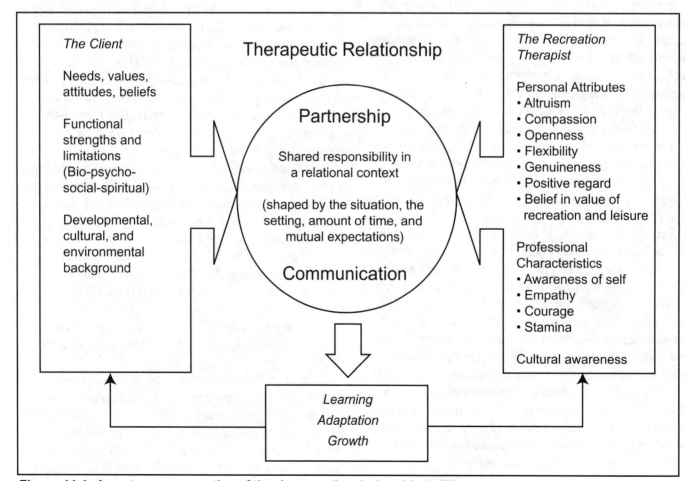

Figure 11.1: A systems perspective of the therapeutic relationship in TR

quality are compelling reasons to become helping professionals. Brammer and MacDonald (1999) contend that many of us come from backgrounds where having compassion for the perceived suffering of others is rooted in a variety of religious and spiritual traditions. Thus, compassion, combined with a desire to care for and serve others is a primary personal attribute of helping professionals.

Openness and Flexibility

Individuals who are open to new experiences and accepting of values and perceptions different from their own tend to be comfortable working with others. Openness stems from a basic curiosity about human behavior and an acceptance that one's own lived experience and subsequent worldview is not the same as it is for others. Being open to new experiences and alternative points of view is also consistent with being flexible, another important characteristic of effective helpers. Flexibility is important because helping professionals need to be adaptable to constant change encountered in their work (e.g., varying settings, clients, TR procedures).

Genuineness

The capacity to be genuine is another personal attribute required for effective helping. Professionals who are genuine behave in an honest manner. Genuineness implies a match or congruence between a therapist's words and actions. Consider for a moment a comment directed at a therapist by a client. "You don't really care; you are only here because you are paid to care." While such a statement might appear to be a hostile expression, it may also imply a valid perception that there is an inconsistency between a therapist's claim of caring and the level of caring that is expressed by his or her actions.

Positive Regard and Respect for Others

Another personal attribute found among people who pursue helping professions is a genuine positive attitude toward and respect for others. Often this emerges from a core set of values instilled in families and promoted in various faith traditions. Positive regard is an attitude of valuing and appreciating others as unique and worthwhile human beings. It is the capacity to suspend judgment and to seek empathy, whether or not we agree with the values and behaviors of the other (Cormier &

Hackney, 1999). Positive regard and respect for others stems from being open and comfortable with diversity, whether related to race, ethnicity, culture, class, gender, spirituality, or sexual orientation. In essence, it is the capacity to be accepting and to find the humanity in others, no matter what their conditions. Positive regard and respect is also reflected in a belief that all humankind is motivated by a desire to live effective and meaningful lives (Egan, 1994). This belief is the basis for wanting to assist others to achieve an optimal state of health and well-being. Even in instances where clients have illnesses that are beyond any possibility of a cure or they may be dying, this belief has relevance. In these situations, the focus is on healing rather than curing. When addressing the ATRA national conference, Rabbi Kuschner (1998) said that true healing had nothing to do with a cure. Rather, healing occurs when our presence gives a person the message that, in spite of minimal chance of recovery, the individual is worth caring about and that their life has meaning. In these cases, Kuschner said, our "medicine" would be the gift of time and concern. This can only happen when we value and respect the dignity of each person.

Belief in the Value of Play, Recreation, and Leisure

An abiding belief in the importance of play, recreation, and leisure to the human experience is a personal attribute that is fundamental to those who work in TR. Perhaps this belief comes from your own life experience, either as an artist, athlete, musician, or outdoor enthusiast. Perhaps it grew from witnessing the important role that play and recreation have in making people feel good about themselves. Or it may have resulted from seeing how play, recreation, and leisure allows people to feel connected with others in a meaningful way. In any event, believing in the potential for play, recreation, and leisure to be a forum for human growth and development and life satisfaction is essential to TR practice. After all, your belief in the value of play, recreation, and leisure may be tested many times. It is likely that you will face situations where you will have to advocate for clients who are denied opportunities for play and recreation because of their illness or disabling conditions, such as in the case of adults with chronic mental illness or incarcerated youth. You may also need to advocate for recognition of these issues as relevant service outcomes for the health and human services system.

Characteristic Skills of Helping Professionals

Altruism, compassion, openness and flexibility, genuineness, positive regard for others, and a belief in the value of play, recreation, and leisure are important personal attributes that TR professionals ought to bring to their work. These attributes are the basis for a trusting relationship with clients. Yet, these attributes alone are not enough. To form and maintain therapeutic relationships that facilitate change and growth for clients there are additional skills needed by helping professionals. These skills are refined through experience and include an awareness and understanding of oneself, empathy for clients, courage, and stamina.

Awareness of Self

Knowing oneself is critical to effective helping. This includes an awareness of significant social and cultural forces influencing personal values and beliefs as well as an awareness of values and beliefs regarding therapeutic recreation. Knowing one's personal and professional values and beliefs is critical to recognizing when they might conflict with the values of those individuals we expect to help. Awareness of self also helps us recognize when our worldview is so strong that we actually project our own set of values onto clients. An awareness of our own emotional, psychological, and social needs can help with recognizing personal motivations to be helping professionals. Knowing what motivates us to be in helping relationships allows us to recognize the possibility that we may be serving our own personal needs through the act of serving others. Self-awareness is not just important when we prepare for and enter a helping profession—it is necessary throughout our careers. Since the TR practitioner's life is constantly changing, there is a need to be aware of how changes may influence your motivation to help. Indeed, one's own development can produce personal needs that conflict with your desire and ability to work in therapeutic relationships. For example, consider how your willingness to work evenings, weekends, or holidays might change as you start your own family.

Ability to Analyze One's Own Feelings

Beyond an awareness of self, therapeutic relationships require practitioners to examine feelings. According to

Brammer and MacDonald (1999) the courage and ability to become aware of and to understand one's own feelings are very important to the helping process. All human relationships, especially those involving careful and deliberate helping, generate many complex and powerful feelings. Feelings created by the act of helping can include pride and gratitude, as well as frustration, disappointment, and insecurity. Feelings of frustration can be aroused when clients resist or reject TR services. Similarly, a client's lack of effort or investment in their own care can produce feelings of anger or disapproval. Sometimes, you will be drawn to certain clients and distance yourself from others. For example, some clients are more "attractive" or make you feel more needed or effective as a therapist. While feeling needed by clients can be gratifying, promoting this can foster dependency in clients. Other clients may be difficult and can make you feel insecure and impatient. For example, the slow progress of a person with a brain injury and the need for repetitive practice using the same cognitive skills can easily test one's patience and skills. Consequently, you may unknowingly avoid these clients in an effort to avoid personal feelings of incompetence or frustration.

Without recognizing, examining, and managing these feelings and emotions, the helping process can be compromised, even to the point of harming clients. It is essential for TR specialists to be willing and able to examine personal feelings aroused in their relationships with clients. This self-reflection will help you to understand how these feelings influence your behavior and subsequent client relationships. It takes courage to examine attitudes, feelings, and values that are unavoidably involved in therapeutic relationships, and courage to seek and use support or clinical supervision to recognize, understand, and manage these responses. Reading and journaling about your work can help you develop this depth of thought and insight.

Empathy

Empathy is the capacity to perceive another's situation and their feelings associated with it. To be empathetic is to be "present" in the moment with the other person and to place oneself into that person's "internal perceptual frame" without losing one's own identity or objectivity (Brammer & MacDonald, 1999, p. 30). This depth of understanding is helped by being perceptively attuned to nonverbal behavior as well as verbal communication. The adage "walking in another person's shoes" captures the essence of empathy. It is fostered by a willingness to think and feel as the other person does. As Falvo

(1994) suggests, empathy involves pausing and asking oneself "How would I feel if I were in the client's situation?" At the same time, the helping professional is constantly open to evidence that would answer "why" questions posed to oneself, such as "Why is this individual feeling insecure?" or "Why is this individual hesitant to join in the group activity?" This is described as "emotionally knowing" by van Servellen (1997) and involves an objective awareness of the client and an appreciation of the world as that person experiences it. This is achieved by identifying what it must be like to be that person. When this is accomplished, the professional has "empathic understanding."

Courage

Courage is one of the most important characteristics of helping professionals. Courage allows you to be more *inventive* and *creative*. While recreation therapists can vary in their creativity with activities, the issue also pertains to creative approaches to assisting clients. A lack of creativity in this regard may have more to do with the reluctance to seek new perspectives or to "think outside the box." Mackelprang and Salsgiver (1999) reported that professionals who were creative and unconventional were perceived to be of the greatest help by people with disabilities. This does not imply disregarding standards of practice or particular clinical practice guidelines that may exist. It does mean, however, having openness to trying new approaches, especially with the most challenging clients or when programs become boring and routine to clients and therapists.

It also takes courage to admit to not knowing how to do something and to seek advice from others. Too often helping professionals believe that they must always demonstrate expertise and so they rush into situations with hasty responses instead of stepping back and accepting their need for guidance or clinical supervision. Sometimes the hesitancy to seek assistance or to admit being uncertain is associated with feelings that are uncomfortable. Yet, having the courage to accept one's limitations is the first step in improving and growing as a professional. Finally, courage is also needed when one's profession is devalued or when play, recreation, and leisure needs of clients are disregarded. It takes courage to speak up on behalf of clients in care meetings or case conferences and to advocate for something when others do not understand, value, or agree.

Stamina

Helping others can be quite demanding, both physically and emotionally. The energy output expected of recreation therapists is often a surprise for new professionals. Your energy and enthusiasm for individual and group programs is usually an important source of motivation for client involvement. This energy, coupled with the physical demands associated with TR practice as an action therapy, requires stamina. Stamina is also required to deal with the constant changes and seemingly unrelenting pressure within health and human service agencies to do more with less. Being emotionally "present" for clients, which means to be fully engaged through compassion and empathy, can also be emotionally draining (Corey & Corey, 2002). Thus, helping professionals need to have stamina to meet the physical and emotional demands of practice and to ward off the risk of burnout.

 • • •Thinking Trigger
Think about the attributes and skills needed as a foundation for therapeutic relationships. How strong is your foundation? How can you build on it? **• • •**

Austin (1999) contends that recreation therapists are at risk for burnout due to the ongoing, repetitive, and intense nature of helping others. To counteract exhaustion and fatigue, he suggests that you have a reliable social support system. Corey and Corey (2002) encourage practitioners to find multiple sources of psychological nourishment and to nurture themselves as well as care for their clients. This nurturing comes from having outside interests and effective social support, both through work relationships and in one's personal life. It also comes from using leisure to renew your physical and mental health. It is not surprising to find that a sense of humor is on Corey and Corey's list of personal characteristics for helping professionals. Of course, humor in this case serves to maintain a reasonable perspective and not take things too seriously. It is also the ability to laugh at yourself. A sense of humor can be a real asset in your work and can help to maintain stamina.

Competencies Needed for Therapeutic Relationships

Relationships between TR specialists and their clients will vary depending on the amount of time they have to work together and the nature of the client's needs. Certainly, there will be circumstances when establishing a relationship will be very difficult. Nevertheless, you should strive to create and maintain therapeutic relationships to every extent possible to facilitate change and growth for clients. In addition to the attributes and skills just presented, effective therapeutic relationships depend on several specific competencies. These include the ability to create partnerships with clients, the ability to practice from a multicultural perspective, and the ability to communicate effectively.

Creating Partnerships

Increasingly, health and human service providers are recognizing that clients want to be partners in their care, whether they are in hospitals or in the community. Affording them opportunities to be partners is consistent with patient-centered care, described in Chapter 2. Allhouse (1993) reported that determining and respecting clients' preferences for involvement in clinical care is an important part of respecting their individuality. Yet, it is nearly impossible to define exactly what it means to be active or involved, since this notion is highly individualistic. Likewise, a preference for involvement varies. "Time, experience, and the course of illness can dramatically affect both the ability and the desire to participate" (Allhouse, 1993, p. 28).

Clients generally do better when they are actively involved in the change process. For example, Falvo (1994) indicated that education-based interventions are more likely to be successful if clients assume an active role in determining desired outcomes, creating action plans, and evaluating progress. Built on a foundation of trust and genuine caring, therapeutic relationships reflect shared commitment to change and growth. Because of this mutuality, a therapeutic relationship is often referred to as a *therapeutic alliance*. This alliance represents a "tacit understanding that both partners share a common purpose, namely, to help the client attain a more satisfactory life" (Kanfer & Schefft, 1988, p. 115). Collaboration is promoted by engaging the client as an active partner in the change process. Recreation therapists motivate clients to identify and use their own strengths and resources, thereby reinforc-

ing their beliefs that they have the potential to change and grow. To whatever extent possible, clients and therapists work together to identify problems, set goals, and monitor progress. Egan (1994) prefers the term *working alliance* because it underscores the hard work that must come from each partner.

A key factor in creating a therapeutic alliance is the client's perception that TR interventions are relevant to their needs. Many clients who receive clinical TR interventions do not necessarily seek them. While you may firmly believe that TR interventions are relevant to your client's overall needs and can complement routine care, ultimately clients must decide whether they want involvement. In some cases, "helping may involve reducing the client's resistance to a therapeutic intervention or building confidence in the ability of the program to assist in meeting his or her needs" (Carter, Van Andel & Robb, 1995, p. 78). However, your zeal to be helpful can actually be intrusive and overbearing for some clients, and can be a form of paternalism. This occurs when "helpful" actions overpower client autonomy. Thus, recreation therapists have to be careful that their belief in the value of TR involvement does not obliterate the client's right to decide where, when, and in what form help should be given.

Client's Perspective on Partnerships

Clients are more likely to involve themselves as care partners if they see the relevance of TR interventions and if they believe the recreation therapist will be helpful. In addition to being trustworthy, honest, and respectful, recreation therapists must be knowledgeable and competent. Clients expect you to have technical skills and abilities that will help them with symptom relief and functional improvement. Clients also rely on you for information, especially that which they believe is useful. They need information about their health conditions and they need to understand the relationship between TR interventions and their overall care needs. Many clients also need information about adaptive and assistive technologies and the wide range of recreation and leisure resources available to them.

Next, clients want helping relationships that provide them with support, especially emotional support. Hospitalized individuals want professionals to take time to listen to their fears and understand their sense of vulnerability and uncertainty. Emotional support is highly desired by clients.

> From the patient's perspective, the first and most important category of support was the expression of positive affect and bolstering

self-esteem. The majority of patients studied found encouragement to talk about feelings to be the *most* helpful support given by *all* providers; but it was the *least* helpful when it was done poorly or not at all. (Edgman-Levitan, 1993, p. 158)

Clients also count on recreation therapists to be advocates, speaking on their behalf in care meetings to ensure that their needs and desires are understood. This is often the case in rehabilitation settings where the emphasis is on functional needs almost to the exclusion of psychosocial needs. Similar support is counted on when changes are needed in the client's environment to minimize or reduce barriers to recreation and leisure involvement.

Finally, clients look to helping relationships for *hope*. When recreation therapists appreciate various sources of meaning in clients' lives and offer opportunities to continue experiencing things that are meaningful, a sense of hope is instilled. Clients also have a greater chance for hope when you convey a belief in what they *can* do, rather than focusing on what they cannot do. When Ted Kennedy, Jr. addressed a gathering of TR professionals, he told of his own experience in rehabilitation and sense of demoralization after losing a leg to cancer. A pivotal experience for him was when his recreation therapist showed a film on adapted skiing. Viewing the film and talking with his therapist rekindled his hope that he could continue to join his family in skiing and other outdoor pursuits. Hope for Kennedy and others like him is not artificial optimism but a realistic and encouraging sense that things can improve or change.

Factors that Influence the Client's Perspective on Partnerships

There are additional factors to consider when forming partnerships with clients. First, there are different cultural perspectives and expectations about client–therapist partnerships. For instance, a Western approach to health promotion and wellness programs expects clients to assume personal responsibility for their health. This includes asking questions of health professionals and asserting their own views about health. However, some cultural groups consider asking questions or stating their opinions about treatment to be disrespectful (Falvo, 1999). Instead, they defer to the opinion of health professionals.

Second, clients and recreation therapists may have different values and beliefs about recreation and leisure. This can influence a partnership. For instance, elderly clients often have backgrounds that emphasized work or other "productive" and worthwhile activities like raising families. Likewise, clients who are poor and live in impoverished communities may view the recreation therapist's emphasis on leisure involvement as an unfamiliar luxury compared to such basic needs as housing, childcare, and meaningful employment. In both these instances, discussions about recreation and leisure involvement may appear irrelevant because it is inconsistent with clients' values and priorities. Clients are more likely to want to assume some responsibility for health-related changes if they value the outcomes and see them as being consistent with their expectations and priorities.

Beyond this, Falvo (1994) advises therapists to explore the costs clients associate with making behavioral change. In addition to financial costs, clients may perceive pain, discomfort, lack of functional skills, and loss of self-esteem as additional costs associated with their effort to incorporate recreation and leisure involvement into their lifestyle.

This concept [perceived costs] has relevance whether it is used in teaching patients about acute illness, chronic disease or preventive practices. Not only must patients believe that the treatment will be effective; they must also believe that the treatment or change in lifestyle will be worth the cost. (p. 206)

Empowering Clients through Shared Responsibility

Partnerships between clients and therapists are based on two fundamental assumptions: respect for clients' right to self-determination, and a belief that clients have strengths that can be used to affect their own desired change. Therefore, therapeutic relationships need to be collaborative. This often means that TR specialists must help clients believe in themselves and express their wishes and desires. A helping professional's ability to empower others is a key facilitative characteristic (Brammer & MacDonald, 1999; Egan, 1994). Empowerment involves helping clients to discover and use their own resources. Even though there are clear situations that require therapists to assume most of the responsibility for the intervention process, a commitment to empowerment and shared responsibility ought to be at the core of all helping actions.

Clinical judgment determines when and how much responsibility can be reasonably expected of clients. A delicate balance exists between urging clients to take an active role in the intervention program and respecting their need and right to reject any help and any responsibility for change. Of course, in some cases, such as with very young children and clients with advanced dementia, shared responsibility is less likely. In most cases though, it is a matter of listening carefully to what clients want and finding ways to reinforce their sense of competence and control. This is a matter of respecting the client's experience, and having a genuine commitment to preserving the client's dignity. A conscious commitment to shared responsibility and partnerships helps health and human service professionals reconcile self-responsibility and social influence. Helping is a form of social influence, and the power ascribed to the professional can unwittingly foster helplessness and dependency (Egan, 1994). It can also intrude on a client's autonomy. This issue has particular relevance to TR practice, and is embedded in TR service models as control.

Client autonomy and control are contained in the various TR service models because they are germane to a client's experience of recreation and leisure. For instance, control is depicted along a continuum in both the Leisure Ability Model (Stumbo & Peterson, 1998) and the Health Protection/Health Promotion Model (Austin, 1998). At one end of the continuum is the use of TR as a treatment or intervention. At this point practitioners function as therapists and assume control of the process. This has the greatest chance for oppressing client autonomy. At the other end of the continuum TR services involve the provision of recreation and leisure opportunities. At this point the client is free to make his or her own decisions.

While these TR service models illustrate some general components of practice, they oversimplify the issue of control in client–therapist relationships. In actual TR practice, therapists can respect client autonomy and self-determination by sharing responsibility for decision-making during treatment. Asking clients a question like "What would your situation look like if things were good?" helps them visualize changes they want and actions needed to achieve them. TR service model presented by Van Andel (1998) includes informed consent to remind practitioners that they must seek client's agreement to be involved in TR intervention programs. Seeking informed consent is also a deliberate way to involve clients in decision making and to ensure that the power exercised in helping relationships is not demeaning nor an unintentional influence on helplessness.

Partnerships can promote shared responsibility in several ways. For instance, Miller (1992) suggests that

clients can exercise personal control by using their preferred coping mechanisms (e.g., watching TV), even if it is not consistent with what therapists think is best. She also recommends involving clients in determining which aspects of their care they would like to learn. Once this is decided, teaching skills in small increments helps to increase a sense of control while the use of "homework" or practice exercises can give clients responsibility. Finally, it is very important that the partnership adheres to an "ecological perspective" and recognizes that there are probably factors in the client's environment or situational context that help or hinder opportunities for change and growth. They may be beyond the client's control, yet equally deserving of attention in the clinical change process. For example, an environmental intervention can involve a recreation therapist talking to group home managers and parents about the importance of giving choices to persons with disabilities as a way to counteract learned helplessness.

☆•••Thinking Trigger

At this point in your TR education, how much has "partnerships" with clients been emphasized? Can you think of an instance when it might be difficult to forge a partnership with clients?   •••☆

Cultural Competence

Earlier in this text we addressed the influence of culture on the individual via the client–system perspective. The client–system perspective implies an appreciation for cultural influences on perceptions of health, illness, recreation, leisure, and quality of life. Increasingly, there has been recognition that effective therapeutic relationships are culturally sensitive, and that helping professionals need a multicultural worldview. The most inclusive approach to multiculturalism pivots on a broad definition of culture, which includes race, ethnicity, social class, gender, religion, sexual orientation, and disability. Obviously, such a broad definition represents the range of diversity that can be experienced by recreation therapists in health and human services.

According to van Servellen (1997), cultural competence refers to the capacity to function within a multicultural context by acknowledging, accepting, and respecting differences, and continuously expanding knowledge about different groups of people. Multicultural competencies are evident in three areas: beliefs and attitudes, knowledge, and skills (Sue, Arrendondo & McDavis, 1992). Each area needs to be addressed as practitioners strive to be culturally competent.

Examining personal attitudes and beliefs includes a willingness to examine your values and attitudes that may be latently prejudiced or racist. This issue extends to professional practices as well. It has been suggested that all helping professionals should explore the relationship between power, privilege, and poverty. For instance, Corey and Corey (2002) believe that mental health practitioners need to recognize the institutional barriers preventing easy access to and use of community mental health services. Brammer and MacDonald (1999) warn that White helping professionals may encounter some resentment from clients who are cultural minorities because of perceived "White privilege." Similarly, Daw (1997) urged helping professionals to take a candid look at the imbalance of power that permeates health care (between provider and patient) and the fact that this can represent an extension of oppression experienced by many people.

A genuine commitment to cultural competence requires TR professionals to develop a personal awareness training program, which would include learning more about cultural similarities and differences, and confronting their own ethnocentrism, racist tendencies, and stereotypic thinking. Exploring the questions and related topics contained in **Table 11.1** (p. 198) is a good starting point. For instance, personal attitudes, beliefs, and behaviors can be examined by asking questions like *How does my gender affect relationships with clients and other staff? What have been my experiences with rejection, isolation, loss, and oppression, and how might these experiences help or hinder my ability to appreciate these same situational experiences of others?*

Cultural biases may also permeate the theoretical and practical approaches used by professionals in their work with clients. For instance, Deiser and Peregoy (1999) contend that individualistic values dominate TR philosophy and practice. An emphasis on individualism and self-sufficiency can conflict with collectivistic cultural values that place greater emphasis on group identity and family involvement. Furthermore, each client's cultural background and frame of reference includes beliefs about health and the expectations associated with seeking and defining help. Each culture has its own way of defining and experiencing health care and the helping process. Such views may not be the same as those taught in formal educational and training programs, which are typically taught from an Anglo or European worldview. Acknowledging cultural differences and making efforts to understand and respect the client's cultural orientation will influence the level of trust, genuineness, and empathy needed in therapeutic relationships. It is a mistake to ignore differences or to pretend that one understands the culture of others. Practitioners should not be afraid to acknowledge unfamiliarity with a culture or to apologize for any faux pax. "Statements such as 'I have little experience with people of your culture, but I would like it if you could help me learn' conveys caring and concern and will be accepted by most people as such" (Falvo, 1994, p. 154).

Communication Competence

Effective helping relationships depend on clear and purposeful communication. Throughout the TR clinical process, you will work to create an open and trustworthy level of information exchange. You seek to understand the client's story, listening carefully to what is being communicated visually, verbally, and kinesthetically. The intent is to hear and feel the client's needs and wants. Beyond knowing facts or details, effective communication requires emotional empathy, which means knowing what it must feel like to be this individual. Each activity-based modality used in clinical practice provides an opportunity for clients to express themselves and a chance for therapists to listen and understand. In turn, therapists communicate therapeutically by responding with information and feedback, offering support and hope (i.e., processing). As you will recall from Chapter 6, processing involves sensitive and skillful feedback that is supportive and encouraging, relevant to the goals that have been established, and directed at reinforcing or altering clients' thoughts, attitudes and behaviors. The entire TR process depends on communication competence, which involves specific skills and abilities described in the following sections. These skills enable you to effectively interact with clients.

Using Active Listening and Responding Skills

According to van Servellen (1997), to be effective as a helper you must possess accurate perceptions and processing and self-expression skills. This involves a core set of functional communication skills involving listening, clarifying, and responding. Most importantly, you must be willing to listen rather than rush in with new questions and quick advice. The core communication skills needed for active listening and responding are listed in **Table 11.2** (pp. 200–201) They are synthesized from several writers, including van Servellen

Table 11.1: Developing multicultural competencies (Adapted from Ivey, Peterson & Ivey, 2001; Peregoy & Deiser, 1997; Sheldon & Dattilo, 1997; and Keller & Stevens, 1997)

Examine Personal and Professional Beliefs and Attitudes

How do my background and personal life experiences affect my worldview as a person and as a professional? How are my interactions with others influenced by my…

- Language?
- Gender?
- Family values?
- Sexual orientation?
- Religion and spirituality?
- Socioeconomic background?
- Education?
- Group affiliation?
- Significant life experiences (e.g., trauma, losses, discrimination, prejudice)?

What personal or professional biases and stereotypes operate in my view of others?

- How do I feel about people who are drug dependent?
- How do I feel about people who are poor and unemployed?
- What is it like to work two jobs?
- What is it like to be a single parent?

How might an emphasis on independence in TR theory and practice conflict with cultural beliefs and practices that value interdependence and group attachment?

Acquire Knowledge about Diverse Cultures

What can I learn about other cultures?
What do I know about…

- Structure and role of the family in diverse cultures (e.g., issues of authority, respect, decision making)?
- Influences of culture, religion and lifestyle on the family unit?
- Dietary practices, both for nutrition, pleasure ("treats"), and healing (e.g., Asian use of herbs)?
- Festivals and celebrations of diverse ethnic and cultural groups (e.g., holy days, holidays)?
- Preferred and symbolic dress (e.g., kimar worn by Muslim women), and the issue of modesty?
- Social rules of diverse cultures (e.g., greetings, contact between men and women, provider–client conduct)?
- Defining characteristics of the communities where clients live?
- Cultural explanations of health and illness based on values and traditions?
- Cultural role of faith healer or shaman and its comparison to Western medicine?

Acquire and Use Multicultural Skills

How can I utilize my knowledge and understanding of cultural diversity in TR practice?
Some possibilities include:

- Encourage more involvement from families, partners or significant others.
- Acknowledge traditional healing methods.
- Acknowledge the role of family and the client's faith community.
- Consider literacy by simplifying written materials and using pictures and graphics as needed.
- Use interpreters.
- Explore community resources that are available for holistic health.
- Use client's language to the extent possible. Have essential terms translated into client's language and keep a two-way dictionary handy.
- Accept silence and lack of eye contact as culturally normative.
- Learn American Sign Language.
- Learn games and social activities popular in other cultures.

(1997), Brammer and MacDonald (1999), and Corey and Corey (2002).

Using Alternative Forms of Communication

Communication exchanges are effective only to the extent that your verbal exchange with clients matches their ability for comprehension and self-expression. Sometimes there is a need to modify one's communication style or format, especially when the client's ability to process information from spoken language may be diminished. For example, young children often require therapists to modify their language so they understand what is being said. This is most clearly evident in medical settings where confusing and frightening technical terminology is used routinely. Consider, for instance, when children are told that they will have an x-ray. More appropriate language would be "having a picture taken." Abbreviated terms such as ICU (intensive care unit) can be interpreted literally to mean "I see you." Also, since play is a child's primary mode of learning and expression, recreation therapists use medical play with hospitalized children so they can understand medical procedures on their own cognitive and emotional level. These are examples of developmentally sensitive practice. Other examples of communication techniques that extend beyond the spoken word include American Sign Language and the range of augmentative and alternative communication devices (e.g., from simple picture boards to computer-assisted voice synthesizers). You demonstrate a genuine desire to communicate and a respect for diverse abilities and communication styles when you become familiar with clients' preferred modes of communication.

Understanding Cultural Aspects of Communication

Culture generally influences communication patterns. Research suggests that cultural variations exist in terms of communication style, eye contact, body language, and voice quality. For example, White Americans generally speak quickly and expect a good deal of eye contact, while Asian Americans speak softly, use less eye contact (especially with people of high status), and respect silence (Sue & Sue, 1990). There are cultural variations with interpersonal space or how close people get to each other when speaking (Ting-Toomey, 1999). In addition, there are cultural variations related to the ease with which people share personal information (Sue & Sue, 1990). An effective helping professional must recognize and respect culturally different communication styles.

You can expect to encounter clients who do not speak English, and you may be unable to speak their language. Consequently, nonverbal communication behaviors can unintentionally compound the communications problem. For instance, care should be taken when using hand gestures since simple gestures can be interpreted differently in various cultures. Likewise, it is important to monitor one's own level of anxiety in these situations because of the tendency to talk louder, exaggerate words, or to equate an inability to speak English with diminished intelligence. Saarmann (1992) recommends the use of picture-boards, dictionaries, and translators when communicating with clients who do not speak English. Progressive health care agencies keep a list of bilingual employees who can serve as translators. Sometimes translators are relatives of the client or a member of his or her community. In these instances, you should realize that translators might have limited vocabulary related to health care. Also, non-English speaking clients may be uncomfortable with an interpreter, especially if the exchange involves sensitive information and the interpreter is of the opposite sex or is the client's child. Of course, it is a good idea for you to learn some key words and phrases of the client's language and to incorporate them into oral and written communication. This conveys respect and a desire to communicate. In some circumstances, clients who use English as a second language can be invited to help TR specialists prepare written instructions and explanations for TR services into other languages.

Using Touch When Communicating

One other communication variable worth mentioning is touch. In many circumstances, communication can be enhanced through physical contact. Simply touching the arm of a client or holding their hand can be calming and reassuring. A gentle hug can be supportive and comforting, too. In pediatric and long-term care settings, physical contact is often the most effective form of communicating care. Many nursing home residents have a pervasive sense of loneliness and have lost opportunities for physical contact. For some clients, words will never be as effective as a touch in communicating empathy and compassion. Of course, all physical contact needs to be used with discretion. Physical touch may be unacceptable or deemed inappropriate in some cultures. Some clients, particularly those who have poor ego boundaries (e.g., a person who is psychotic) and those who have been physically or sexually abused may

Table 11.2: Communication skills

1. Listening

Listening is an active process in which you take in information (verbal and nonverbal expressions, and the affective qualities of the message and messenger) and respond in ways that elicit clear communication. Effective listening is being "present" for a client, both physically and psychologically. Listening has four subskills: attending, paraphrasing, clarifying, and perception checking.

Attending	Eye contact should be direct, but it does vary according to sociocultural norms. Posture should be relaxed, open, and you should squarely face the person. Facial gestures should convey interest, and verbal statements should encourage the other person to keep talking (*I see. Mm-hmm*).
Paraphrasing	Restating the content of the message (perhaps in fewer and simpler terms) to test the accuracy of what you heard and understood. This involves repeating concisely only the client's message without adding any new ideas. Paraphrasing communicates your effort to understand the basic message. Consequently, the client may feel understood and more competent in his or her ability to communicate. Also, paraphrasing encourages the client to continue talking because you are really listening.
Clarifying	Seeking to make vague or confusing messages clear. Unlike paraphrasing, you make a statement that "guesses" about the basic message, or admits to confusion and asks the client to give more information or to try and restate his or her message. Clarifying can help to focus or center the conversation. (*I'm confused; Would you go over that again? I'm afraid I am not following you.*)
Perception checking	Seeking to be sure that communication is clear. This involves three things: paraphrasing what was heard, seeking confirmation of your perceptions, and allowing the client to correct your perceptions. (*You seem to be worried about discharge; is that right? You've been smiling a lot. Does this mean you are enjoying this art activity?*).

2. Leading

Leading assists the client to communicate more fully. It involves anticipating where the client is going and encouraging him or her to explore thoughts and feelings in a way that helps the client to understand rather than just provide more information. Leading involves questioning, probing, and focusing.

Questioning	Closed-ended questions phrased to evoke a narrow range of possible responses, or that elicit one-word or yes/no responses. (*Do you ever feel bored?*) Open-ended questions phrased to evoke a wide range of possible responses; frequently begin with "what" phrases. (*What would it be like if you weren't bored?*) Multiple-choice questions phrased to evoke a response to simultaneously presented choices. (*What are you more likely to do when you get bored: complain, watch TV, sleep, or talk on the phone?*)
Probing	Searching for additional information with an invitation to "tell me more about that." (*Please tell me more about your past experiences with using recreation to deal with stress*).
Focusing	Honing in on a particular topic, issue, or feeling. May be done by selecting one word for the client to focus on. (*You mentioned several issues about your overall health. I'd like us to talk about your views on being physically active.*)

Table 11.2: Communication skills (continued)

3. Reflecting
 	
Reflecting is a process of affirming a client's feelings and affective quality of his or her experiences in an attempt to convey that you perceive the experience as the client does. Reflective statements serve as a "mirror" for the client's feelings and emotions, which can encourage further awareness and exploration of feelings.
 	
Similar to paraphrasing, reflecting involves giving back to the client his or her total message at three levels:
    • Feelings (*It sounds like you are excited about going home.*)
    • Experience, including reference to accompanying body language (*That big grin on your face tells me you're excited to go home.*)
    • Content (*The activities you mentioned for your weekend and the big smile on your face tell me you're excited about going home.*)

4. Interpreting Interpreting involves making statements that offer some possible explanation for thoughts, behaviors, or feelings in an attempt to add new perspective to a client's understanding. For example, a client says, *I don't want to go on that community re-entry outing.* You respond, *Since you are just getting to feel comfortable with your prosthesis, you may be worried about keeping up with the group when we're at the mall.*
5. Confronting Confrontation occurs when you challenge discrepancies in a client's words and actions and shed light on apparent inconsistencies. This allows the client to examine mixed feelings or ambivalence honestly. For example, a confronting response could be, *You say you are ready to leave the rehab program, but you have refused to go on the last two outings you signed up for. What's going on?* (*Note*: Confronting involves risk, and should not be used until a therapeutic relationship has been established. The client may value the honest feedback, but may also feel threatened and shut down in the conversation. Consider the timing of the confrontation and the readiness of the client to receive feedback).
6. Informing Informing occurs when a recreation therapist provides factual information to the client without suggesting or stating what she or he should do. Informing also involves providing suggestions and advice based on clinical experience (e.g., The recreation therapist says to a client, *Here is a list of suppliers of adaptive gardening tools. Other clients with gardening interests have found the tools to be inexpensive and easy to use.*)
7. Summarizing This occurs when you pull together the important and central ideas and feelings of the client. The intention is to synthesize what's been communicated, to give clients a feeling of progress in learning and problem solving, and to have a direction for the next session or next part of the interview/conversation.

be troubled by touch or may misinterpret the meaning of the gesture. Yet the value of touch may, on balance, outweigh the potential harm. Therefore, it is worth learning about the meaning of touch in various cultures.

Obviously, communication is a complex exchange process, and becoming competent at it takes time and effort. Despite the pressures from large caseloads and constant paperwork, a genuine commitment to communication competence needs to be reaffirmed continuously. You will need to seek out opportunities to learn about cultural styles of communication, and you will have to self-evaluate your efforts to maintain a client-centered communication style.

Issues in Therapeutic Relationships

Therapeutic relationships are complicated by a variety of factors generic to all helping professions that have specific relevance to TR practice. Thus, we end this chapter with a discussion of several challenging issues that you will face in your relationships with clients. These issues include, but are not limited to, time constraints and timeliness, managing emotional closeness, self-disclosure, terminating relationships, and relationships with people in clients' lives.

Time and Timing

Developing and maintaining a therapeutic relationship takes time. Unfortunately, in many care situations the focus is on expediency. Practitioners experience real pressure from administrators to provide effective care in the shortest amount of time possible. Consequently, you may have very limited contact with a client even though you are expected to assess needs, plan and deliver interventions, and document the outcomes of your services. The pace of care and shorter lengths of stays often leaves many recreation therapists feeling as if they barely had enough time to learn the client's name. However, this does not eliminate the need for you to establish a relationship—it merely alters the depth of the relationship. As we explained earlier in this chapter, helping relationships are based on trust, empathy, and respect. Even though the length of time with a client may be brief, any amount of helping must emerge from a commitment to provide care for the person who has the symptoms rather than the symptoms alone. We must take the time to communicate with clients so we understand them. Otherwise, our practice runs the risk of adding to the dehumanization of health care.

Perhaps no other area of practice has experienced the challenges of limited contact time more than psychiatric or behavioral health care. Brief hospitalizations have made it necessary to have a solution-oriented approach guided by clearly defined outcomes. Brief treatment requires a high level of client–therapist interaction where trust and rapport are established quickly. Hoyt (1995) characterizes brief treatment as having clearly defined client and therapist responsibilities and a working relationship that is marked by flexibility and creativity. Frequency and length of treatment varies according to client needs, and there is a significant expectation for client work (e.g., homework assignments outside of scheduled sessions). Using client strengths and abilities to the extent that is possible, interventions are considered merely springboards for changes that can occur in real life. That is, brief treatment operates on the premise that the intended change will occur in the client's life, not during intervention sessions. For example, inpatient programs utilize recreation therapists to run stress management, exercise, and communications groups that are brief, self-contained sessions in which clients receive, examine, and apply information. The expectation is that the clients will ultimately decide whether to incorporate these elements into daily routines. Despite the brevity, helping clients invest themselves in the intervention depends on a therapeutic relationship.

Effective therapeutic relationships also reflect good *timing*. That is, practitioners learn to recognize verbal and nonverbal cues from clients that indicate a readiness for certain interactions. This comes from being empathetic. Even though a recreation therapist has a focused agenda—for example, to conduct an assessment or provide information about adaptive equipment or community resources—the therapist strives to be attentive to client concerns. Forging ahead with little or no sensitivity to client readiness can be alienating and can render intervention meaningless. This is particularly relevant to education-based interventions where the purpose is to give clients information that they can use to support their health and well-being.

Clients have many legitimate reasons why they may feel the time is not right for TR interventions. For some, the issue may be pain or other forms of physical discomfort. For others the lack of receptivity to clinical TR services at a particular time may be due to anxiety or other forms of emotional upset. It may also be that recreation and leisure issues are not a priority for the client. High and low levels of receptivity are an expected part of therapeutic relationships. Effective therapists are flexible enough to take these variations in stride. If they find a client to be unreceptive at one time, they recognize that a return visit may find the individual once again receptive to interaction. Most importantly, recreation therapists ought to stand ready to put aside their own agendas and tune in to what is pressing the client. Often this sensitivity increases the client's trust in the relationship and subsequent receptivity to TR interventions.

The timing of certain interventions can also be built into overall care, as is the case with clinical pathways. For instance, inpatient physical rehabilitation programs often confine clinically based TR services to the predischarge phase of care. At this time, clients are most ready for and receptive to addressing issues about community reintegration and resuming recreation and leisure involvement. Not only does this help to streamline overall care, it helps with the client–therapist relationship since the purpose, focus, and overall relevance of the interaction is clearer and more relevant to the client.

The Rewards and Risks of Emotional Closeness

One of the great pleasures TR specialists can experience is a sense of closeness with their clients. This closeness often results because of the playful nature of recreation activities and the emphasis on what clients *can* do rather than limitations or inability. Also, activity-based interventions often reveal qualities of clients that other professionals rarely see. Consequently, within the context of these activities, clients tend to feel comfortable enough to openly share their thoughts and feelings. Most importantly, helping clients focus on things they enjoy doing and find meaningful reaches beneath their diagnostic labels and touches the spirit of these individuals. This can lead to a level of emotional closeness between you and your clients that can be very gratifying and rewarding.

Clients are also curious about the person behind the professional title, and sometimes want to know what you think and feel about certain issues or life experiences. They may want to share in the excitement about an impending marriage or birth. They may be curious about your recreational interests and wonder whether you practice what you preach. In essence, some clients expect therapists to be their friends. After all, friendships are often formed on a basis of shared experiences and genuine concern for the welfare of another.

Helping relationships and friendships do share some commonalties, yet there are differences. Friendships are based on mutuality. That is, a friend can

expect that the other person will reciprocate his or her warmth and concern. Friendships also have no time constraints or artificial boundaries imposed on them. These same expectations do not easily fit therapeutic relationships. Still, all therapeutic relationships can have genuine warmth and caring and an appropriate amount of personal sharing without the complications that friendships imply to some clients.

Just how close you ought to get with your clients generally depends on the basis of the relationships, client needs, and the service delivery setting (e.g., psychiatric day program, nursing home, independent living program for adults with head injuries). In some instances, clients seek relationships with TR specialists after discharge, or in the case of community-based service delivery, while the program is continuing. In the case of nursing home residents, TR specialists are permanent parts of the residents' social world and can be considered by residents to be within their new circle of friends. It is difficult to state an unconditional stance that you ought to take on this matter—each case needs to be addressed individually. Overall though, serious consideration should be given to the meaning a friendship would have for both you and your clients. It is important to clarify the boundaries of this friendship and to prevent any false or unrealistic expectations from being developed. You should rely on rules of ethical conduct and guidance from clinical supervisors. Certainly, it is inappropriate and unethical to form an intimate relationship with a client. Beyond that, therapists should weigh the benefits and liabilities emotional closeness has for client care.

Emotional closeness poses some risks for recreation therapists, as well as rewards. First, it is not uncommon for beginning therapists to overidentify with clients, especially when they are close in age or share other similar circumstances. Overidentification can interfere with staying client-focused and objective. You will recall reading earlier in this chapter about the importance of analyzing one's own feelings that arise in practice. Personally identifying with clients is very common yet it can interfere with effective helping. Clinical supervision can help you become aware of and understand the impact of your thoughts and feelings on client care.

Second, closeness usually happens as a result of a therapist's willingness to be open and genuine and to share personal information with clients. Yet you must realize that therapeutic relationships sometimes require more careful consideration of openness and the role and function of self-disclosure, an essential skill for effective therapeutic relationships.

Self-Disclosure

Self-disclosure involves knowing when, where, and how much to share about oneself. According to Egan (1994), helping professionals are always involved in indirect self-disclosure through facial expressions, body language, and other emotional responses. Direct self-disclosure, on the other hand, is a more explicit and direct sharing of personal experiences, behaviors, and feelings. Self-disclosure is revealing nonobvious aspects of self, such as thoughts, feelings, attitudes, or experiences through a distinct and meaningful self-reference. These are true statements intentionally made by the therapist to a client with a therapeutic aim in mind (van Servellen, 1997, p. 137). Used judiciously they can elicit more information or engage the client in mutual problem solving. They can be used to build trust and to establish a common link with a client. Self-disclosure can validate a client's feelings and experiences a client is having or to provide concrete examples to help a client grasp an idea or make a connection. In some therapeutic intervention programs, self-disclosure is used routinely to contribute to the therapeutic process. For instance, Egan (1994) indicated that counselor's self-disclosure is generally the norm in alcohol and drug addiction programs. Carruthers and Hood (1994) also believe self-disclosure is appropriate for TR interventions as long as it is aimed at helping clients address their issues and not those of the recreation therapists.

Consider the following example. Nicole, a CTRS working with Linda, a woman who had an exacerbation of MS, finds Linda quite demoralized about her current health status. Especially upsetting is the fact that her diminished energy level interferes with her ability to care for her two school-age children, tend to household duties, or interact with her husband. Linda refuses to work on the leisure lifestyle action plan with Nicole, claiming "What's the use; I just can't do it all." Nicole decides to disclose some personal information. She tells Linda that she understands her sense of overwhelming demoralization, as she experienced a similar situation trying to care for her new baby, who could not sleep through the night. Nicole tells of her own struggle with sleep deprivation, the resulting fatigue, and the difficulty she had with her husband as she tried to involve him in household and parenting responsibilities. Nicole's decision to self-disclose was made with the hope that her personal information would validate Linda's feelings, convey support and understanding, and lessen Linda's self-criticism.

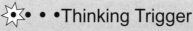

Thinking Trigger

Do you think that Nicole was correct to self-disclose? How would she know if her disclosure helped?

Just as it is probable that personal sharing conveyed a sense of empathy, it is also possible that a client could reject the implied comparison between the client and the therapist. Self-disclosure can have both positive and negative effects on helping relationships, and this must be considered when you are making decisions about self-disclosing. van Servellen (1997) has identified several therapeutic and nontherapeutic effects of self-disclosure, which are found in **Table 11.3**.

Inevitably, you will be in situations where you have to decide when and how much to disclose about yourself. This is a normal part of client–therapist relationships. Not long ago, training programs for counseling-oriented professions maintained that practitioners should avoid sharing personal information. Today, that view is challenged as being too rigid. If practitioners are too guarded about sharing personal information and rebuff any overtures from clients in this vein, the distance created between client and therapist can be counterproductive. Again, the issue requires thoughtfulness and care. **Table 11.4** (p. 206) presents a list of guidelines for using self-disclosure therapeutically. These guidelines are based on a review of literature on therapeutic self-disclosure (Brammer & MacDonald, 1999; Cormier & Hackney, 1999; Egan, 1994; van Servellen, 1997).

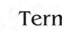 Termination

Just as it is important to develop a working relationship with a client, it is also important to properly end the relationship. Typically, the evaluation phase of the clinical TR process is considered the last stage of the relationship. However, we believe that there is another phase in the clinical process, termination, which involves bringing the helping relationship to meaningful closure. Unfortunately, in some cases the nature of health care service delivery poses barriers to this process. Too often, for example, recreation therapists come to work and find that their clients have been discharged abruptly, and their chance to provide discharge guidance and to terminate the relationship is lost. Despite such possibilities, you must try to bring a fitting end to the client–therapist partnership. Ending relationships does not only pertain to clients who are served as inpatients and are going to be discharged. Termination is a matter for all relationships regardless of service delivery setting. For example, in-home services or clinical intervention programs that occur where there is no formal discharge have their own predetermined or natural ending. In these cases as well, relationships must be terminated appropriately.

Ideally, proper termination of a therapeutic relationship begins before the last scheduled encounter with a client. Terminating the relationship involves reflecting together on the work done as partners, progress made, and hopes for the future. In some cases, clients feel grateful for the help they received but worry about losing this support. They mention how the therapist's encouragement and emotional support helped them to cope and to adapt. Consideration needs to be given to resources that can replace this support. Finding a substitute can be difficult for some clients, reinforcing the need for thoughtful and caring termination. It is also important to realize that many clients have a tendency to attribute any improvements in their condition to the skills and dedication of their therapists. In an effort to revise self-efficacy beliefs, therapists ought to correct these misperceptions during termination and provide valuable feedback that underscores the role of the client in effecting change.

In some cases, termination or the act of saying goodbye is ritualized through parties, gifts, or other tokens that represent the relationship and celebrate accomplishments. The chance to mark the occasion with something tangible is very important to many clients. Therapeutic recreation activity can be used in these rituals as a symbolic way to mark changes that have been made and to say "thank you" and "goodbye." For example, mental health and alcohol treatment programs sometimes use "trouble boxes" made in arts-and-crafts programs to symbolically store the discharged client's written messages pertaining to their "old" self. In other instances certificates, medallions, or framed pictures of the client with particular staff are used to formalize discharge or note the successful completion of a program. Craft projects or potted plants that might have been used in recreation therapy sessions can also be used to ritualize beginnings and endings.

Reunions for groups of clients can also be an effective way to help clients manage termination and any losses that are associated with it. These reunions are commonly used in health promotion programs where clients developed lifestyle action plans, which are difficult to maintain and require periodic support and reinforcement. Client reunions are also common in rehabilitation programs. Reunions provide a chance for a refresher course on recreation and leisure topics since clients may now be more aware of their needs and the importance of healthy and satisfying lifestyle.

Of course, termination is not always filled with positive feelings. In some cases there is disappointment that goals were not reached or that clients never really connected with the therapist. Fiscal constraints have resulted in

Table 11.3: Therapeutic and nontherapeutic effects of self-disclosure (Adapted from van Servellen, 1997)

Therapeutic Effects	Nontherapeutic Effects
Sense of being understood. When a therapist shares brief, pertinent, and well-timed personal information, clients gain some reassurance that the therapist is listening carefully, is empathetic, and understands at a human level.	***Decreased understanding.*** Disclosure unrelated to the client's experience or current frame of reference can be distracting and counterproductive. It can interrupt a client's thinking and make the client feel that the therapist is not listening.
Enhanced trust. When a client senses that a therapist understands the situation or the context of their experience, they are more likely to trust the therapist.	***Role reversal.*** Self-disclosure is counterproductive when it results in an exchange of roles between the client and therapist. This occurs when the therapist's disclosure shifts the focus to the therapist and away from the client. This can place the client in a position of trying to help, guide, or support the therapist.
Decreased loneliness. Self-disclosure communicates sharing an experience, which tends to reduce the sense of isolation that clients often feel.	
Decreased role distance. Self-disclosure can modify the distance the client feels from the therapist, which increases the likelihood that mutual, collaborative problem solving will occur.	

clients being discharged before their rehabilitation is complete, which leaves care providers feeling frustrated and worried for the client's future. This frustration sometimes leads to cynicism because health professionals know that they will soon see the client returning to the hospital as part of a "revolving door" of treatment and discharge. Regardless, termination should be handled professionally and in the best interest of the client. When that individual does get readmitted, a necessary therapeutic relationship must be reestablished without resentment toward the client.

Finally, termination can be experienced around a client's death. In some cases, such as in hospice care, recreation therapists may actually have an integral part in helping the client pass from this life in a dignified manner. Despite impending death, and indeed because of it, recreation therapists have an opportunity to help clients live fully to the very end. In hospice and AIDS programs, for instance, recreation therapists can use their compassion and skill to help clients creatively express themselves to those they are leaving behind, or to create living legacies of their lives. One example is making a video or audiotape recording of the client's message to friends or grandchildren.

In other instances recreation therapists and other staff are caught by the unexpected nature of death, or they can witness a very painful ending of a person's life. Death can be difficult to handle emotionally. It is a loss that recreation therapists must acknowledge, and they must turn to others for support so that their capacity to give to other clients will not be compromised (Cappel & Mathieu, 1997). Additionally, a client's death often affects other clients. It might represent a loss of a peer or a reminder of their own mortality. As grief and loss counseling becomes more prevalent,

Table 11.4: Guidelines for using self-disclosure

Consider your motivation. Ask yourself: *Why do I want to share this information? How can disclosure help? What is my client-centered goal for disclosing?* Use disclosure to help clients open up, not to meet your own needs for attention or reassurance that you are making a difference.

Consider the stage of the relationship. Disclosing too early (and too much) can make clients uncomfortable and can turn them off.

Keep disclosures short and focused. Do not distract clients with long stories about yourself. Do not disclose more than is necessary to help facilitate therapeutic aims. Do not assume that your experience is the same as the client's experience.

Keep disclosures relevant to the client's needs and goals. Tie the disclosure to the client's issues or situation.

Use disclosure as a form of sharing and feedback. Share your present feelings in relation to the client's behavior. (*Right now, watching you do this activity, I am feeling optimistic that you can master the use of these adaptive devices*).

Give brief and direct responses when asked for personal information. When asked for personal information (e.g., *Are you married?*), be sure to return the focus back to the client. If the client requests information that is intrusive and makes you feel uncomfortable, say so. Express curiosity with a response (*I'm wondering why you are asking me this.*).

Be flexible in your approach to using self-disclosure. Consider the situational context by making decisions about disclosure according to each client and situation individually.

Evaluate the usefulness of the disclosure. Did it enhance client cooperation, learning, and insight? Was it perceived as supportive? Therapeutic self-disclosure depends on good timing, the right amount of information, and a client-centered objective.

Use clinical supervision to review your use of self-disclosure. Recognize that there are cultural differences regarding self-disclosure and that some persons from other cultures may find your disclosures indiscreet and a violation of privacy. Review how frequently you use self-disclosure. If disclosing is a frequent occurrence then it is probably being used inappropriately.

bereavement support is being initiated in some agencies. Recreation therapists can investigate death education resources as a way to manage personal feelings as well as discovering ways to foster comfort among surviving family, friends, clients, and colleagues (Murray & Simpson, 2001).

Relationships with People in Clients' Lives

Throughout this chapter we have addressed therapeutic relationships in terms of your interaction with clients. However, the personal attributes, characteristics, and competencies you read about will also be needed in forming and maintaining therapeutic relationships with important people in a client's life. In many cases, relationships with parents, spouses, and other significant people in your clients' lives can be extremely important and a primary focus of your work. For example, recreation therapists are sources of information, support, and hope for parents who are dealing with a sick child. The ability to help parents cope bears directly on a child's well-being. Likewise, spouses who share with their loved one the challenges associated with managing chronic illness and other disabling conditions learn through TR how to support functional recovery and adaptation. After all, these individuals often determine the day-to-day success of rehabilitation and ultimate lifestyle changes you encourage through TR interventions.

Summary

The client–therapist relationship is perhaps the most important part of clinical TR practice. It is an opportunity to use yourself as a tool in helping clients. Even when there is too little time to get very involved, or the client's motivation or level of investment is limited, you have a duty to form a therapeutic relationship that is genuine, reliable, and respectful. Therapeutic relationships are challenging, especially in situations where the pressure for expedient functional interventions or symptom reduction is emphasized and the demand for outcome evidence is high. In these instances, it is easy to overlook the importance of promoting client dignity through shared responsibility for care. Yet, clinical practice aimed at promoting client dignity and the capacity to change and grow must be based on a therapeutic relationship between client and therapist.

TR clinical practice requires that you commit yourself to developing skills and abilities that are instrumental in facilitating clients' learning, adaptation, and growth. These include an awareness of yourself as a person and a professional. Additionally, you need to develop both communication and cultural competence so you can form partnerships with clients. These skills and abilities take time to develop, and require ongoing education, and solid clinical supervision.

The importance of supervision cannot be overemphasized. It will maximize the chance that you will become a reflective practitioner who is deeply aware of the pivotal role of therapeutic relationships in quality TR practice. Ultimately, you benefit, as well, from your work with clients. O'Keefe (2000) described the unique spiritual transaction that can happen in TR.

> It seems to me that we do our best work when we, as professionals, allow our own spirits to enkindle hope in our clients. The great and wonderful mystery to those of us who see with spiritual eyes is that we, too, are touched and made better as human beings by the very people we serve. (p. 14)

References

Allhouse, K. (1993). Treating patients as individuals. In M. Gerteis, S. Edgman-Levitan, J. Daly, and T. Delbanco (Eds.), *Through the patient's eyes: Understanding and promoting patient-centered care* (pp. 19–44). San Francisco, CA: Jossey-Bass.

Austin, D. (1998). The health protection/health promotion model. *Therapeutic Recreation Journal, 32*(2), 109–117.

Austin, D. (1999). *Therapeutic recreation: Processes and techniques* (4th ed.). Champaign, IL: Sagamore Publishing.

Brammer, L. and MacDonald, G. (1999). *The helping relationship: Process and skills*. Needham Heights, MA: Allyn & Bacon.

Cappel, M. and Mathieu, S. (1997). The grieving process. *Parks & Recreation, 32*(5), 82–85.

Carruthers, C. and Hood, C. (1994). *A model leisure education program for substance abusers: Implementation and evaluation*. Paper presented at the annual conference of the American Therapeutic Recreation Association, Orlando, FL.

Carter, M., Van Andel, G., and Robb, G. (1995). *Therapeutic recreation: A practical approach* (2nd ed.). Prospect Heights, IL: Waveland Press.

Corey, M. and Corey, G. (2002). *Groups: Process and practice* (6th ed.). Pacific Grove, CA: Brooks/Cole.

Cormier, S. and Hackney, H. (1999). *Counseling strategies and interventions*. Needham Heights, MA: Allyn & Bacon.

Daw, J. (1997). Cultural competency: What does it mean? *Family therapy news, 28*, 8–9, 27.

Dieser, R. and Peregoy, J. (1999). A multicultural critique of three therapeutic recreation service models. *Annual in Therapeutic Recreation 8*, 56–69.

Edgman-Levitan, S. (1993). Providing effective emotional support. In M. Gerteis, S. Edgman-Levitan, J. Daly, and T. Delbanco (Eds.), *Through the patient's eyes: Understanding and promoting patient-centered care* (pp 154–177). San Francisco, CA: Jossey-Bass.

Egan, G. (1994). *The skilled helper: A problem-management approach to helping* (5th ed.). Pacific Grove, CA: Brooks/Cole.

Falvo, D. (1994). *Effective patient education: A guide to increased compliance*. Gaithersburg, MD: Aspen.

Falvo, D. (1999). *Effective patient education: A guide to increased compliance*. (2nd Ed.). Gaithersburg, MD: Aspen.

Hoyt, M. (1995). *Brief therapy and managed care*. San Francisco, CA: Jossey-Bass.

Ivey, A., Peterson, P., and Ivey, M. (2001). *Intentional group counseling: A microskills approach*. Belmont, CA: Wadsworth/Thomson Learning.

Kanfer, F. and Schefft, B. (1988). *Guiding the process of therapeutic change*. Champaign, IL: Research Press.

Keller, C. and Stevens, K. (1997). Cultural considerations in promotion of wellness. *Journal of Cardiovascular Nursing 11*(3), 15–25.

Kuschner, H. (1998, September). *What heals?* Paper presented at the ATRA Annual Conference, Boston, MA.

Mackelprang, R. and Salsgiver, R. (1999). *Disability: A diversity model approach to human service practice*. Pacific Grove, CA: Brooks/Cole.

Miller, J. (1992). *Coping with chronic illness: Overcoming powerlessness*. Philadelphia, PA: F. A. Davis Co.

Murray, S. and Simpson, E. (2001). What is bereavement support? Facilitation techniques for grief and loss counseling in therapeutic recreation. In G. Hitzhusen and L. Thomas (Eds.), *Expanding horizons* (pp. 18–35). Columbia, MO: University of Missouri.

O'Keefe, C. (2000, October). *Spirituality and the ethics of caring*. Paper presented at the NTRS Institute, Phoenix, AZ.

Peregoy, J. and Dieser, R. (1997). Multicultural awareness in therapeutic recreation: Hamlet living. *Therapeutic Recreation Journal, 31*(3), 174–188.

Saarmann, L. (1992). Communication: The vital connection. *Topics in Emergency Medicine, 44*(4). Gaithersburg, MD: Aspen.

Sheldon, K. and Dattilo, J. (1997). Multiculturalism in therapeutic recreation: Terminology clarification and practical suggestions. *Therapeutic Recreation Journal, 32*(2), 82–96.

Stumbo, N. and Peterson, C. (1998). The leisure ability model. *Therapeutic Recreation Journal, 32*(2), 82–96.

Sue, D., Arrendondo, P., and McDavis, R. (1992). Multicultural counseling competencies and standards: A call to the profession. *Journal of Counseling and Development, 70*, 477–486.

Sue, D. and Sue, D. (1990). *Counseling the culturally different: Theory and practice* (2nd ed.). New York, NY: John Wiley & Sons.

Ting-Toomey, S. (1999). *Communicating across cultures*. New York, NY: Basic Books.

Van Andel (1998). TR service delivery and TR outcome models. *Therapeutic Recreation Journal, 32*(3), 180–193.

van Servellen, G. (1997). *Communication skills for the health care professional: Concepts and techniques*. Gaithersburg, MD: Aspen.

Chapter 12
Using Intervention Groups in TR Practice

Guided Reading Questions

After reading this chapter, you should be able to answer the following:

- What are the characteristics of TR intervention groups?
- What are four broad categories of TR intervention groups?
- What structural and process elements must be considered in TR intervention groups?
- What are the functions of an intervention group leader?
- What are positive and negative aspects of co-leading intervention groups?
- What is processing and how does its use contribute to client outcomes?
- What techniques are used in processing intervention groups?
- What are therapeutic factors and how do they contribute positively to intervention groups?

Introduction

Recreation therapists have always used groups as a primary way to deliver intervention services to clients. Intervention groups can be efficient and practical because several clients can be gathered in the same place to do the same or similar activities with a supervising recreation therapist. Recreation therapists can alternate their attention and interactions among clients in the group, thereby providing services in an efficient and effective manner. Such efficiency is important in the current climate of managed care: however, this is not the primary reason for using groups in clinical practice. Intervention groups provide opportunities for interactions among clients, and recreation therapists use these interactions to facilitate therapeutic outcomes. This chapter examines the structure and process associated with intervention groups and explains leadership skills and techniques essential to group facilitation.

Characteristics of an Intervention Group

Although groups are formed in every service delivery setting, simply creating an aggregate of clients does not constitute a TR intervention group. Intervention groups have certain defining characteristics that contribute to their potential to promote change and growth in clients. To begin, intervention groups combine *two energies*:

1. Tasks or activities that group members do together

2. Interpersonal dynamics associated with group process that meet social and emotional needs of clients (Posthuma, 1999)

Intervention group leaders decide how to blend these energies so that both individual and group goals can be reached. The balance between the energies depends on the group's purpose, the clients' abilities, and the time available.

Another characteristic of intervention groups is the *common identity and shared purpose* that clients experience as members of a group. For instance, members of a community reintegration group share a common identity, as each person is preparing for discharge. While each client maintains his or her own identity during group interventions, a group identity emerges. They also share the common purpose of the group: learning to deal with returning to the community. This shared identity and purpose serves as validation that individuals are not alone in their feelings. Consequently, a basic level of trust is built around feelings of acceptance and support.

Building on this common identity and shared purpose, group activities or tasks become catalysts for meaningful interactions among group members. In some instances, these *group dynamics* occur spontaneously, as in the case of a group of clients working together to successfully pass through a "spider web" during an adventure–challenge group. At other times, the group dynamics result from reflective discussions where clients explore concerns and use each other as a benchmark for comparing thoughts, feelings, and behavior. These interactions allow clients to learn from each other and experiment with new perspectives and behaviors important to making changes in their lives (Corey & Corey, 2002). Processing tasks and interaction dynamics helps group members to draw something positive and useful from the group experience. Ultimately then, intervention groups have a level of involvement that fosters *cohesion*. Group members develop a sense of "we-ness" because of the acceptance and empathy expressed in the group and because of the work they do together to achieve common goals (Posthuma, 1999).

Intervention Groups Used in TR Practice

While TR practice is quite diverse, several common categories of intervention groups are used in clinical TR practice, including educational groups, functional skills groups, support groups, and psychoeducational groups. Many of the activity-based interventions (see Chapter 9) can be used in any of these groups. The distinctions made here have to do with the intended purposes and outcomes of the groups.

Educational Groups

Educational groups are primarily used to provide information. This can include information on a variety of topics pertaining to health, disability, or leisure. For example, clients can be provided with health promotion information related to recreation and leisure's contribution to wellness and a healthy lifestyle. An example of such an educational group would be a leisure education group that provides participants with information on leisure resources, the benefits of social contact, and the importance of regular exercise. In addition, education groups provide information that enables participants to examine their existing knowledge, values, and attitudes about health and leisure.

Functional Skills Groups

Functional skills groups improve clients' abilities to interact with their environment, manage their illness or disability, and engage in daily living tasks, including recreation. Skill enhancement groups are most effective when there is enough time for clients to practice applying skills to daily life. In some care settings, recreation therapists use group activities with clients whose illnesses or disabilities impair their ability to

focus on an activity or interact with others. Group activities stimulate attention to the tasks and the presence of other group members. With higher functioning clients, group interventions improve and enhance existing skills. Mental health agencies, for example, use skill enhancement groups to assist clients with developing and using assertiveness skills and stress management techniques. Social skills training groups are used with children and adults who have developmental disabilities or at-risk youth (Stumbo, 1999).

Support Groups

Support groups provide consistent and reliable social and emotional support for clients dealing with health crises (e.g., cancer treatment) or managing daily living issues that are secondary to a primary health condition. For example, outpatient mental health clinics offer clients ongoing support groups that help with needed coping resources. Client interactions center on discussions about medication compliance, current events, social relationships, and leisure. Also, many rehabilitation hospitals offer ongoing socially supportive "peer counseling" groups to individuals who have been discharged from rehabilitation programs. These groups usually have open agendas covering a wide range of issues, including social and emotional issues related to health maintenance, leisure interests and opportunities, and self-advocacy challenges.

Psychoeducational Groups

Another type of intervention group used in TR is a psychoeducational group, which combines education, skill enhancement, and social support. Psychoeducational groups are structured around a topic or theme relevant to clients' overall health and well-being. They are psychoeducational because they combine education about a topic or theme with opportunities to examine underlying psychological issues that affect participants' intentions and abilities to use the information provided. Psychoeducational groups typically have preset agendas and use formats that allow clients to share useful information. For example, clients who need to develop a more physically active lifestyle following cardiac or stroke rehabilitation can learn about the importance of exercise and can explore a variety of ways to incorporate physical activities into their overall recreation and leisure routines. However, behavior change is rarely just a matter of having information. You will recall that, theoretically, changing health behaviors involves consideration of the values and beliefs individuals hold about a particular health behavior (e.g., physically active recreation). Therefore, an important part of psychoeducational groups is exploring issues related to personal motivation, competence, efficacy beliefs, and the role of social support in behavior change.

Many leisure education or health promotion programs use psychoeducational groups that focus on a particular theme or issue. Activities such as games, worksheets, and group discussion are used so members' interactions can help them learn from each other and develop insights into their own perspectives on health and leisure. Clients develop concrete plans for behavior change. "Homework assignments" are used to apply what may have been learned in the group sessions to group members' current situation and personal goals. **Table 12.1** lists examples of theme-oriented psychoeducational groups used in TR clinical practice. At first glance, you might think that the intervention groups on Table 12.1 could be educational or skill enhancement groups. What makes them psychoeducational is the additional focus on psychological or social issues that interfere with clients using the information or applying the skills in efforts to make changes in their lives.

The combined approach of providing information, developing skills, and examining psychological issues in an emotionally and socially supportive environment is effective (Corey & Corey, 2002). Such an approach was illustrated in the program designed to increase the health and wellness of women with physical disabilities described in Chapter 6. The group's structure and process was integral to helping women gain information, learn skills, and exchange social and emotional support with one another.

There are other examples of similar groups. Consider a support group for individuals caring for persons with Alzheimer's or Parkinson's disease. These groups can provide basic information about illness, new advances in medical and psychosocial care, adaptive equipment, and recreation's role in health and life quality. Caregivers can also gain skills in using recreation activities to structure time and interactions with their loved one. Additionally, group members can exchange emotional support around their common experiences related to loss, anger, and frustration, and their own need for recreation and leisure.

Elements of Intervention Groups

All TR intervention groups involve a number of key elements that influence the intervention's effectiveness. These elements comprise the structure or inputs to the group and the process or dynamics of the group. Together the structural and process elements produce specific outcomes. Ideally group outcomes match original goals set for the intervention program. **Table 12.2** (p. 214) displays various structural and process elements that shape intervention groups. The remainder of this chapter discusses the structure and process of intervention groups, as well as the importance of monitoring outcomes derived from them.

Structural Elements

Patterson and Melcher (2000) identified several key factors affecting intervention groups used in mental health agencies. These include clients, group design, and leaders' competencies. While Patterson and Melcher focused on mental health groups, all intervention groups are structured around these elements regardless of setting.

Table 12.1: Examples of TR psychoeducational groups

Stress Management group for clients with chronic mental illness living in a supervised community setting

Assertiveness Training group for young women with mental retardation transitioning from school to community and adult life

Coping Skills group for clients learning to manage alcohol addiction

Wellness through Leisure group for adults attending an adult day care center

Caring for the Caregiver group for spouses of people with Alzheimer's disease living at home

Community Reintegration group for clients getting ready for discharge from a physical rehabilitation hospital

Weekend Leisure Planning group for clients with developmental disabilities who attend a community center for adult education and skills training

Group Format

Intervention groups vary in size and membership. Certainly, size will influence the level of interaction and cohesion that can be expected. Grouping clients with similar needs or functional levels is sometimes the basis for creating membership. Groups can also be described as either closed or open.

Closed groups generally begin with a fixed number of participants (e.g., 8 members). No new members are added after the group starts. Closed groups are generally better for creating cohesion, but the rapid turnover of clients that occurs in most settings makes closed groups impractical.

Open groups allow clients to join at any time and to remain for however many sessions as possible. In some settings, clients choose from among the available or recommended intervention groups, rather than being assigned. Open groups do not have any membership restrictions. Clients join or are added at any time regardless of what is being discussed or done in the group sessions. Open groups are used most often in practice, which means that recreation therapists need to motivate clients to attend. If clients understand the benefits that can be derived from attending, and if these benefits are consistent with their needs and concerns, they are more likely to attend. A flyer announcing or advertising a group and its benefits is a practical way to promote open groups.

Open groups also require you to be prepared to accommodate a diverse mix of clients. While such diversity challenges the most skilled therapists, clients usually have common issues despite differences in diagnoses, age, and gender. Spira (1997) identified several common issues and themes that can be addressed in a psychoeducational group for persons with medical illnesses, including:

- Adjustments to physical and psychological changes imposed by illness or disability and the subsequent changes in self-image
- Relationships with care providers, family and friends
- Resuming an active engagement in life

Similar client concerns include adjusting to treatment and side effects; changes in mood, energy, self-image, and priorities; altered levels of functioning and lifestyle; and recreation and leisure involvement.

Group Duration

Circumstances can dictate how long intervention groups will last. In some cases, groups are time-limited in that they are comprised of a specific number of sessions occurring over a limited period of time. For example, an assertiveness training group in a psychiatric day treatment program might be limited to four to six sessions. Once these sessions are concluded, a new cycle of the program begins. *Open-ended groups* tend to be ongoing with no particular end point, as might be the case with a weekly caregiver support group offered at an adult day center. Another example is a *discharge-*

Table 12.2: Elements of intervention groups

Structure (Input)	Process	Outcome (Output)
Clients Age, gender, culture, literacy level, reason for involvement, perceived comfort with being in a group	*Session structure* Opening, body, closure	*End result of session* Intended outcomes resulting from planned session
Group format Closed or open, time limitations, purpose, size, expectations (norms or rules)	*Session content* Tasks or activities structured to facilitate individual and group goals	Unintended consequences resulting from session dynamics
Leadership Training and experience, belief in group process, number of leaders	*Session process* Member–leader interactions and member–member interactions (facilitated and spontaneous)	
Environment ("climate") Privacy, degree of distraction, physical arrangements (e.g., space, seating), mood of participants	*Group dynamics* Subgroups or cliques, adherence to norms, therapeutic factors	

planning group that meets once a week for any client preparing for discharge at that particular time. The agenda is flexible enough to accommodate diverse members and issues pertaining to general discharge concerns.

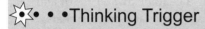
☼• • •Thinking Trigger

What is the distinction between an open group and an open-ended group? • • • ☼

Group Leadership

Intervention groups depend on effective leadership. This begins with an awareness of the factors that define and give meaning to groups, and an appreciation of the leader's influence on the therapeutic potential of intervention groups. Several leadership skills are fundamental. Therapists must be able to structure group experiences to help individuals achieve their goals and contribute to the group as a whole. Leaders engage clients in activities and discussions relevant to individual and group goals. This necessitates being able to create a climate of trust, respect, and acceptance within the group. It also means having an understanding of clients' needs, including developmental issues important in age-specific groups (see Corey and Corey, 2002). Finally, managing group dynamics by tracking verbal and nonverbal communication, and monitoring your own impact on the group are additional skills needed when leading intervention groups.

Function of Group Leaders

Group leaders have several general functions that have an important influence on the group. First, enthusiasm for and belief in the value of groups helps to motivate clients and sets a positive tone for learning and growth. The ability to motivate clients is critical throughout intervention programs. **Table 12.3** (p. 216) contains some suggested leadership techniques for client motivation.

Second, leaders act as unifying and stabilizing force in the group. This includes serving as a link between clients, making sure new members feel welcomed and accepted, and promoting feelings of cohesion and accomplishment through group experiences. Leaders also make sure that rules or norms are maintained (e.g., beginning on time and respecting others), thereby giving the group a sense of stability. Leaders are also

technical experts. As a leader you must be able to guide clients in doing activities or tasks and accessing and using information and resources. Finally, leaders must model desirable behavior, such as respect for others and a willingness to participate in activities. Modeling also includes recognizing and acknowledging the "positives" displayed in the group. For example, leaders can model giving positive feedback to individuals for their contributions to group activities, call attention to strengths, and acknowledge the accomplishments of the group as a whole.

Co-Leading Intervention Groups

Increasingly TR specialists collaborate with other professionals in designing and implementing intervention groups. Groups are co-led with social workers, occupational therapists, nurses, and others. In mental health agencies in particular, co-leadership is used to train young and inexperienced staff. This is an excellent way to learn necessary skills without the added pressure of being solely responsible for outcomes. Particularly in situations where open-ended groups are used and when diverse backgrounds and functional abilities complicate group membership, co-leadership may be the best approach. However, these arrangements should never be entered into without thoughtful consideration of the strengths and limitations associated with co-leadership.

Strengths of Co-Leadership

Certainly, there are many benefits to co-leadership, including the chance for leaders to learn from each other and to share responsibilities for planning, implementing, and evaluating group interventions. Each leader's strengths can add to or complement the other, which may also offset weaknesses. Co-leadership doubles the potential contribution leaders make to group process, including heightened observations of group members' reactions and attention to group dynamics. In some cases co-leaders can model appropriate interpersonal behaviors and can provide children and adolescents a chance to reenact parent–child issues.

Limitations of Co-Leadership

Co-leadership can have its problems, as well. Sometimes less experienced group leaders take passive roles due to fear of making mistakes. They defer to the senior therapist and so they pass up opportunities to learn by attempting to facilitate the group. This imbalance of responsibility can become confusing and uncomfortable for clients. Also, competition can surface between leaders in terms of primary authority and control. These power struggles can center on leading and managing sessions, but competition can also reflect petty rivalries and turf issues between disciplines. For example, physical rehabilitation programs frequently place primary value on physical functional outcomes over psychosocial outcomes. Consequently, community reintegration programs that are co-led by PT and TR may experience conflict around skills to be taught and issues to be covered. Above all, the primary problem or limitation associated with co-leadership is lack of time for leaders to talk with each other about the group and to share their views and experiences.

Co-leadership must start with a conscious and deliberate commitment to maximizing its positive aspects while minimizing potential problems. This begins with developing a genuine awareness of and respect for each other as people and professionals. Discussions ought to include each other's beliefs and perceptions about group interventions, leadership styles, and facilitation techniques. Before initiating an

Table 12.3: Leadership techniques for client motivation

Motivate by Building Anticipation

- Make programs special and something that clients will look forward to. For instance, stir up some anticipation or excitement with advertisements that promote an event. "Coming soon…" or "This week only…" connotes something special about to happen. Highlighting benefits from attending and participating can also be a creative and intriguing part of your advertisements.
- Create a welcoming environment with pleasant sights and sounds using decorations, music, lighting, table cloths, costumes, posters, and other props.
- Give personal invitations to these events. Invitations can be verbal or written. For example, ask staff to give you used greeting cards from holidays and birthdays. Use the reverse side of the card cover, which is usually blank, to write special invitations or announcements.

Motivate by Inclusion

- Provide activities familiar to clients. Involve them in identifying possibilities and making plans for events.
- Create situations that have minimal expectations for skills or active involvement.
- Make everyone feel included. Have a name for the program or group and use signs, cards, banners or customized shirts that indicate clients belong.
- Find something for everyone to do. Ask for assistance—have clients help by setting up supplies, giving out materials, serving refreshments, holding something, or keeping track of something during the activity.
- Use the great equalizer and fail-safe motivator—food. Regardless of ability level, everyone enjoys a tasty snack or refreshment, and food has been shown through research to influence attendance.

Motivate through Pleasant Recollection

- Provide opportunities for clients to receive something for their participation (e.g., prize, certificate). Similarly, provide a memento that they can keep to remind them of their involvement. For example, a Polaroid picture can be shared with others and can be examined long after the program is over.
- Make a video of clients participating in a program and show it occasionally. Like home movies, clients and their family members can enjoy recollecting past events.

Use Yourself as a Motivating Force

- Be inquisitive about your clients. Seek out their stories. Acknowledge their abilities and have them teach you.
- Be an enthusiastic participant. Your enjoyment of an activity or event can be contagious.
- Use laughter and humor, the gentle, humble kind that can be shared with others, but never at their expense.

intervention group, co-leaders need to discuss how to share leadership responsibilities and blend their areas of expertise. As the intervention group proceeds, co-leaders need to talk about any problems with contrasting leadership styles, as well as things that make co-leadership enjoyable and effective. Such conversations are unfortunately often sacrificed due to overall demands in today's work environment; however, this level of communication is absolutely necessary for the success of co-leadership (Corey & Corey, 1997).

> ☆ • • •Thinking Trigger
>
> What would be your preference: leading a group alone or co-leading a group? Why?　　　　• • •☆

Process Elements

Process elements refer to what happens during an intervention group. How a group session is implemented will certainly affect the energies mentioned earlier that contribute to intended outcomes. However, all groups will have certain dynamics that reflect human interaction. These can also have a significant effect on the experiences participants have in intervention groups.

Session Structure

While intervention groups are structured around a specific purpose and a combination of people, each group session is most productive when implemented in a consistent or structured manner. Some intervention groups are structured as several interrelated sessions; others involve a single stand-alone session. Whether stand-alone or interrelated, each session follows a systematic process from beginning to end.

There are three essential parts to every session in an intervention group. The *opening* portion concentrates on building rapport among group members, and helping them to feel at ease and to be aware of what to expect. The body or *structure* portion refers to the session's content and process (i.e., what occurs during the session and how it is conducted). Finally, the ending or *closure portion* concentrates on summarizing what was done in the session and drawing connections that generalize to life outside the group. **Table 12.4** (p. 218) contains a format for conducting group sessions. This format also includes pregroup and postgroup tasks of group leaders.

Session Content

Content refers to activities or tasks that will be used as the focus for group action and as an essential basis for achieving group goals. Content can include a variety of activities (e.g., games, group challenges, role plays, creative–expressive tasks), as well as discussions about particular topics. Familiarity with various activity interventions and their potential to meet clients' needs and the group's purpose is critical. There are several considerations to keep in mind as you select content for your intervention groups.

First, the content selected must match the overall purpose of the group intervention. In some cases activities are the primary content chosen for achieving group goals. For instance, activities are often selected because they promote cohesion by offering opportunities to experience fun and enjoyment. Group games and problem-solving exercises are chosen because they can be used to emphasize what clients can do, and to challenge them to be creative and appreciate the feelings of belonging and group success. With clients who have limited functional abilities, activities are a primary way to motivate them to engage with their surroundings. In the case of health promotion and leisure education groups, activities are purposely selected for their potential to help clients achieve concrete and tangible outcomes. For example, a stress management group often involves activities that allow clients to examine their typical, and sometimes irrational, responses to stress, and practice with using humor, deep breathing, and imagery to manage tension and anxiety.

Content can also be used as a catalyst for eliciting thoughts, feelings, and behaviors that clients can reflect on and generalize to their present situation. For instance, self-esteem groups with adolescents frequently use poetry or the lyrics of popular music to stimulate self-discovery and self-expression. Additionally, activity content can be a catalyst that stimulates group interaction. All levels of group interaction—from basic ones like sharing materials for a group art project to complex ones such as achieving consensus on a group problem-solving strategy—can help clients learn about themselves and learn from each other. Kees and Jacobs (1990) recommend selecting group activities that generate discussion focused on a common topic or issue, thereby providing opportunities for exchanging useful information and experiential learning.

Session content should also match the abilities of clients to function as a group. Carefully chosen activities can help build understanding and acceptance as

Table 12.4: Structure of group sessions

Presession Preparation
- Examine goals.
- Make sure session goals reflect overall group goals.
- Gather materials and supplies needed for session content.
- Determine any adaptations needed to accommodate variations in physical, cognitive, and social functioning.
- Prepare physical space (e.g., seating, tables, lighting, privacy).

Opening the Session (Introduction)
- Greet participants warmly and enthusiastically.
- Consider who is present and acknowledge any group members who are absent.
- Observe clients' moods, energy levels, and other "readiness" cues that could influence participation.
- If there are new participants, ask a returning group member to comment on what the group has been doing/learning.
- If members have had previous sessions together, discuss what happened previously and link it to what you intend for this session. Invite comments about thoughts and feelings that may have carried over from past session. Check participants' frame of mind. Consider asking, "What were you thinking and feeling before coming to today's group session?" If the group is relatively small, you might say, "As a way of beginning today, let's go around and have each of you say what you'd like to accomplish or feel by the end of this session."
- Use a simple and fun "warm-up" activity to get energy going and to set a positive mood.

Content (Activity or Task)
- Introduce session content with simple, step-by-step explanations and directions.
- Use attractive handouts or large poster boards for written directions and displaying information.
- Use visual examples and demonstrations as needed.
- Use activities that engage participants visually, auditorily, and kinesthetically.
- Use activities that can involve everyone (no matter how simple).
- Have back-up plans in case your planned activities need to change.

Process/Processing
- Use word rounds or questioning to begin a discussion about the session activities or learning tasks. See Table 12.6 for various processing techniques.
- While it is good to have some preplanned questions to guide your processing, avoid any "rapid firing" of one question after another. Allow group members time to think about and respond to questions posed, and listen carefully to form new questions based upon their responses.
- Facilitate discussion among group members by using specific communication techniques (e.g., clarifying, redirecting, linking, and summarizing).
- Consider which therapeutic factors ought to be facilitated through the discussion (e.g., universality, guidance, cohesion). See Table 12.7 for explanation of therapeutic factors.

Closing the Session
- Bring the session to a close by summarizing what has occurred in the session.
- Provide reinforcement for cooperation of members or individual efforts that added to the success of the session.
- Consider posing questions for members to think about outside of the group as a way to encourage further reflection.
- If appropriate, assign "homework" for members to complete between sessions.
- When possible, provide information that would help members anticipate the next session. If there are members who will not be returning to future sessions, acknowledge this and allow them time to comment on what they have learned.

Postsession
- Write a "process note" on the session, including brief comments on individuals, the overall group, and impressions of content and process. Include any suggestions or recommendations for the next time the session is conducted.
- Follow up with individual clients on "homework" or issues that came up for them in the session.

well as willingness and ability to collaborate among members. Ultimately, session content is instrumental in building cohesion within groups. Of course, activities must be used carefully so that the required level of interaction matches the level of group development. For example, implementing an activity that requires clients to disclose personal views and values when they have had very little contact with each other can be counter-productive.

Finally, session content should be selected according to a sequential approach to learning. When a therapeutic group has a particular theme carried over several sessions, the content should be presented with a logical progression in mind (Posthuma, 1999). For instance, leisure education sessions generally follow a sequence of awareness, understanding, and application. Each session's content builds on previous sessions. Similarly, group initiative activities, a core of adventure-based counseling programs, follow an important risk-taking sequence that reflects increasing amounts of group comfort and increasing capacity to cooperate and communicate. Schoel, Prouty, and Radcliffe (1988) recommend selecting activities that progress from ice-breaker/acquaintance activities, to trust and communication activities, to problem-solving activities, and then to social responsibility activities.

Processing Session Content

While the activity content of TR interventions is important, it is the process involved in doing an activity that contributes most to learning, adaptation, and growth. Therefore, when activities, games and other structured experiences are used in clinical practice, recreation therapists must carefully monitor client's thoughts, feelings, and behavior within the total context of the activity. This helps you *and* your clients determine whether progress is being made toward intended goals, and increases the chance that clients can extract all they possibly can from their experiences in TR. Processing is an important part of all clinical practice, whether conducted with a single client or with a group of clients. Therefore, the following overview of processing pertains to TR interventions used with individual clients as well as groups.

Processing Defined

Processing is a therapeutic technique primarily involving verbal discussion of client behaviors, as well as their thoughts, feelings, and other external factors that relate to the behavior. Recall from Chapter 6 (Figure

6.1, p. 84) that processing helps clients become aware of their behavior, the decision making that shaped their behavior, and the connection between specific behavior and their wants and needs. Unlike verbal-oriented counseling interventions that focus on past behaviors, processing within TR practice focuses on here and now behaviors evident in activities. It also helps clients to generalize from the present activity to life beyond the TR intervention. Processing is essential to the appropriate and effective use of activities targeted at facilitating behavioral change among clients.

Processing is important, yet it can easily be ignored or overlooked in TR clinical practice. It is easier and emotionally safer to simply do the activity without talking about it or trying to make sense from it. Also, many TR specialists, especially those with limited clinical experience, are preoccupied with finding and using interesting activities. Beyond that, clients may not expect to discuss their thoughts and feelings about recreation. However, when the intent of activities is to serve as a means to achieving intervention goals, selecting and processing content appropriately is critical.

Processing increases the likelihood that clients will benefit from TR interventions by not allowing the conclusion of the activity to be the end of the learning experience. Specifically, processing:

- Assists clients in making connections between thoughts, feelings, and behavior
- Consolidates learning derived from several activities
- Helps therapists to understand more completely what is being learned or experienced by clients
- Promotes group cohesion
- Presents opportunities to receive useful feedback or input from others, as well as the chance to learn from others

Because therapeutic relationships are predicated on shared responsibility for goal setting and goal attainment, processing helps clients and therapists review together the relevance of the activity interventions to goal attainment, and to identify evidence of progress. Furthermore, the clients' self-assessment and opinions about their progress can be used in written progress notes. Processing, therefore, supports clients' choice and control.

Luckner and Nadler (1995) identified the theory of constructivism as a relevant framework for understanding the important role processing plays in learning and change.

Constructivists posit that learning is a process whereby new meanings are created (constructed) by learners within the context of their current knowledge. They believe that knowledge is constructed in the process of reflection, inquiry, and action, by learners themselves.

People are always trying to make sense of their own lives and the things they experience around them. The process of making sense of things involves a never-ending search for and construction of personal meaning. (p. 177)

In a similar vein, Mobily (1985) suggested that an existential view of clients searching for meaning in life was an appropriate philosophical base for therapeutic recreation practice. Whether our view is constructivist or existential, clients must be active participants in learning, discovery, and meaning making. Processing facilitates clients' involvement in finding meaning in their experiences.

Processing during Individual Client Sessions

Processing is not restricted to the end of an activity intervention session. It probably occurs most often at the end because the completed activity serves to focus the dialogue. Processing can occur at the beginning, middle, and end of a session. Beginning an individual intervention session by checking in with your client and explaining what will be happening is a helpful strategy. This *prebriefing* (Priest & Gass, 1997) or *frontloading* (Hutchinson & Dattilo, 2001) helps to focus clients on the purpose of the session before it begins. This is an opportunity to reinforce the session's goals and its relevance to overall treatment objectives. The client's thoughts and feelings regarding the impending activity session are also pertinent. At this point, therapists can get some idea about their client's level of motivation and readiness for the session. Given this check-in, you may decide to scrap the planned activity and alter the session's content.

Processing can also occur during TR interventions. It can happen during a break in the activity or during a rest period built into the activity. For example, when a recreation therapist involves a client who has a brain injury in a community reintegration activity, therapist and client can periodically stop and examine what's going on within the activity itself. The recreation therapist can ask about feelings being stirred by being in the community, and how the client is assessing his or her performance and confidence to proceed. This is an opportunity to help clients become aware of how attentive they are to environmental cues and their use of cognitive or visual compensatory strategies.

Processing during the session can also happen spontaneously, such as when the therapist notices behavior that represents a teachable moment for the client. Behavior can be used as feedback to help the client become more aware and to make adjustments before continuing on with the activity. Feedback can be used to reinforce strengths and abilities exhibited by the client. It can also be used to seek clarification about any nonverbal client expressions (e.g., body language), or explore thoughts and feelings clients may have regarding the activity itself. Consider, for example, stopping a session to seek some clarification from the client about his sudden silence and sad affect. This processing might result in refocusing or modifying the intervention to make it more relevant and helpful for the client.

> ☆• • •Thinking Trigger
>
> What are some nonverbal mannerisms to be attentive to when working with clients? What interferes with nonverbal communication? • • • ☆

While it is appropriate to process before and during an intervention session, processing certainly should happen at the end of the session. The session can end with a brief review of what occurred, its relevance to the client's path of progress, and ways to build on each step of success. Processing at the end of a session can also help set the stage for subsequent sessions. Ultimately, processing is used as a barometer to judge whether the client is getting as much as possible from the activity, and whether perceptions of mastery, competence, and overall self-efficacy are occurring. **Table 12.5** contains some sample processing questions that can be used with a client at the beginning, middle, and end of an intervention session.

Note that processing does not always occur in an intervention session. Therapists need to develop good clinical judgment regarding processing because it can be overdone and clients can be left feeling that their activities are overly "therapized." It is more effective to find teachable moments where processing actually enhances the therapeutic potential of your interventions. Take cues from clients and process from their frame of reference rather than your own agenda. It takes practice to become perceptive about the client's thoughts and feelings and to use that to ignite the processing dialogue. Some clients are limited in their abilities to verbalize their thoughts and feelings, so it is essential that leaders develop a keen sensitivity to nonverbal communication as well.

Processing Group Activities

Processing group activities increases the likelihood that clients will benefit from their interaction. Through processing, clients can learn from the perspectives of others and can feel acceptance and support. They can get feedback about their behavior, and their feelings

Table 12.5: Processing throughout individual sessions

Processing Phase	Sample Processing Questions
Before the activity intervention Check in with the client to get a sense of energy level, mood/affect, and overall readiness. Prepare the client for the session by describing what will be occurring, and clarifying the relevance of the session's content to intervention goals.	How are you feeling since our last session? Do you have anything on your mind or anything you want me to know about? How are you feeling about what we did in our last session? Any questions or concerns? What would you like to accomplish during today's session? Now that you know what we are going to do today, can you tell me how this could help you with goals that are important to you?
During the activity intervention Monitor and use verbal and nonverbal behavior of the client to explore reactions during the session (e.g., enthusiasm, hesitance, effort) and as indications of progress.	Your mood seems to have changed since we started. How come? You look concerned; what's going on? You seem to be having an easier time today. Why do you think that is?
After the activity intervention Review what was done in the session and relate this to overall intervention goals. Connect this session to past and upcoming sessions to reinforce the idea of small steps on the path to success.	Tell me one thing you feel you've accomplished in today's session. Which of the following best describes how you are feeling about what you did today: challenging, frustrating, successful, enjoyable, or would you describe it another way? How did today's activity relate to what we have done together in past sessions? If a friend (e.g., spouse, favorite nurse) observed you today doing this activity, what would they have noticed about your abilities? How would you evaluate yourself today? What did you learn that you can use at other times or in other situations?

and self-perceptions can receive a reality check from other group members.

Dattilo and Murphy (1991) developed a sequential approach to running leisure education groups, and processing (debriefing) is an important step in the sequence. Learning activities are followed by debriefings, which consists of a series of questions posed to the group to guide their reflection on the learning activity. "The debriefings encourage the participants to consider the relevance of the learning activity and identify accomplishments and barriers experienced in the learning activity" (p. 39).

Sometimes clients wonder why they are asked to participate in certain group activities during their intervention sessions. Postactivity discussions or debriefings help clients to connect their activity experience to larger and perhaps more important learning outcomes. Kees and Jacobs (1990) suggested that postactivity discussions focus on a review of what group members did, their feelings about the experience, what they noticed about their own behavior and that of others, and what they learned about each other. Most importantly, they suggested that discussions include connections clients can make between the session's activities and their life outside of the group.

A similar debriefing or postactivity processing approach is at the core of adventure-based counseling programs. Adventure-based programs follow a three-part sequence:

1. Brief (leader explains the activity)
2. Activity (group engages in a structured activity)
3. Debrief (reflective discussion of the activity and its implications)

Debriefing is the reflective part of the sequence. Schoel, Prouty, and Radcliffe (1988) presented a useful sequential approach to debriefing adventure activities in groups that has relevance to other activity-based intervention programs as well. For example, a stress management group for clients with addictions can be designed with several activities to facilitate self-exploration and social support. Processing the activities helps group members communicate, learn, and grow. Schoel and his colleagues developed a sequential path to guide processing, which moves from *What happened?* to *So what?* and concludes with *Now what?*

What Happened? Debriefing discussions begin with an overview of factual information. Clients are asked to describe what happened in the activity without any interpretation as to why. Clients can share immediate reactions to the activity, such as what they found to

be easy or difficult, and they can share behavioral observations they made of themselves and others during the activity.

So What? This part of the processing makes sense of what was done, observed, or said during the activity, as well as during the "what happened" part of the debriefing. This is an opportunity for clients to consider and discuss the consequences the activity had for them individually and as a group and the meaning of the experience overall. They can reflect on what they became more aware of, and what they learned. This is a shift from the descriptive to the interpretive. Group members "are abstracting and generalizing what they learned from the experience" as well as relating the experience to their personal goals (Schoel et al., 1988, p. 173). This part of the debriefing allows clients to consider why the activity was relevant and how they might be able to use the same skills and behaviors in real life.

Now What? The final phase of debriefing involves transfer of learning and generalization to personal situations and life beyond this group experience. New goals, referred to as *spiral goals* can be set by clients, with the intention of using new knowledge and insights derived from this experience in other areas of their lives.

Ellmo and Graser (1995) developed and applied the adventure model to a head injury rehabilitation program. They contend that processing is the most important phase of adapted adventure programs with clients who have disabilities.

> The activity phase, with all its experiential learning, can be worthless without the debrief to help integrate the experience. Just because you saw wonderful (or terrible!) things taking place during the activity, do not take it for granted that the group saw the same things. Even if they were aware of some of it, take this opportunity to integrate it further. (p. 24)

Ellmo and Graser's program represents a successful application of the adventure-based counseling model to clients who have cognitive and communication impairments. They simply adapt the procedures to fit the limitations of their clients. For instance, they make sure the activities are highly structured and that clients receive written directions and many cues during the activity. They encourage clients to take notes or use other recording methods to help them communicate and remember. Processing often involves having clients explain their decisions and behavior to reinforce memory and to make sure that all their options were considered and a safe and rational action plan was formulated. Finally, Ellmo and Graser utilize videotapes to enhance processing. They find that videotaped activities help clients compensate for memory deficits and self-monitoring problems and assist with accurate assessing of their own behavior. The concrete evidence of behavior contained in the videotapes circumvents any challenges to recollection, and can also be used to compare with future performance.

Methods and Techniques for Processing with Groups

Processing is not limited to the debriefing stage of a group activity. It can occur prior to, during, or after the activities, just as it does in individual client sessions. Processing can be used to help raise awareness about issues associated with an impending activity or event. As mentioned before, processing requires clinical judgment regarding how and when to engage clients. It is an art and a science. There are several methods for processing group activities (see **Table 12.6**, p. 224). The primary intention of all methods is to stimulate thinking, reflection, and discussion. Some processing techniques often become activities in themselves. Lane (1997) referred to a *tracking bag* that contains various props used to stimulate group conversation and discussion. For example, she passes out coins that members can use to hear what others are thinking ("penny for your thoughts"). She also passes around the group a polished stone, called a *bragging stone*. Upon receiving the stone, the individual tells the group what behaviors in the group activity they can brag about.

Chiji Cards, developed at the Institute for Experiential Education at the University of Wisconsin-LaCrosse, can also be used in processing group activities. *Chiji* is a Chinese word meaning "significant moment." As a processing tool, the images on the cards are used by group members to represent their feelings subsequent to the group's activities and any metaphor that can be associated with the member's learning or insight gained through the activity.

A Note of Caution and a Plea for Sensitivity

Table 12.6 contains a variety of methods drawn from the work of Luckner and Nadler (1997) on experiential learning and a review of the topic by Hutchinson and Dattilo (2001). Most are used widely in adventure-based counseling groups but have relevance to other TR

group interventions as well. While these and many other creative techniques can be used, we want to caution indiscriminate use of processing techniques. Placing an emphasis on verbalizing feelings, whether in individual sessions or within groups reflects a western, Euro-American approach to counseling and psycho-education. Thus, group activities and exercises that involve writing and discussion that expect clients to share thoughts and feelings freely may create cultural conflict. Interventions that have a strong cognitive component and involve examining and perhaps challenging thinking and beliefs may not fit with some clients from nondominant cultural groups (Cormier & Hackney, 1999). Leaders need to be sensitive to this potential conflict and respect the right of clients to abstain from participation. Silence or a refusal to complete some of the processing exercises contained in Table 12.6 should not be automatically interpreted negatively. Be flexible with approaches and sensitive to client reactions.

Processing Skills

While Table 12.6 presents a diverse mix of processing techniques, most require group conversations. Thus, good communication skills are called upon continuously when leading intervention groups. The same skills presented in Chapter 11 are needed to facilitate group discussions, especially questioning, paraphrasing, clarifying, and reflecting. In addition to these communication skills, several other microskills have particular relevance to leading intervention groups, including focusing, redirecting, blocking, linking, and summarizing (Ivey, Pederson & Ivey, 2001).

Focusing. During processing discussions, clients often focus on the activity and overlook behaviors that may be more important to the intended purpose of the group. For example, sports are commonly used with at-risk youth to help them learn appropriate social behaviors. Often youth want to talk about the outcome of the game and who has superior talents. The recreation therapist must focus the attention on the social behaviors evident when the game was played.

Redirecting. Sometimes group members' comments make the discussion drift from the topic or the session's main focus. At other times, individuals' comments are so self-focused that other group members lose interest. When this happens, you must sensitively steer the individual's comments and attention back toward a more productive direction for the entire group. Also, redirection is often needed to facilitate group interaction. For example, group members have a

Table 12.6: Group processing techniques

Processing Technique	Illustration
Large and Small Group Discussion	
Open Forum: The leader provides an opening statement as an invitation for members to volunteer their observations and perceptions.	I am interested in hearing your reactions to this session's activities.
Questioning: Leader poses preplanned sequence of questions intended to structure and focus group discussion. Questions should begin with simple, concrete matters and then move to more challenging ones. Consider the sequence of What Happened? So What? and Now What?	Would someone summarize for the group what we just did together? How does the interaction we had in this activity relate to your interactions at home, school, and work?
Rounds: Rounds focus participants by giving them a chance to think before responding. They also allow leaders to quickly assess members' thoughts and feelings before moving on with new session content. There are three types of rounds: (a) designated word or number round, (b) word or phrase round, and (c) comments round.	(a) Were you a leader or follower in today's session? (a) On a scale of 1–10, (1 is not at all, 10 is a great deal), how much did you enjoy today's activities? (b) State one word or a short phrase that describes your reaction to the session. (c) Let's go around the group and have everyone say a few comments about today's activity.
Dyads and Small Group Discussions: This involves mixing group members into pairs or small groups for focused discussion on a common experience, concern, or issue. Pairings can be based on similarities or differences such as age, type of disability, gender, or life circumstances.	Now that you are in pairs, take a few minutes to discuss how what we did in today's session relates to your hopes for the future.
Metaphors: These are symbolic ways of relating the individual's experience in the group activity to another situation in that person's life. Metaphors help group members generalize or transfer learning and insight from the group experience to life beyond.	The box in the center of our circle contains several objects, like keys, a cane, credit cards, eyeglasses. As we go around the group, pick an item from this box and explain how this object represents the experience you are having in this group.
Techniques to Prepare for Processing Discussions	
Written Activity Sheets: Activity sheets allow members to formulate their responses to what was experienced before any group discussion occurs. They often take the form of making lists or completing sentences.	Before we begin our discussion, make a list of 5 feelings you had while participating in today's activity. Based on the activity we did today, complete the following sentences: *My biggest concern about being part of a team is…* *I feel good about myself when I….*
Journal Writing: Journals can be used for members to write freely or to respond to specific processing questions posed ahead of time by the leader. Members can write about their thoughts and feelings, goals, concerns for the future, and so forth. Members can be asked to share their writing with others in the group.	Now that we decorated the cover of these notebooks, use it as a journal and write or draw your reactions to what we have been discussing about anger and getting along with others. Before you come back to group next week, ask someone else to write or draw in your journal about how they think you are doing in getting along with your peers.
Videotaping: Group members use the content of videotapes to stimulate discussion. Videotapes can be of them engaged in an activity, or of other clients that depict behaviors relevant to issues and concerns of the group.	Let's watch the videotape to find examples of cooperation and teamwork when we were completing the tower-building activity.

tendency to direct all their comments toward the leader. This can interfere with effective group communication. When this happens you can redirect the interaction with comments like *What you are saying is important to everyone; talk to the group, not just me*, or *Bill, your comments relate to Jim; how about telling Jim directly what you just said*. Unless you believe such interaction is premature or might make a group member uncomfortable, this sort of redirection helps reinforce an expectation for member-to-member interaction.

Blocking. It is also possible that some members' comments and behaviors will not be helpful to the group experience. Group leaders must make sure group intervention programs are safe places for people to learn and grow. Therefore, be prepared to block any behavior that is unnecessarily intrusive, rude, or hurtful. This can include blocking behaviors that breach confidence or violate another client's privacy. In many situations TR intervention groups involve a mix of clients with varying functional abilities. Out of frustration or impatience, higher functioning clients can make insensitive comments or simply ignore group members who are less capable. It is up to the leader to block any hurtful comments or criticisms. This can be done by redirecting the focus back to a topic that is useful to the group, or extracting something positive from members' behavior so that any personal attacks are avoided and dignity is preserved.

Linking. One of the greatest values of intervention groups is the chance for clients to feel understood, accepted, and supported by each other. This sense of connection is fostered when you link members to each other and to themes or issues raised in group discussions. Alert group leaders listen for common concerns, similar perspectives, or lived experiences and point out how members are connected. This encourages communication, which builds group cohesion. Consider how

Exhibit 12.1: Linking—A processing skill

> Even though Fred and Joe were twenty years apart in age, they had similar leisure interests prior to their injuries and hospitalization: Fred enjoyed boating and Joe enjoyed fishing. However, their tendency to only see differences between them interfered with group discussions about feelings of loss and the need to find renewed motivation. Their CTRS, Lamar, skillfully used their common interest in water activities as a focal point for discussing activity adaptations, and encouraged them to use the Internet together to find information on adaptive equipment for their common interests.

Lamar, the recreation therapist in **Exhibit 12.1**, linked two seemingly dissimilar group members.

Summarizing. This skill is used throughout group sessions, especially during processing and at the close of a session. Summarizing involves pulling together essential parts of the session and tying them together in ways that highlight main points related to program or session goals. Intervention groups that have multiple sessions should begin by having a member or the leader summarize what occurred in previous sessions. This is then used as a bridge to the current session. Summarizing is also used to transition from one activity to the next so clients can understand how the activities, individually and collectively, relate to the session's focus. During processing discussions, group leaders summarize various thoughts and feelings that were expressed so that the group's attention can move to the next topic. Finally, when a session ends, closure summaries are used to prepare the group for the next session.

Group Dynamics and Therapeutic Factors

Group dynamics are the essence of what makes groups uniquely beneficial in clinical practice. *Group dynamics* refer to everything happening within the group, including verbal and nonverbal behavior and the energy that exists during group activities. Intervention groups also have a pattern of interaction among group members, which is often referred to as *group process*. Group dynamics and group process are often used interchangeably. Both relate to the potential for people to learn, adapt, and grow through intervention groups.

Yalom (1983) identified specific beneficial factors associated with group process, which he originally labeled *curative*. Today, experts on clinical groups (Corey & Corey, 1997; MacKensie, 1997; Yalom, 1995) consider these therapeutic factors to be interrelated and mutually reinforcing. Some factors create group cohesion, which is essential for change and growth. Other factors are actual mechanisms of change (e.g., guidance, modeling). Recreation therapists should learn to recognize and facilitate these factors in intervention groups. They are an integral part of helping clients to benefit from groups. While some factors might happen spontaneously, skilled recreation therapists deliberately foster the presence of these factors by using a mix of activities and processing discussions.

MacKensie (1997) grouped therapeutic factors into four clusters based on their primary functions (see **Table 12.6**, pp. 226–227) The first cluster, *supportive* *factors*, includes universality, acceptance, altruism, and hope. Supportive factors promote a sense of involvement and connection among group members. These factors are effective in addressing feelings of low self-esteem and demoralization commonly experienced by many clients. These factors emerge rather quickly and can help motivate clients to remain involved with the group.

The second cluster, *self-revelation factors*, includes self-disclosure and catharsis. These factors allow individuals to share their stories and relate their feelings to the feelings of other group members. For some, this sharing can be risky, but it also provides an opportunity for individuals to receive feedback from others that indicates acceptance and support.

The third cluster of therapeutic factors, *learning factors*, includes modeling, vicarious learning, guid-

Table 12.7: Therapeutic factors associated with groups (Adapted from MacKensie, 1997)

Therapeutic Factor	Definition	Example
Supportive Factors		
Universality	Sense of commonality and shared experience, resulting in feelings that one is not alone in his or her situation.	At the end of the session, Tom realized that other group members also struggled with substance abuse and really understood his fear of losing control in his life.
Acceptance	Feeling that the group accepts the individual because the group validates the person's feelings and experiences.	Tiesha is very self-conscious about her weight, but she feels that the group appreciates her struggle to be happy despite social biases against obese people.
Altruism	Opportunity to help oneself by turning attention from self to others and acting in ways that help others.	Lydia offered words of encouragement and support to other women in her group, and felt good that she was able to be helpful.
Instillation of Hope	Restoration of self-worth that comes from group acceptance and support, and a renewed belief that change and self-improvement is possible because one sees improvement in others.	Jim has a renewed commitment to dealing with the rigors of rehabilitation after hearing a former client describe his ability to resume involvement in sports and family life.
Self-Revelation Factors		
Self-Disclosure	Verbal sharing of information about one's past and present as well as thoughts and feelings. It encourages others to react and perhaps to challenge these thoughts and feelings with greater objectivity.	Hearing himself talk about leisure boredom actually helped Hakim recognize that he had a hard time identifying things he enjoyed doing in his free time.
Catharsis	Expression of deeply felt emotion that promotes a sense of relief and an opportunity to form stronger bonds with others in the group.	The laughter and humor shared by members of the caregiver support group during a discussion of their common frustrations reflected greater closeness and comfort among group members.

ance, and education. These factors represent various ways clients can learn from others, which is an essential principle in cognitive–behavioral clinical TR practice (see Chapter 6).

Supportive, self-revelation, and learning factors are common to all intervention groups. In contrast, the fourth cluster, *psychological factors*, contains dynamics that typically occur in therapy groups where highly trained and experienced therapists have sufficient skill

to help clients receive and use feedback from others, and make connections between their thoughts, feelings, and behavior. This cluster includes factors such as interpersonal learning and insight.

Note that all of the therapeutic factors do not occur in every group. Their presence varies according to the type of group and the level of interaction among group members. For example, most TR intervention groups have the potential for members to experience at least

Table 12.7: Therapeutic factors associated with groups (continued)

Therapeutic Factor	Definition	Example
Learning Factors		
Modeling	Emulating or copying the behavior of others in the group (including the leader). Group leaders model behavior and call attention to exemplary behavior of others so it will be copied.	After watching his teammate apologize for his unsportsmanlike behavior, and seeing the leader's positive reaction, Tom tried to remember to apologize to others as well.
Vicarious learning	Similar to modeling, group members learn from watching others with whom they identify.	Watching her roommate in a role-playing exercise gave Jane some ideas on how to speak to her friends when offered drugs.
Guidance	Advice and suggestions exchanged among members.	The women in the leisure group exchanged ideas about ways to entertain friends with low-cost activities.
Education	Information and skill instruction provided through structured group sessions aimed at helping members change attitudes and behavior.	Members of the stress management group learned specific steps in progressive muscle relaxation.
Psychological Factors		
Interpersonal Learning	Learning about oneself through interactions with others in the group. Member's behavior elicits responses (feedback) from others. Feedback allows member to understand how he or she affects others. This feedback, coupled with support and encouragement, is a basis for members to find more productive ways to interact with others.	The need to be first in all activities and to dominate group discussions became more apparent to Steve after the group confronted him during the debriefing discussions. From then on Steve tried to adjust his behavior so that others would want him in group activities rather than getting mad at him.
Insight	Internal psychological process of making connections between thoughts feelings, and behaviors and gaining a greater sense of one's needs, motivations, fears, and hopes. Gaining perspective on one's past, present situation, and expectations for the future.	After group discussion, Tyra realizes that her unwillingness to join the aftercare social club and her tendency to do a lot of negative "self-talk" came from past disappointments in making friends.

some level of acceptance and commonality (i.e., universality), but only those designed for deeper psychological work will have the potential to help clients gain insight. Generally, TR intervention groups do not address issues at this level. TR intervention will usually help clients experience most of the therapeutic factors within the supportive, learning, and self-revelation clusters.

One additional therapeutic factor not included in Table 12.7 has been identified in the literature on group work and has special relevance to TR practice—*humor*. Humor is present in two ways. Humor can be an attribute of a recreation therapist and can be important in forming relationships with clients. The ability to keep things in perspective and not take oneself too seriously helps clients approach the challenges of learning and adaptation with a lighter mood and reasonable perspective (Posthuma, 1999). Also, laughter and humor can relax people and can bring people closer together. There is plenty of evidence that humor and laughter is healing, and so it ought to be used to build trust and cohesion in intervention groups. Enjoying sessions, despite the seriousness of their conditions or circumstances, fosters feelings of comfort and connection, which motivates clients to want to participate in a TR intervention group.

Monitoring Outcomes

As indicated in Table 12.2 (p. 214) outcomes are the end result of a group's structure and process. Group leaders monitor whether the sessions are implemented according to plan, and whether the sessions are adjusted as needed to achieve both individual and group goals. Although intervention groups have predetermined goals, other outcomes invariably result from group dynamics. Outcome monitoring should not happen only at the end of a group intervention program. It is best to use both formative and summative evaluation strategies.

Formative evaluation occurs while the program is happening. This might involve keeping brief process notes. These notes, which therapists write after each session, include brief narratives about each member, any alterations to session content and process (or recommendations for next time), and any issues pertaining to the group as a whole. Process notes are also very handy references for documenting client progress in their charts. Another type of formative evaluation occurs when co-leaders meet before each session to reaffirm the session's goals and review any carry-over from previous sessions. Co-leaders should also evaluate after the session as they debrief what happened in the session.

Summative evaluation occurs at the conclusion of the group intervention. This includes the use of client satisfaction questionnaires and/or self-reports on goal attainment, as well as any other evaluation data that can be used for ongoing quality improvement. Ultimately, both evaluations can help with revising and improving interventions.

Summary

Increasingly clinical TR interventions are provided through group formats. More than a mere gathering of clients in the same place at the same time, the interactions that occur in intervention groups foster common identity and cohesion among members. Recreation therapists leading intervention groups use a combination of activities and group dynamics to help clients learn important and useful information, enhance their functional skills, and experience social and emotional support. Many intervention groups used in TR practice are designed to be psychoeducational. In these groups clients obtain information useful for achieving and maintaining health, while also receiving support to understand and deal with psychological factors that influence their needs, motivations, hopes, and intentions related to making change. The interaction and support group members experience with each other contributes most to positive change and growth.

This chapter provided a basic overview of many key elements associated with intervention groups and the necessary knowledge and skills associated with group leadership. While this information can serve as a framework for understanding and using groups in clinical TR practice, real understanding and skills come from conscientious application of the knowledge. Learning about groups and developing your leadership (and co-leadership) competencies depends on your willingness to seek out mentoring from more experienced group leaders and supervisors. Even though structuring and managing intervention groups are among the bigger challenges in TR clinical practice, the potential gains for clients make the effort well worth it.

References

Corey, M. and Corey, G. (1997). *Groups: Process and practice* (5th ed.). Pacific Grove, CA: Brooks/Cole.

Corey, M. and Corey, G. (2002). *Groups: Process and practice* (6th ed.). Pacific Grove, CA: Brooks/Cole.

Cormier, M. and Hackney, C. (1999). *Counseling strategies and interventions*. Needham Heights, MA: Allyn & Bacon.

Dattilo, J. and Murphy, W. (1991). *Leisure education program planning: A systematic approach*. State College, PA: Venture Publishing, Inc.

Ellmo, W. and Graser, J. (1995). *Adapted adventure activities: A rehabilitation model for adventure programming and group initiatives*. Dubuque, IA: Kendell/Hunt.

Hutchinson, S. and Dattilo, J. (2001). Processing: Possibilities for therapeutic recreation. *Therapeutic Recreation Journal, 35*(1), 43–56.

Ivey, A., Pederson, P., and Ivey, M. (2001). *Intentional group counseling: A microskills approach*. Belmont, CA: Wadsworth/Thomson Learning.

Kees, N. and Jacobs, E. (1990). Conducting more effective groups: How to select and process group exercises. *The Journal for Group Work Specialists, 15*(1), 21–29.

Lane, S. (1997, September). *Back to basics*. Paper presented at the American Therapeutic Recreation Association Annual Conference, Nashville, TN.

Luckner, J. and Nadler, R. (1995). Processing adventure experiences: It's the story that counts. *Therapeutic Recreation Journal, 29*(3), 175–205.

Luckner, J. and Nadler, R. (1997). *Processing the experience: Strategies to enhance and generalize learning*. Dubuque, IA: Kendall/Hunt.

MacKensie, K. R. (1997). *Time-managed group psychotherapy: Effective clinical applications*. Washington, DC: American Psychiatric Press.

Mobily, K. (1985). A philosophical analysis of therapeutic recreation: What does it mean to say, "We can be therapeutic?" Part I. *Therapeutic Recreation Journal, 19*(1), 14–26.

Patterson, R. and Melcher, S. (2000, July/August). Mental health treatment network: Proactive team building. *ATRA Newsletter 16* (4).

Posthuma, B. (1999). *Small groups in counseling and therapy* (3rd ed.). Boston, MA: Allyn & Bacon.

Priest, S. and Gass, M. (1997). *Effective leadership in adventure programming*. Champaign, IL: Human Kinetics.

Schoel, J., Prouty, D., and Radcliffe, P. (1988). *Islands of healing: A guide to adventure-based counseling*. Hamilton, MA: Project Adventure, Inc.

Spira, J. (1997). *Group therapy for medically ill patients*. New York, NY: The Guilford Press.

Stumbo, N. (1999). *Intervention activities for at-risk youth*. State College, PA: Venture Publishing, Inc.

Yalom, I. (1983). *Inpatient group psychotherapy*. New York, NY: Basic Books.

Yalom, I. (1995). *Theory and practice of group psychotherapy* (4th ed.). New York, NY: Basic Books.

Part 4

Documenting Practice
and
Ensuring Competence

Chapter 13
Documenting Practice

Guided Reading Questions

After reading this chapter, you should be able to answer the following:
- What are the primary ways that recreation therapists communicate with clients, families, and colleagues about clinical TR services?
- What barriers impinge upon effective team communication and how can such barriers be minimized?
- What purposes and functions does the written client record serve?
- What are key rules for effective clinical writing?
- What are the similarities and differences between various charting formats for progress/service notes?
- What information must be included in a client's discharge summary?
- What are some of the legal issues and concerns to be considered when documenting client care?

Introduction

Previous chapters discussed clinical TR services and the manner by which therapists interact with clients to help them learn, adapt, and grow. In each of these chapters we have underscored the importance of communication.

Each day you will be involved in numerous communication exchanges in the workplace. Some of these exchanges will be casual, impromptu, and brief while others will be more formal. Communication exchanges occur with clients in the context of conducting assessments and planning and leading interventions. With families, communication occurs most often during education sessions or discharge activities. With staff, it transpires through oral reports in team or care conferences or written reports in the client record. A more formal process of communicating about TR practice involves submission of a case report for publication. Collectively, these exchanges form an important foundation for effective working relationships among staff, clients, clients' families, and professional colleagues. This chapter discusses the role of recreation therapists in these exchanges with an emphasis on how information about clinical TR services is exchanged among colleagues.

Communicating with Clients and Their Families

Much of this text has focused on the communication exchanges that occur between recreation therapists and clients. The majority of Chapter 7, Chapter 8, and Chapter 11 addressed many issues that influence effective client communication. In addition to communicating with clients, recreation therapists also communicate with clients' families. Clients do not exist in isolation—their families or immediate social networks influence their recovery, adaptation, and growth. Recreation therapists must be skilled at communicating compassionately with their clients' families. They must work with families and significant others in a caring manner to address fears and concerns and provide factual information and adequate follow-up. This communication should occur throughout the clinical process. Families can be informants in the assessment process, co-decision makers in the planning process, caregivers in the implementation phase, and reporters in the evaluation phase.

Communicating with Colleagues

In addition to communicating with clients and families, TR specialists will interact with colleagues. The agency's administrative structure influences the manner by which recreation therapists communicate with colleagues. Each agency will develop its own structure and guidelines for oral and written communications about client care. Often, these will result in the formation of a team of service providers responsible for providing services to particular clients.

Working in Teams

Chapter 8 identified the types of treatment teams in health and human service organizations, including multidisciplinary, interdisciplinary, and transdisciplinary teams (see Table 8.1, p. 132) as well as person-centered teams. While each of these teams may differ in their orientation to practice, all teams share in the process of planning and delivering services to clients.

Teams function like task groups, as they have a primary purpose for each meeting. This involves planning clinical services and problem-solving difficulties that occur in the course of client care. To achieve their purpose, teams develop their own method of communicating. Smooth communication among team members is essential. To be effective team members need to assess the team's formal and informal patterns of communicating and understand the potential barriers that can impede successful team communication.

Barriers to Successful Team Communication

According to Rothberg (1981) conflicts often occur within teams and interfere with their efficiency and effectiveness. These conflicts can arise from three overlapping barriers: interpersonal, interprofessional, and practice. *Interpersonal barriers* refer to personality and leadership styles that impair effective communication. These occur due to the individuals involved and not as a result of organizational or discipline issues. *Interprofessional barriers* "encompass attributes that are characteristics of a profession and are not unique to a work setting" (Smith, Perry, Neumayer, Potter & Smeal, 1992, p. 32). Examples include a lack of trust in the professional judgment of other disciplines; a lack of understanding about training experiences, or capabilities of another profession; or status differences between professions. *Practice barriers* are traditionally role related and may vary from one work environment to another. They can occur from *role ambiguity* in which disciplines do not have clearly defined boundaries, or *role overlap* in which responsibility for a specific task overlaps two or more disciplines. Recreation therapists are particularly vulnerable to interprofessional and practice barriers for two reasons. First, many of the

modalities used in TR clinical interventions are also used by other disciplines. Second, many health-related professionals do not understand the training or capabilities of recreation therapists.

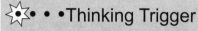

Thinking Trigger

How would you explain clinical TR services to a colleague? How would you handle this person's response if it challenged your qualifications to provide such services?

To minimize potential barriers to effective team communication, you must adequately express the intent and outcomes of your services. You must also advocate for client needs that the team may neglect to consider, such as recreation and leisure involvement. Having a thorough understanding of your professional identity and being able to explain it to your colleagues helps the team clearly understand the role of TR in clinical services. In addition, it helps to present information using the style and language typically used by the team. Of course, what works in one team may not work in another team because no two teams are alike in terms of their social climate.

Being Part of a Team

The social climate of a team "refers to the distinctive 'personality' of a team and is a cause and consequence of team activity" (Strasser & Falconer, 1997, p. 65). Each team's social climate influences team members' behavior (Moos, 1994). This is important for you to recognize, as your effectiveness will be influenced by how comfortable you feel interacting with other team members. Respecting and earning the respect of your colleagues will enhance your comfort level within a team. As a team member you will earn respect and recognition as a valued team member when your clinical TR services are thoughtful, focused, and based on identifiable client needs and wants. You can show respect to colleagues by recognizing their roles and functions and respecting their clinical judgment. As a team member, you must also be able to collaborate and coordinate your services and, most importantly, effectively communicate with colleagues. This communication typically occurs via oral and written reports.

Oral Reports

Oral communication is a skill often overlooked by TR specialists. Oral communication takes place through face-to-face or telephone conversations. It is used extensively in clinical practice because it is quick, it is personable, and it provides immediate feedback from others involved.

Oral Reporting in Teams

Oral exchanges about clinical practice often occur during team or care conferences. When involved in team meetings, recreation therapists typically share information. Factors influencing successful oral communication include colleagues' motivation to hear what is said and presentation style. The degree to which the content of your report is consistent with or contradictory to your colleagues' knowledge about a client or a related topic also influences success.

When providing oral reports during team conferences, begin by recalling information already shared and building from this point. Integrate information about a client with colleagues' knowledge or reports. Use explanations and illustrations to assist colleagues in understanding the report. Finally, be aware of nonverbal communication. Generally, nonverbal behavior influences the social climate of the team and the receptivity of colleagues to the information shared.

☼• • •Thinking Trigger

Think of times when your nonverbal behaviors helped or hindered your ability to communicate. What were you doing? What are some strategies that can be used to monitor your nonverbal behaviors in team meetings? • • •☼

Effective oral communication takes work. Many recreation therapists report experiencing anxiety when providing oral reports in team meetings or when their reports or perspectives differ from their colleagues. While it may seem easier to sit silently in team meetings rather than confront this anxiety, remember that professionals are ethically bound to contribute to the team planning and decision-making processes. By not discussing your perspective, you have shortchanged your clients and may be withholding important infor-

mation that could change the course of care. You may also encounter situations during your clinical practice when TR is overlooked in team rounds. In such instances you will need to assertively request permission to provide relevant information that may be of use to the team. Such assertiveness, if tactfully done, will enhance your respect among team members and decrease the likelihood that your colleagues will overlook you in future meetings.

While effective oral reporting challenges and occasionally provokes anxiety, it is important to invest energy in developing good oral communication skills and making a commitment to be an effective and active team member. Remember the following points adapted from the work of Galanes and Brilhart (1997):

- *Effective group communication is the responsibility of every member*. You have a responsibility to let your colleagues know when you don't understand something. The communication process must be monitored to make sure it is working and if problems occur they need to be resolved.

- *Perfect understanding among group members is impossible*. The communication process can break down and be confusing. Meaning is ascribed based on perceptions of how we read the speaker's nonverbal behavior. Therefore, some differences in understanding always exist between two or more people. Make certain that you understand what was communicated well enough so that you can coordinate your actions toward the team's goals for a client.

- *Disagreements will occur and do not necessarily signal a breakdown in a group communication*. While it is true that some group conflicts are due to misunderstandings resulting from poor communication, many conflicts are the result of differing values, goals, and beliefs among group members. Recreation therapists need to recognize the source of the conflict, articulate it, and then persuade the team to work toward a compromise that is in the client's best interest.

Written Reports

In addition to oral reports, written reports are used to detail services provided to clients and clients' responses to the services. Written reports are the primary method by which therapists document the outcome of their services. Federal and state laws and TR Standards of Practice often mandate these reports, which are placed in the client's clinical record. Additional mandates requiring written reports about client care and its outcomes come from third-party sources, such as insurance companies who need documented evidence for reimbursement.

The function of written reports in the client's record depends on the perspective of the person reading the report. For example, insurance companies use the record to verify services that qualify for reimbursement. Accrediting bodies expect the record to reflect compliance with standards for care. Team members expect the record to inform them about the client's response to care. Written reports, especially progress notes and discharge reports, evaluate the effectiveness of clinical services.

Generally, two primary perspectives guide the use of client records. One perspective focuses on client care. The other perspective focuses on the business and legal needs of the agency. **Table 13.1** profiles various ways that written reports can be used from each of these perspectives.

Clinical Writing

Written communications made by recreation therapists in the client's record must be completed in a timely fashion with clear, precise, and succinct *clinical writing*. Unlike general correspondence writing, clinical writing requires you to be cognizant of the varied audiences who read and use the information in the client record. Therapists must understand the legal aspects of documentation and have good writing skills related to grammar, syntax, and spelling. They must also be aware of the style and structure of clinical writing. Audiences who read therapists' notes expect written entries to follow a certain style and structure and often disregard those entries that fail to follow the appropriate format. A number of useful rules for clinical writing, offered by Baird (2002), are detailed in the following sections. These will help you develop excellent clinical documentation skills.

Rule #1: Simplify the Writing but not the Client

Trying to document a client's progress, emotional state, or interactions is a complex task. Humans are complex beings who use nonverbal language as much as verbal language to convey critical pieces of information in

their daily exchanges. Unfortunately, nonverbal language can often be lost when an interaction or exchange is translated into a written format. The result can often be an oversimplification of the exchange or the client. While good clinical writing is clear, precise, and succinct, it should still provide the reader with a vivid image of the person. This is especially true with initial assessment reports. As a general rule use specific, descriptive words that convey the complexities of the client's progress, emotional state, or interactions.

Rule #2: Omit Needless Words

Effective clinical writing is concise. Avoid stock phrases, vaguely defined clinical terms like "inappropriate," or value-laden words like "manipulative," "resistant," or "dependent." Revising and rewriting can help therapists' written communications by removing redundant and filler phrases so that writing is clearer and more concise. The checklist in **Table 13.2** (p. 238) can help to critique clinical writing.

Rule #3: Have Clarity in Words, Syntax, and Organization

Clarity is essential in clinical writing. The likelihood that your writing is clear can be enhanced by making certain that you choose words that best fit what you are trying to say, use proper grammatical syntax in your writing, and organize your thoughts prior to writing.

Select the Best Words. To be an effective writer, you will need to pay close attention to the multiplicity of meanings that a word may have and choose your words carefully. Many words, depending on the context in which they are used can have multiple meanings. For instance, the word "denial" can mean a declaration that a statement made is untrue as in "the agency issued a *denial* of all wrong doing" or "denial" can mean a refusal to admit a truth as in "the *denial* of his illness." Likewise, there are many words that have similar but not always the same meaning like "cooperative" and "sociable." Understanding these variations and choosing words that give your writing clarity is important. Value-laden phrases and words should also be avoided and replaced with more precise words or description.

Professional jargon can also cause documentation problems. Often therapists use words in their clinical reports that are widely used in practice such as "appropriate" or "bizarre." However, practitioners are usually unable to clearly and consistently define these words. Other times, therapists choose to include clinical descriptors of functional limitations like "aphasia," "hemiplegia," or "delusion" in their documentation. Unfortunately, these terms are sometimes used incorrectly, especially by beginning therapists. Be sure that clinical terms are used correctly in documentation (e.g., delusions are different from hallucinations, hemiparesis is different from hemiplegia, aphasia is not apraxia).

Know what you want to say and choose the best word. A medical dictionary may be especially helpful in choosing the correct word.

Strive for Clarity in Syntax. Good writing requires that sentences have proper syntax and structure. Often in the haste of writing a quick note, therapists omit key

Table 13.1: Uses of the client's record

Function	Purpose	Examples
Client Care Perspective		
Communication	Record is used for staff correspondence about client care, especially when staff is unavailable for oral exchanges.	Physician orders for medications, diagnostic tests, or specific treatments, test or assessment results, progress notes, incident reports
Intervention Planning, Implementation, and Evaluation	Information in record is reviewed to design treatment plan. Attendance and performance in rehabilitation program is recorded and evaluated.	Progress notes, intervention plans, discharge summaries
Informed Consent	Information is recorded regarding consent to treatment and client wishes regarding life-sustaining measures.	Informed consent documents, living wills
Agency Perspective		
Standard of Care	Client record is evidence of the nature, extent, and quality of care provided to a client in a facility. It is the only objective means by which the care given to a client can be compared to minimum standards, such as those suggested by accrediting bodies.	Chart Audits
Business Document	Services recorded in the client record form the basis for reimbursement requests of third-party payers such as Medicare, Medicaid, Health Management Organizations (HMO) or Prospective Payment Organizations (PPO). In this function, the medical record serves to detail the type and quantity of services provided to a client.	Chart Audits
Staff Development and Research	Client records can indicate areas of practice not being completed in a timely fashion or whether staff failed to address client progress when writing progress notes. Client records can be reviewed for research purposes, for the development of clinical practice guidelines, or as a resource for practitioner education.	Chart Reviews

structural elements that would give more clarity to their writing. They fail to group related words together, misplace prepositional phrases, use pronouns without a reference noun, or write run-on sentences. Such syntax errors increase the likelihood that the written report can be interpreted in more ways than intended.

Have Clarity in the Organizational Structure. Most clinical reports follow a structural outline. Yet authors still have freedom to decide what information should be included under each structural heading and in what sequence to present the information. It is imperative that writing follows a logical sequence and that the purpose is clear.

Rule #4 Know the Audience

Clinical writing communicates specific, detailed information about a client to a reader so that the reader is better able to understand and work with the client. "Reports are for the reader not the author" (Fisher, 1985, p. 115).

While it is true that many diverse audiences read client records, ultimately they serve the purpose of communication among team members. Reports, therefore, should be useful to colleagues in their work with clients. Understanding which information would be useful to colleagues provides the foundation for writing excellent reports and notes. This is not to say that clinical writing will not be influenced by the needs of other audiences beyond immediate colleagues. Clearly, information critical to other priorities in your agency (e.g., risk management, utilization review) must be

Table 13.2: Checklist for clinical writing

- ☐ Do all words in this report serve a function?
- ☐ Can any words be changed for more clarity (e.g., shorter words for longer words)?
- ☐ Are all words used correctly?
- ☐ Has the passive voice been avoided?
- ☐ Have I switched pronouns or tense in mid-sentence?
- ☐ Are any adverbs redundant with the verb (e.g., sadly crying)?
- ☐ Are any adjectives unnecessary?
- ☐ Are there any prepositions added onto verbs (e.g., stood up)?
- ☐ Are there any qualifiers (e.g., sort of) included in the sentence that can be removed?
- ☐ Are there any stock phases that can be deleted or replaced (e.g., due to the fact that)?

included. Ultimately, however, the primary audience will be team members who expect clear, succinct information.

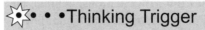

Thinking Trigger

What concerns you about clinical writing? Which rules will be the most challenging for you?

Types of Written Reports

TR specialists make many different types of documentation entries in the client record. The type of agency (e.g., nursing home, psychiatric hospital, rehabilitation hospital, outpatient clinic, school district) influences the format and frequency of documentation. For instance, in educational settings the entries made by recreation therapists into students' educational records would most likely be limited to consultation, assessment, or annual summary reports.

In contrast, recreation therapists employed by health care agencies make numerous entries into a client's record. These entries follow the clinical reasoning process (detailed in Chapter 4) and include assessment notes, intervention plans, progress/service notes, and discharge notes (see **Figure 13.1**). While some generic rules and components are required for the various types of documentation entries, the specific format and frequency for each entry will be influenced by the particular agencies' policies and procedures. In instances where TR is provided through nonprofit recreation programs (e.g., United Cerebral Palsy Association, public recreation departments) record keeping is usually left to the professional discretion of the recreation therapist. Regardless of setting, TR's *Standards of Practice* obligate documenting all aspects of the clinical process. Thus recreation therapists who provide clinical services are obligated to develop some type of documentation system.

Documenting Assessment Findings and Intervention Plans

One of the more frequent entries made into the clinical record involves communicating about assessment findings and intervention plans. Typically, an *Assessment Summary Report*—which includes baseline data identifying client strengths and limitations, information on the process used to collect data, a summary of the client's performance in the functional areas assessed, and mutually agreed upon goals and interventions—is written and entered into the client's record.

The major content headings of the Assessment Summary Report are fairly standard from agency to agency. Some agencies will require a written narrative report similar to the one contained in Exhibit 8.1 (p. 133), while other agencies will develop specific forms on which therapists detail assessment findings and intervention plans. For instance, Project PATH, a community-based TR transition program in New Hampshire for clients with spinal cord injury, uses a standardized form to document their assessment findings. Major content areas included on the assessment report include the client's:

- *Preinjury leisure history*, including leisure patterns, obstacles to leisure/community involvement, satisfaction with leisure time, and leisure interests

- *Postinjury attitudes toward leisure*, including perceived obstacles to leisure pursuits, social support for leisure, attitude toward return to community, and community awareness

- *Functional/educational skills*, including knowledge of SCI-related risk factors, stress management techniques, and functional skills related to transfers, wheelchair mobility, weight shifts, and ambulating

- *Personal client goals* for Project PATH involvement

- *Identified problem areas* related to leisure skill development, community access, social support, knowledge of risk factors and health promotion, knowledge of resources, and functional skill development

Project PATH's assessment reporting form also emphasizes assessing the client's knowledge of health promoting behaviors, spinal cord injury risk factors, and wellness. **Exhibit 13.1** (p. 240) contains some of the components found on the form.

Agencies also differ in terms of where the Assessment Summary Report or Form is placed in the client record, because agencies may use different types of recordkeeping. For instance, some agencies use *source-oriented records*, which divide client records according to discipline-specific sections (e.g., a social history is filed behind the index for social work). In source-oriented records, the Assessment Summary Report would be entered in the TR section of the chart. Other agencies use *problem-oriented records*, which organize client records so that information from all disciplines is grouped categorically. In these agencies, the Assessment Summary Report would be entered in the consultation, assessment, or database sections of the client's chart.

Evaluating Interventions in the Documentation Process: Progress/Service Notes

Progress or service notes are the second most frequent entry made in the client record. These entries link the provision of clinical services and the evaluation of those services. Written progress/service notes represent the evaluation phase of the clinical process, as they focus on documenting client outcomes or observed changes in client's status as a result of TR interventions and interactions. The process of writing a progress/service note allows therapists to evaluate the outcomes derived from their services for a particular client. Within the clinical process, evaluation is client-focused and occurs when therapists determine whether the outcomes identified via client goals and objectives have been achieved. While evaluation is a distinct phase in the clinical reasoning process, it is embodied in the process of written progress/service notes. Not only do progress/service notes evaluate the outcomes of services with a client, but also they inform other staff about the client's performance in relation to goals established during the planning phase. In addition to information about clients' progress and outcomes, these entries can contain other information about the client, including:

- Appearance (e.g., facial, posture, clothing)

- General attitude toward the task, therapist, or other clients

Figure 13.1: Documenting clinical practice

Clinical Reasoning Process	Documentation Entry
Assessment	⟶ Assessment summary reports
Planning	⟶ Goals, objectives, intervention strategies
Implementation and evaluation	⟶ Progress/service notes
Termination	⟶ Discharge summaries

Exhibit 13.1: Excerpts from Project PATH assessment form

I. LEISURE HISTORY (preinjury)

A. Preinjury patterns		B. Preinjury obstacles		C. Preinjury satisfaction with leisure time
Hrs/Wk				
	Work		Time	Satisfied
	School		Work demands	Somewhat satisfied
	Volunteer		Family demands	Neutral
	Leisure out of home		Money	Somewhat dissatisfied
	Leisure in home		Lack of partners	Very dissatisfied

D. Leisure interest (Use data from Project PATH leisure battery)			
Category	Preinjury interest	Redevelop skill	New skill interest

II. POSTINJURY ATTITUDE TOWARD LEISURE

A. Perceived obstacles to leisure pursuits (Check those that apply)

Medical concerns		Time		Work demands
Physical ability		Money		Lack of social support
Lack of equipment		Transportation		Lack of programs

III. FUNCTIONAL/EDUCATIONAL SKILLS

A. Knowledge of SCI-related risk factors (circle one)   None   Limited   Full

Identified following risk factors: _____

B. Stress Management (circle one)   Not used   Used often

Following stress management techniques identified: _____

C. Functional Skills

Transfers	Inpatient level	Current level	Even/Uneven	Date completed
Car				
Floor				
Furniture				
Wheelchair mobility				
Home environment				
Community				

IV. PERSONAL PROJECT PATH GOALS (check those that apply)

	Complement skills learned in rehab
	Use leisure as coping mechanism
	Explore alternative to preinjury lifestyle

V. IDENTIFIED PROBLEM AREAS (check those that apply)

Leisure skill development		Community access
Social support		Knowledge of risk factors and health promotion
Knowledge of resources		Functional skill development

Note: This exhibit contains excerpts from each of the PATH assessment headings. It is not the complete assessment form.

- Work habits
- Attitude toward instruction
- Motor activity and coordination
- Emotional reaction to task, therapist, or peers
- General affect/mood
- Behavior during unstructured time
- Hopes, concerns, or queries expressed by client, family, or support systems
- Explanation of events that prevented participation with intervention plan

In long-term care settings, progress/service notes also verify quarterly and annual ratings given to a client on the Minimum Data Set (MDS). When used in this manner, they are considered a "proof source" for the MDS rating. It is important, therefore, that progress/ service notes in these settings include information on the amount of time that the client is awake; the client's involvement in activities, interests, and preferred participation settings; and any observed changes in the client's preferred routine.

Recreation therapists use the information compiled for a progress/service note to evaluate their interventions. This evaluative process may result in three outcomes:

1. Identifying new goals for the client because he or she has achieved original goals
2. Discharging the client from TR services because he or she has achieved his or her goals and does not need any further interventions at this point
3. Identifying new goals or interventions because the client has not achieved the targeted goals or the client has set new goals for himself or herself

The frequency with which progress/service notes are written is influenced by agency guidelines, accreditation standards (e.g., JCAHO, CARF), and regulatory agencies (e.g., CMS) with which the agency complies. In addition, documentation entries can be made using a variety of formats. Some of the more common charting formats include narrative charting, SOAP (subjective, objective, assessment, plan) charting, PIE (problem, intervention, evaluation) charting, focus charting, and charting by exception.

Narrative Charting

Narrative or *free-form charting* is typically used in long-term care, adult day care, behavioral health care, residential settings, and community agencies like Easter Seals. These notes are also common in community recreation centers that provide TR clinical services, such as a health promotion program for weight management or cardiac health and fitness. A narrative note does not have any structure or format. Clinicians are free to organize their information in a logical, sequential manner; however, the content must reflect the client's progress toward goals. Narrative notes are often used with source-oriented record keeping.

For example, Mr. Marko (a 35-year-old admitted to a behavioral health care facility due to auditory hallucinations and aggressive outbursts) and his recreation therapist identified these initial TR goals as a focus for their work together:

Client will sustain focus on task for 15 minutes

Client will verbalize aggressive impulses without becoming threatening or physically abusive to others

The TR intervention plan had Mr. Marko attending a sports group 3 times per week and a craft group 3 times per week. In addition, the use of a behavioral contract was agreed to by Mr. Marko to encourage his attendance at groups. Additional techniques were introduced including the use of a heavy bag as a cognitive behavioral strategy when Mr. Marko was beginning to feel agitated. (See Chapter 6 for a review of cognitive behavioral strategies used in the intervention planning process.) Following the first week of interventions, the recreation therapist entered the following narrative note in Mr. Marko's chart.

4/28/2001   Recreation Therapy Note

Client attended 33% of scheduled recreation therapy intervention groups (sports 4/23/2001, crafts 4/24/2001). Concentration is improving as client is able to focus on task for 10 minutes during both groups. Auditory hallucinations continue to be a problem as client reports reason for nonattendance at other intervention groups—"My voices told me not to come." During verbal exchanges, some hostility displayed with peers and staff (e.g., told staff "Leave me alone!") but physical aggressiveness was not present. Client did request to use the heavy bag 5 times this past week when feeling agitated. Will continue with current intervention plan and incorporate daily reminders to increase attendance at intervention groups.

Signature, CTRS

A progress note about a client who had a cerebral vascular accident (CVA) and was in treatment at a physical rehabilitation center is found in **Exhibit 13.2.** Notice it is written on an agency-developed form. **Exhibit 13.3** is a quarterly progress note written about a client (Mary) in a long-term care facility. In each note, the therapist comments on the progress the clients made toward achieving their goals. However, the quarterly progress note for the long-term care setting also contains information that will be used as evidence for Mary's quarterly MDS evaluation ratings, such as the amount of time Mary was involved in activities. Because the quarterly note contains such information, it would be considered a "proof source" for the MDS ratings.

SOAP Charting

SOAP is an acronym for a charting style developed for use in problem-oriented medical records. Each letter in the acronym reminds the therapist to include necessary information in the progress/service note. *S* stands for *subjective data*. Subjective data would include a quote from a client related to his or her perceptions of progress or problems. In instances where clients have not made any comments about their progress or care, the S portion may be left blank. Some agencies allow variation in the recording of subjective data so that statements from family or friends may be included in the S portion of the note. This often occurs when you are working with nonverbal clients. When such statements are included, the written entry must attribute the statement to the person making it and not the client.

O stands for *objective data*. This represents factual information gathered by the therapist about the client's performance. These observations must be written using specific behavioral terms that describe the client's performance in relation to the client's goals. *A* stand for the *analysis* or *assessment* made by the therapist based upon the subjective and objective data presented. This section of the progress note contains the therapist's evaluation of how the client is doing based on the data presented. *P* represents the intervention *plan* being proposed based upon the information presented. The therapist may suggest continuing with the current plan or revising it. In either instance, the plan must relate to client's goals. If the SOAP format was used to chart Mr. Marko's progress, the following documentation entry would be made in Mr. Marko's record:

4/28/2001   Recreation Therapy Progress Note

S: "When I come to recreation, I don't hear the voices as much."

O: Attended 2 of 6 scheduled intervention groups (i.e., sport group 4/23/2001 and crafts 4/24/2001). Pacing, able to focus for 10 minutes during craft and sport groups. Hostile with staff telling them to leave him alone. No hostile behaviors with peers, muttering to self most of the time during activities. Requested use of heavy bag 5x during the week.

A: Client continues to respond to auditory hallucinations, has difficulty with concentration and with interactions with staff and peers.

Exhibit 13.2: Narrative progress note for physical medicine and rehabilitation setting

TR Progress Note

Weekly Goals	Status Last Report	Status This Report	Goal Next Report
Memory	2 (Max verbal cues)	3 (Mod verbal cues)	4 (Min verbal cues)
Endurance during functional task	5 minutes	15–20 minutes	20–25 minutes
Verbal expression of 1–2 word phrases	2 (Max verbal cues)	3 (Mod verbal cues)	4 (Min verbal cues)
Date:12/6	**Type and unit of Service: Individual Tx 4 units**		**Group 0 units**

Progress/Goals/Comments: Pt. performed FM tasks c̄ L UE. Pt. required HOH assistance for 25% of trials 2° decreased motor initiation and increased anxiety. Pt. required mod verbal cues to recall familiar game rules within tx. session. Pt. provided 1 word response within structured task with mod verbal cueing.

Signature, CTRS

Some progress made with controlling aggressive outbursts and task attention. More comfortable with social groups.

P: Continue with TR intervention plan, begin daily 1:1 sessions for 15 minutes to facilitate trust relationship, review activity schedule each AM following morning meeting to facilitate attendance. Provide firm limits for aggressive outbursts, praise self-initiated use of the heavy bag for self-control, and review behavioral contract for attending intervention groups.

Signature, CTRS

Sometimes, recreation therapists will work in agencies that utilize a hybrid form of SOAP charting. For example, Project PATH recreation therapists document *action plans* following every client visit. Subjective and objective information is combined in the *action* section of the note while the *plan* portion identifies future goals and actions for the client and therapist (see **Exhibit 13.4**, p. 245).

PIE Charting

Another acronym used in some facilities to facilitate accurate documentation is *PIE charting*. PIE stands for *Problem*, *Intervention*, and *Evaluation*. In this documentation style, staff would enter information in the *P* portion of their note that indicated the problems that were occurring. The *I* portion would include the staff's response or interventions related to the problems identified in the note. The *E* portion would include the staff's assessment of how effective their intervention was and future plans that might be used. While similar to SOAP charting, this documentation format differs in that it exclusively focuses on problems. Unlike SOAP charting—where all subjective and objective data is presented separately—the PIE charting format combines subjective and objective data and presents only problematic information. Recreation therapists who use this form of documentation might write Mr. Marko's note as follows:

4/28/2001   Recreation Therapy Progress Note

P: Attendance at groups sporadic (attended 2 of 6 intervention groups: sports 4/23, crafts 4/24), mumbling during groups, and hostile with staff telling them to leave him alone.

I: Spoke with client about consistent attendance, utilized refocusing techniques when client was mumbling, and set firm limits for hostile behavior.

Exhibit 13.3: Narrative progress note for long-term care setting

---

12/6   *Quarterly TR Progress Note*

Mary has made progress toward both of her TR treatment goals since her last note. She is adjusting to the facility, continues to maintain her admission fitness levels, and has not had any falls during activity programming. Mary has received 15-minute individual room visit each day to assist with her adjustment to the facility. These visits have focused on establishing a therapeutic relationship, orienting Mary to the facility and activity programs available, and engaging Mary in a productive task (e.g., crossword puzzles). Mary's preferred recreation setting continues to be her room; however, in the past week Mary has identified facility-sponsored activity programs in which she is interested. These include religious services and the horticulture program. Although interested, Mary continues to express uncertainty about leaving her room to attend these activities. To assist Mary with maintaining her current level of fitness and reduce her risk for falls, she has been participating in the afternoon exercise program on a daily basis. In addition, Mary takes a 30-minute walk outdoors each day with a family member. Initially, Mary's husband accompanied her to the exercise group, but she now attends the exercise group on her own. During the program Mary mimics the leader 50% of the time but requires verbal cueing to stay on task. While Mary does participate in the activity, she is eager to leave and return to her room to await her husband's visit. The exercise program and the individual room visits are the only facility-sponsored activities in which Mary is currently involved. While Mary continues to need assistance to structure her free time, it is apparent that she is more comfortable with her new surroundings. She is awake most of the day with a noted exception of an afternoon nap from 1:00 to 2:30 p.m., and has maintained her current level of fitness. TR will begin to introduce horticulture activities during individual room visits and encourage Mary to escort staff to the greenhouse to gather supplies with the intended goal of having Mary join the horticulture group. Will also encourage Mary to attend available religious services.

Signature, CTRS

E: Client responded to firm limits, apologizing for behavior and requesting use of heavy bag. With cues, client can focus for 10 minutes on task. Client agrees that he needs reminders to attend intervention groups due to confusion created by auditory hallucinations therefore will establish daily contact to facilitate trust and increase attendance at intervention groups.

Signature, CTRS

Focus Charting

In *focus charting* the concerns—which can be a problem, a current behavior, or an event—are central. Staff must provide a categorical heading or focus for each documentation entry. According to Peterson and Stumbo (2000), categorical headings can include:

- Key words related to diagnostic categories (e.g., hallucinations, activity tolerance)
- Identified client problems from the intervention plan
- Current client behaviors or concerns (e.g., pain, blurred vision, aggressive outburst)
- Changes in symptoms or health status (e.g., incontinence, fever, suicide threat, falls)
- Significant event in the client's care (e.g., family visit or absence, change in medication)
- Key words related to standard care procedures (e.g., assessment, patient education session)
- The discipline making the entry (e.g., therapeutic recreation/community reentry note)

The categorical heading for the focus note is recorded to the left of the entry and helps the reader easily identify entries related to a specific topic. The narrative portion of the entry is organized for each identified focus to include data, action, response and plan for future interventions. The *data* portion of the narrative includes subjective and objective information related to the focus of the note. The *action* portion indicates what the therapist did in the form of interventions, supports, or programs. The *response* portion summarizes the client's reaction to the actions taken and the *plan* portion indicates the future focus for interactions/interventions with the client. This format assists both the reader and the writer in grouping relevant information together. A focus charting entry for Mr. Marko might read as follows:

4/23/2001   Recreation Therapy Progress Note

FOCUS: Hallucinations

D: Mumbling to self during intervention groups on 4/23 and 4/24, pacing, unable to focus on task.

A: Provided verbal cues to remain focused, utilized concrete markers to maintain focus (e.g., "When 5 minutes have passed, you can take a break.")

R: Able to focus for 10 minutes with support but becomes agitated if additional time demands for attention are made.

P: Continue involvement in intervention groups to facilitate focusing on external stimuli. Gradually increase time requirements for maintaining focus. Provide positive reinforcement for sustained attention.

FOCUS: Aggression

D: Aggressive with staff telling them to leave him alone, verbally nonresponsive to peers' requests, responds to repeated attempts at interaction by pacing or asking to use the heavy bag (5 times in past week).

A: Set firm limits and reminded client of consequences for aggressive behavior, praised client for requesting use of heavy bag.

R: Remorseful when confronted about behavior and limits set.

P: Continue to set firm limits and review behavioral contract to incorporate positive rewards for appropriate social behavior, encourage client to disclose source of agitation prior to using heavy bag.

Signature, CTRS

Charting by Exception

Charting by exception (CBE) is used when standardized, detailed clinical pathways for clients in a particular diagnostic category have been identified by an agency. These standardized clinical pathways have clearly defined rehabilitation activities that must occur within a specified amount of time and the anticipated outcomes that will result from these rehabilitative activities. The clinical pathway reflects the activities of all disciplines working with a particular diagnostic group. In agencies using clinical pathways, charting only occurs when an exception to the established plan of care exists, or a particular outcome is not achieved or is achieved sooner than expected. In these instances, there is a *variance* or *exception* from the anticipated course of recovery that had been projected by the agency. When a particular outcome is achieved sooner than expected, it is labeled a *positive variance*. When a particular outcome is not achieved by the time it was anticipated, it is called a *negative variance*. Both positive and negative variances must be documented and explained. The variance or CBE note must include the date, what the intended or projected outcome was, an explanation of why the variance (either positive or negative) may have occurred, and a plan to deal with the identified variance. This variance note is typically signed or in some agencies initialed if a signature log is used in the front of the client's chart. In the case of Mr. Marko, his care plan projected that he would be able to maintain self-control throughout the day and attend all of his intervention programs after the first week of hospitalization. Given his behavior and attendance record, a variance note such as this would be required for Mr. Marko:

Variance Statements

4/24/01 Client attended 1 of 2 scheduled intervention groups, identifying auditory hallucinations as reason for nonattendance. Unable to maintain self-control when he did

attend intervention group, expressing feelings of hostility toward staff when prompted to focus on task. Relayed information about behavior and attendance to case manager. Will provide daily cues to facilitate attendance.

Initials

Documenting the Final Phase of the Clinical Process: Termination

In Chapter 5 we identified termination as the final phase of the clinical process. Typically termination is mutually agreed upon by clients and staff. Often termination is signaled when goals have been achieved. Other times services may be terminated or redirected to another setting (e.g., home with hospice care) because of changes in the client's condition or the client's lack of ability or willingness to comply with the care plan. Typically recreation therapists document this phase of the clinical process through a written discharge summary that signals the end of services and the therapeutic relationship. While termination is the final phase of the clinical process, planning for it should actually begin within the first few days of services. In this way forethought is given to the environmental issues and needs that ought to be addressed if clients return to their homes, or transfer to another facility, such as a skilled nursing facility, boarding home, independent living center, or hospice care.

Exhibit 13.4: Project PATH documentation

June 20, 2001

A: Met with Susan in home. Reviewed the results of the WRAP assessment and provided her with a copy. Susan complains of increased spasticity and had a few episodes of urinary incontinence this past week. "My spasms are really bothersome. I didn't have a very good week." Increased spasticity may be result of skin breakdowns; CTRS encouraged Susan to continue with pressure relief schedule and monitor skin breakdowns closely with help of her husband. Referred to section in wellness manual on "spasticity." Discussed catheterization schedule and volumes—all within normal range. CTRS suggested decreasing caffeine intake. Referred to section in wellness manual on "bladder issues." Susan has been out of the house for doctor's appointment and out to eat with husband once this week. Susan reports that she is independent pushing her wheelchair on flat terrain, but she needs assistance on uneven and hilly terrain. Discussed accessibility issues of the restaurant and the doctor's office. Susan and husband were able to problem-solve solutions to table height issue at restaurant. Susan notes increased fatigue on days she goes out. "All those transfers to and from the car and all the pushing around makes me tired." CTRS encouraged continued involvement in home fitness program; Susan currently uses her Thera-Band for upper extremity strengthening 2–3 times/week; UBE for cardio training 2 times/week.

P: Next meeting scheduled for June 27th. Follow-up on bladder incontinence and spasticity issues. Monitor fitness log. Review community access issues and suggest outing with CTRS to work on wheelchair mobility skills.

Signature, CTRS

Successful discharge planning requires full client and family involvement to ensure success. At minimum the written discharge plan should contain the criteria for discharge, resources, equipment, and contacts required before and after discharge. Formats for discharge summaries and plans will vary from agency to agency. Some agencies will require narrative notes, others will use the SOAP format, while others will use standardized forms or checklists. In each instance, the TR discharge summary should include:

- Reason for admission or referral to TR clinical services
- Significant findings from TR assessment
- Summary of TR services provided
- Response to procedures and interventions rendered
- Condition of the client on discharge, including remaining problems or concerns
- Any specific instructions/information/ referrals given to the client or his or her family (e.g., handouts, adaptive equipment, resource contacts)

TR discharge summaries are not legally required; however, professional standards of practice highlight their importance. Their inclusion in the client's chart is an indication of the quality of care that was rendered to the client.

☆• • •Thinking Trigger

What are the advantages and disadvantages associated with writing discharge summaries? How can discharge summaries be used to evaluate the effectiveness of services? • • •☆

Using Technology to Communicate about Practice

Pressures to contain costs, to deliver clinical services in diverse settings, and to manage information effectively, along with technological advances, have caused health and human service facilities to embrace the use of computers, especially with client records. While the use of computerized records is not yet widespread, many facilities have begun to utilize such recordkeeping. For

instance, at Magee Rehabilitation Hospital, the Delaware Valley Regional Spinal Cord Injury Center, recreation therapists use computerized records for documenting routine client care. A computerized medical information system is also in use at the Clinical Center of the National Institutes for Health. At these agencies, once recreation therapists have accessed the computerized medical information system, they indicate the type of entry or inquiry they want to make in the system. For instance, TR staff may ask to see admissions for a particular unit; make a charting entry on a particular client, review the charting entries made on a client, display the clinical orders for a particular client, or any number of other functions.

As is the case with written medical records, agencies create their computerized medical information systems to conform to their documentation structure. Consider the differences between the format for computerized progress/service notes at Magee Rehabilitation Hospital versus NIH's Clinical Center (see **Exhibit 13.5**, p. 248). While both agencies use computerized documentation systems, both differ in the frequency and format of entries. At Magee Rehabilitation Hospital, TR documentation occurs after each clinical session and utilizes a narrative charting format. In contrast, NIH completes documentation weekly. In addition, NIH uses a structured charting format called GEAP. Similar to a SOAP note, the GEAP charting system requires therapists to structure their notes to convey information on client *G*oals, *E*vents associated with client care, therapists' *A*ssessment of these events, and future intervention *P*lans.

The use of computers for documentation will continue to expand, necessitating that recreation therapists of the 21st century be computer literate. This is apparent in long-term care facilities that require recreation therapists to complete various sections of the MDS using a computer, including Section N on Activity Pursuit Patterns and Section T Therapy Supplement for Medicare PPS.

Another technological advance used by TR specialists to communicate with colleagues is e-mail. When e-mail is used to relay client information to a colleague, steps must be taken to assure the confidentiality of the information, such as using encryption and message verification. At a minimum therapists should utilize identification and passwords with their e-mail system to minimize the likelihood of someone inadvertently accessing confidential client information. In addition, therapists should be sure that they do not leave e-mail messages open when not they are not at their computer. Because of widespread use of e-mail within clinical settings, many agencies and departments have developed policies and procedures to guide therapists in the use and retention of e-mail. Be certain to review these policies if you intend to use e-mail for communicating about client care.

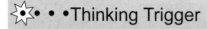

• • •Thinking Trigger

Can you think of a particular risk in using e-mail to communicate about work issues? **• • •**

Legal Issues in Documenting Client Care

Whether using computerized or handwritten entries, practitioners need to be cognizant of the legal issues associated with documenting client care. Legal concerns can arise from illegible and inaccurate entries in the client record. Therapists documenting in the clinical record must also take care to note the authenticity and timeliness of their entries. Other legal issues that arise in the course of documenting client care include confidentiality, privacy, and/or failure to follow mandatory reporting guidelines (e.g., child abuse, elder abuse). **Exhibit 13.6** (p. 249) details some general guidelines to assist recreation therapists in minimizing legal concerns associated with their documentation entries. Before making any documentation entries, check with the agency about acceptable abbreviations and other policies related to documenting in client records. For instance, some agencies require the use of black ink for all documentation entries.

A particular area that TR specialists must be aware of involves correctly completing incident reports. These reports are required after any incident in which an employee or client was injured or encountered a risk of injury such as a fall, an accident, a physical altercation between clients, or an elopement from a facility. Because of the activity-based nature of TR service provision, you will encounter instances when you will need to complete incident reports. These reports document what occurred and how it occurred so that the agency's administration can review and make changes to minimize future risks and/or legal liability.

Each agency will have its own form for incident reports. These forms must be completed within 24 hours of the incident and should include the date and time of the incident and any key witnesses who can verify the events that occurred. When completing incident reports, TR specialists must document the incident that occurred, paying close attention to providing sufficient information to clarify concerns regarding negligence and/or supervision. Information related to the *who*, *what*, *when*, *where*, and *how* of the incident must be recorded, along with any contributory acts on the client's or staff's part. In addition, care provided to the client prior to and following the incident and any additional staff notified of the incident (e.g., charge nurse, attending physician) should also be included in the incident report. Some agencies include these reports in the client record while others do not.

Other Venues for Communicating about Practice

TR specialists can also communicate about practice by submitting manuscripts for publication in professional journals, participating in online bulletin boards and/or discussion groups about practice, or presenting at professional conferences. Each of these venues allows TR practitioners to communicate about clinical TR practice with a broader audience of colleagues. Engagement in such tasks reflect a commitment to *self-enhancement*—a process in which a professional commits to seeking new knowledge, skills, and sensitivity so to make himself or herself a better person and a better professional. Such efforts allow practitioners to share the vast amount of knowledge and information acquired in day-to-day clinical practice. As Negley (1995) wrote, the desire to share information about clinical practice "is rooted in respect for the clients and the positive life changes they accomplish using recreational therapy as the vehicle for those changes" (p. 251).

Summary

One of the most critical tasks for TR specialists involves communicating with clients, their families, and colleagues about the purpose, process, and outcomes of clinical TR interventions. Clear oral and written communication abilities are fundamental prerequisite skills needed for successful practice. New TR practitioners are often overwhelmed with the amount of documentation required in practice. This pressure is compounded by the technical challenges associated with clear and succinct writing. The only way to improve and to become more efficient is to seek out feedback. Documenting TR interventions is not about convenience for you; it is about communicating necessary information to ultimately benefit clients.

Effective communication assures that clients receive quality services. It facilitates coordinated client care and serves as means for professional accountability and self-regulation for recreation therapists (Peterson & Stumbo, 2000). This chapter reviewed aspects of oral and written communication in providing quality clinical TR services to clients and discussed the multiple audiences with whom recreation therapists communicate, including clients, their families, team members,

Exhibit 13.5: Computerized TR progress notes

Magee Rehabilitation Hospital Computerized Progress Note

{CAT}: THERAPEUTIC RECREATION

01/28/98 [1351] Charted by: Signature, CTRS

WHEELCHAIR SKILLS TRAINING

PT. ATTENDED 1:1 REC THERAPY SESSION—ACTIVITY: BILLIARDS. USING CUE STICK W/NO ADAPTATIONS, PT. WAS ABLE TO SUCCESSFULLY MANEUVER POWER W/C AROUND BILLIARD TABLE. PT. EXPRESSED SURPRISE AND PLEASURE WITH BILLIARD SKILLS. SOME DIFFICULTIES WITH BALANCING CUE STICK WHEN MANUEVERING OBSERVED. WILL EXPLORE ADAPTATIONS TO ASSIST WITH BALANCING AND INCREASE INDEPENDENCE.

NIH Clinical Center Computerized Progress Note

THERAPEUTIC RECREATION NOTE:

03/02 08:26 a.m.	THERAPEUTIC RECREATION PROGRESS NOTES—TREATMENT NOTE	DDJ
03/02 08:26 a.m.	G: 2. TO BE AWARE OF & RESPECT PERSONAL BOUNDARIES. B.O.2.1. MAINTAIN AT LEAST ARMS LENGTH DISTANCE FROM OTHERS 90% OF THE TIME.	DDJ
03/02 08:26 a.m.	E: ATTENDED RT 6/6XS, PARTICIPATED IN HI.AD., CARING CANINES, S.S., PHYS. FITNESS, CREAT. COR., ART TX & FREE TIME ACTIVITIES. THERE HAS BEEN NO SPONTANEOUS HUGGING FROM PT. THIS WEEK AS WELL AS NO CROWDING, SITTING, OR STANDING DURING STRUCTURED ACTIVITIES. PT. IS STILL PUSHING AHEAD OF OTHERS TO BE FIRST IN LINE.	DDJ
03/02 08:26 a.m.	A: PT. HAS REGAINED SOME OF HER PREVIOUS GROUND & HAS DEMONSTRATED SIGNIFICANT PROGRESS TOWARD HER B.O. EXCEPT FOR HER COMPETITIVENESS. SHE IS MORE AWARE OF HER AND OTHER'S PERSONAL SPACE.	DDJ
03.02 08:26 a.m.	P: CONTINUE W CURRENT PLAN FOR 1 WK—RT WILL TALK MORE TO PT. ABOUT HER COMPETITIVE NEED TO BE FIRST IN LINE AND ITS IMPLICATIONS FOR RESPECTING BOUNDRIES OF OTHERS.	DDJ

administrators, and accrediting and regulatory agencies. Communication of the purpose, function, and outcomes of clinical TR practice was explained, focusing primarily on ways that recreation therapists exchange information with their colleagues through oral reports or written documentation.

Information on different types of client care teams, sources of conflict that hinder effective team work, and approaches that can be used when providing oral reports in client care or team meetings were discussed, as well as the role of written communication in the provision of quality clinical TR services. Various types of documentation entries were profiled that accompany each phase of the clinical reasoning process. Information about appropriate content and various methods of documenting client care, including narrative, SOAP, PIE, Focus, and CBE charting were presented with examples of each. Information was also provided on legal issues associated with documentation and the increasing use of technology for client documentation.

Exhibit 13.6: General documentation guidelines

- ☐ Correct mistaken entries properly (e.g., cross out entry with a single line, label as error, initial and date correction, do not use correction fluid)
- ☐ Do not tamper with the record (e.g., do not sign a record after the fact, do not change the sequence of notes)
- ☐ Don't leave any blank spaces on forms (e.g., place a single line through any blank space preceding your entry)
- ☐ Record only services provided
- ☐ Avoid using document to criticize others or implicate other disciplines
- ☐ Eliminate bias from written descriptions of the clients
- ☐ Document comments that clients make about a potential lawsuit against the agency or other drastic measures (e.g., suicide, harming others, leaving against medical advice)
- ☐ Document client behaviors that affect outcomes of services (e.g., noncompliance with intervention, ambulating without supervision, leaving an activity during an off-campus trip)
- ☐ Precisely document any information you orally report to the doctor or unit staff
- ☐ Sign the note including one's position, title, and date of entry

References

Baird, B. (2002). *The internship, practicum, and field placement handbook: A guide for the helping professions.* Upper Saddle River: NJ: Prentice Hall.

Fisher, C. (1985). *Individualized psychological assessment.* Monterey, CA: Brooks/Cole.

Galanes G. and Brilhart J. (1997). *Communicating in groups: Applications and skills.* Boston, MA: McGraw-Hill.

Moos, R. (1994). *The social climate scales: A user's guide.* Palo Alto, CA: Consulting Psychological Press.

Negley, S. (1995). Preparing a case history for publication. *Therapeutic Recreation Journal, 29*(4), 251–252.

Peterson C. and Stumbo, N. (2000). *Therapeutic recreation program design: Principles and procedures.* Needham Heights, MA: Allyn & Bacon.

Rothberg, J. (1981). The rehabilitation team: Future directions. *Archives of Physical Medicine and Rehabilitation, 62,* 407–410.

Smith, R., Perry, T., Neumayer, R., Potter, J., and Smeal, T. (1992). Interprofessional perceptions between therapeutic recreation and occupational therapy practitioners: Barriers to effective interdisciplinary team functioning. *Therapeutic Recreation Journal, 26*(4), 31–42.

Strasser, D. and Falconer, J. (1997). Linking treatment to outcomes through teams: Building a conceptual model of rehabilitation effectiveness. *Topics in Stroke Rehabilitation, 4*(1), 15–27.

Chapter 14
Pursuing Competence: The Role of Reflection, Ethics, and Clinical Supervision

Guided Reading Questions

After reading this chapter, you should be able to answer the following:
- What is professional competence, and how is it acquired?
- What does it mean to be a *reflective practitioner*?
- What various ethical issues and dilemmas might TR professionals encounter in practice?
- What resources are available for TR professionals to examine ethical issues?
- What is clinical supervision? How can it help you to become a reflective and competent practitioner?
- Around what topics or issues can clinical supervision be structured?

Introduction

The clinical practice of TR is a complex and dynamic process. It is constantly challenged by client needs and ever-changing conditions within health and human services. Thus, TR clinical practice will always require flexibility, creativity, and recreation therapists who have the courage to examine what they do and why. The willingness to examine one's work is a mark of professionalism and reflects a commitment to seeking competence. No textbook, coursework, or college degree fully prepares someone for the challenges found in practice. Nor will this educational foundation assure competence. Competence is a lifelong pursuit guided by a commitment to being a reflective practitioner.

Not all TR practitioners, however, are "reflective practitioners" (Schon, 1983). Some prefer convenient approaches that demand little thought, effort, or reflection. Their services are routine and lack variation. Others are so self-assured that they rarely question their perspectives, relying primarily on standard methods and past experience. For others, uncertainty and confusion about TR clinical practice outweighs confidence and undermines their beliefs in the purpose and value of practice. To be reflective practitioners, these individuals would need to question their everyday decisions and behaviors and ask: *Am I doing the best I can? How can I be sure I am practicing with integrity? How are my thoughts, feelings, and beliefs influencing my ability to be present with client(s) and virtuous in my actions? Am I competent in what I am doing?* By being reflective, they open the possibilities of becoming *enlightened*

practitioners (Dattilo, 2000). By being reflective, they continue their journey toward competent practice.

Chapter 1 presented the Pew Commission's 21 competencies for health professionals of the 21st century. Two of these competencies—*Demonstrate critical thinking, reflection, and problem-solving skills* and *Continue to learn and help others learn*—have relevance in this chapter. A commitment to professional competence distinguishes the TR practitioner who has a sense of professionalism from another TR practitioner whose work is merely a job. Professionals understand that the context of practice is constantly changing and that they can always improve their knowledge, skills, and insights.

What kind of professional will you be? Long after your TR degree has been earned, how will you have charted your course toward professional competence? This chapter provides a framework for pursuing professional competence. We begin by defining professional competence and describing what it means to be a reflective practitioner. Then we discuss ethics and the role of clinical supervision in supporting the pursuit of competence.

Professional Competence

Professional competence relates to one's obligation to develop and maintain knowledge and skills necessary to practice proficiently. It also involves the development of *clinical judgment*, which is a combination of theoretical and practical knowledge as well as the art of knowing what to do, when, with whom, and why. Professional competence also involves knowing the limitations of your methods and techniques and the boundaries of your training and expertise (Haas & Malouf, 1989).

The pursuit of competence begins with acquiring knowledge and skills through education. To some extent professional competence in TR is reflected through earning national certification from NCTRC. Of course, certification eligibility requirements and the written competency examination are based on *minimum* standards necessary to enter practice. The pursuit of competence cannot end here, but rather it must be maintained and advanced through continued training and education. Commitment to competence is evident in your deliberate and conscientious attempt to self-monitor change and growth.

Certainly, professional conferences, workshops, or in-services provide opportunities to update and refresh knowledge and skills as well as learn new perspectives and approaches for practice. But these experiences will only be effective when the new information is incorporated into practice. When these experiences fail to provide new learning, finding more effective learning opportunities becomes a priority in your journey toward professional competence.

Concern about your professional competence from supervisors or administration is often limited to those instances where you have caused a problem or have the potential to do so. For example, some agencies have procedures for evaluating practitioners' competence to use specialized equipment and perform certain interventions (e.g., aquatic therapy). Based on such evaluations, agencies develop performance improvement plans to help practitioners improve their abilities to deliver safe, effective, and beneficial services to clients. However, objective performance evaluations of one's full scope of practice can be too costly and time-consuming for many agencies. When recreation therapists work alone in an agency, they cannot rely on others to evaluate their specific TR competence. Therefore, significant responsibility to evaluate and enhance performance competence often falls on the practitioner (Sneegas, 2001). "Self-assessment becomes an important component where professionals may reflect on their work and determine how they are doing relative to any existing standards of practice or peer group" (p. 130).

Two documents help with self-monitoring. ATRA's *Guidelines for Competency Assessment and Curriculum Planning in Therapeutic Recreation: A Tool for Self-Evaluation* (Kinney & Witman, 1997) contains seven major content areas to periodically assess learning. Content areas specify knowledge, skills, and abilities related to the TR process (e.g., assessing, planning,

implementing, evaluating). ATRA's *Revised Standards of Practice and Self-Assessment Guide* (Riley, West & Van Andel, 2000) is another excellent tool for monitoring compliance with practice standards.

Competence, however, involves more than knowledge and technical skills. It involves being a fully informed therapist—cognitively, emotionally, and contextually. *Emotional competence* stems from your willingness and ability to understand and appreciate the transaction between your own humanity and that of the people you serve. It involves understanding how your personal needs and feelings affect your work. "Competence is more than the acquisition of factual knowledge. It implies the ability to synthesize all the virtues into practice that is both morally and skillfully exemplary" (O'Keefe, 1994). Pursuing competence is a journey that involves examining what you do and the reasons why. It is a journey of reflection, and the motivation must come from within you. Pursuing competence, as O'Keefe described it, is far more challenging than earning a degree, NCTRC certification, or enough continuing education credits to maintain your certification.

Becoming a Reflective Practitioner

A competent recreation therapist must display integrity. More than being honest or consistent in your actions, *integrity* means behaving with a sense of purpose and an awareness of your values, beliefs, and motives. Thus, practicing TR with integrity requires deliberate reflection. Perhaps you have been asked to express your philosophy of TR as a class assignment or as part of your internship experience. While this may seem to be a rather heady intellectual exercise, it is actually very important to the development of professional character. The reflection required for such an assignment, however, should not be associated only with academics. Throughout practice all TR professionals ought to reach beyond mastering skills and techniques and strive to acquire insight and wisdom. Professional competence depends on insight and wisdom, which comes from having the integrity to reflect.

Insight and wisdom can be achieved when we consider how our values, beliefs, and reasoning processes (decision making) influence our actions, which in turn impact our clients' health and well-being. Charles Sylvester (1986) invited TR practitioners to wonder, to doubt, and to be thoughtful. He encouraged us to *wonder* about the central tenets of TR, what makes it work, and why. For instance, since all TR models are based on assumptions and values, he urged TR practitioners to think critically about these assumptions. Critical wonder encourages healthy skepticism or *doubt.* The greatest danger to the TR profession, Sylvester said, comes from "dogmatism, the arrogant, inflexible brand of myopic thinking that looks no further because it believes the answers have been found absolutely" (p. 8). Thus, when we raise questions about what, how, and why, we have the greatest chance to be *thoughtful* about our work.

Gerald Fain (1989) put it another way. He warned about the tendency in TR to tout only the abilities of TR to *help* clients. Fain argued that such thinking is myopic. Fain asserted that if TR services are strong enough to help, they must be strong enough to *harm.* This insight can only be gained from an honest examination of TR practice. **Exhibit 14.1** is a case in point for one of us (Shank).

Exhibit 14.1: Was he really helped, after all?

> Early in my career I had several years of experience using adventure-based counseling programs with adolescents and adults in a psychiatric hospital. I became a firm believer in its potential to positively impact clients' self-esteem. I published an article on the program in the *Therapeutic Recreation Journal* and wrote of a client's "breakthrough" experience on a high ropes element. After being stuck midway across the tension traverse and unable to move for close to an hour, Michael was finally cajoled into overcoming his fear and moving to the end of the wire and down to the ground. Of course, I was convinced that this was a "success" experience for 15-year-old Michael. Actually, he never said much to me about this ordeal after it was over. Months after the article was published I received a letter from a reader. He congratulated me on the interesting article and raised a question. "How do you *know* that this experience was a positive one for Michael? How can you be sure that he would not look back on that experience with any negative thoughts and feelings or that he was not emotionally traumatized by it?" I closed the letter quickly, and for a long time never had the courage to acknowledge this confrontation. Yet, now that I have acquired some practice wisdom I can ponder this stranger's questions and admit that even with the best of intentions, I may have risked harm in my attempts to help.

Ethics

Any discussion of competence and reflective practice ultimately leads to the topic of ethics. Ethics is a branch of philosophy that examines moral values and individual and collective obligations to others and society at large. While laws tell us what we can and cannot do, ethics tell us what we *ought* to do. Ethics provides a foundation for the moral reasoning, demanded in our personal and professional lives. Morality is associated with the values and beliefs operating when we interpret and interact with the world. Reflecting on what is morally acceptable behavior as a TR professional is an essential component of *ethical competence* (Shank, 1996). "This process of ethical and moral deliberation involves sharpening personal ethical awareness and conducting a conscious examination of one's values and choices" (p. 33).

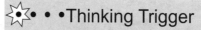

☼• • •Thinking Trigger

What stands out in your mind as a moral or ethical issue associated with TR practice?   • • • ☼

Fain (1989) contended that determining the moral foundation of your professional work is the basis for reflective practice. He suggested using practical, day-to-day experiences with clients to understand the moral imperatives of TR practice. "Those interested in learning more about the moral meaning of their work need look first at what they did yesterday" (p. 201). His examination of the profession led him to conclude that two fundamental social issues inform the moral basis for TR practice: the injustices of discrimination experienced by people with disabilities and the need to ensure that all people have opportunities for normalized recreation to promote health and contribute to the healing process.

Ethical Issues and Moral Dilemmas

Throughout this text certain principles and ideals have been identified that anchor TR practice. These include maintaining a holistic perspective of health (bio/psycho/social/spiritual) and of the client as a system (the whole person in relation to his or her physical and social environment, community, and culture). TR practice also has a deep respect for clients' self-determination and right to be active partners in their own care. While such principles ought to guide TR practice, constantly changing health and human service environments and the complex nature of caring relationships challenge our ability to adhere to these principles and ideals.

Many issues raise moral and ethical questions for health-related professions, including TR. At the broadest level, TR professionals confront *foundational ethical issues* (Collopy, 1996) such as the meaning of autonomy, health, health care, leisure, and quality of life. Understanding these concepts has a direct bearing on TR practice. Consider the following:

- What do *freedom* and *autonomy* mean? Does giving a nursing home resident a choice in recreation activities promote autonomy?

- What does *health* mean to a person who is dying of AIDS?

- What is *quality of life* for people who have Alzheimer's disease?

Some ethical issues are *systemic* (Collopy, 1996) since they pertain to the health care system's regulation and distribution of resources. This is similar to what O'Keefe (1999) labeled *macroethical* issues. Such decisions are not easy, nor can you expect to be insulated from needing to participate in making them. For example,

- What are the social obligations to poor people and their need for quality health care?

- Who is more deserving of health care resources: children with chronic illnesses (e.g., cystic fibrosis) or elderly persons with chronic illnesses (e.g., amyotrophic lateral sclerosis)?

- How do continuous rehospitalizations of persons with drug and alcohol addictions affect attitudes and compassion of health care providers?

- On what basis should a pediatric TR department decide who will be considered priorities: age, degree of illness, or the ability to respond to TR interventions?

The greatest array of systemic ethical issues within the health and human service system comes from managed care. As discussed previously, the economic constraints imposed by managed care have challenged rehabilitation professionals to balance the system's need for cost-effectiveness with clients' needs for compassionate care based on their needs, not economics. While managed care demands evidence of outcomes, there needs to be an equitable way to evaluate moral outcomes in relation to functional outcomes (Salladay, 1996). Only reflective practitioners will have a reasoned response from an ethical as well as economic perspective.

Current health care constraints have also created an unacceptably large proportion of people who cannot access health care. Such inequity ought to challenge one's sense of fairness or justice. This has direct implications for health promotion programs. Consider, for example, the failure of insurance companies and the federal government to provide sufficient financial support for all people to experience health empowerment, a fundamental tenet of health promotion. People who are poor and illiterate are less likely to access health information or be supported in learning to practice preventive health care (Last & Woolf, 1996).

Finally, there are *clinical* (Collopy, 1996) or *microethical issues* (O'Keefe, 1999) that emanate from caregiving relationships. These issues pertain to obligations to be respectful, fair, and helpful to clients. Recreation therapists are also ethically bound to ensure that their own needs to be liked or to feel important and powerful do not result in exploiting clients. In the course of caring, many situations arise with competing ethical obligations and we are forced to choose between two equally unacceptable alternative actions. These conflicts are called *moral dilemmas* and occur when there are good reasons to support opposing courses of action (Sylvester, Voelkl & Ellis, 2001). Chapter 11 mentioned several ethical conflicts faced by recreation therapists. For example, sometimes clients share information with us that they do not want others to know and we feel caught in a dilemma between our duty to share information with other staff and our duty to protect clients' privacy and preserve trust. Consider the dilemma that a recreation therapist faces in **Exhibit 14.2**. Tanya must deal with both systemic and clinical issues that are ethically difficult to resolve.

Code of Ethics

One option Tanya has is to review her professional code of ethics—the core values and ethical principles of the profession that provide guidelines for ethical conduct. The code "provides rules of duty and principles of responsibility to clients, the employer, peer professionals, the profession as a whole, and society at large" (Shank, 1996, p. 32). Both ATRA and NTRS have published codes of ethics. Visit www.atra-tr.org and www.activeparks.com for current versions of each organization's code of ethics.

These codes both articulate obligations to clients based on common principles of *autonomy* (respecting a person's right to self-determination), *beneficence* (acting in ways that benefit clients), *nonmaleficence* (preventing, removing, and doing no harm to clients), and *justice* (treating clients fairly and without discrimination on matters of services and other resources). Both codes specify obligations of TR professionals to be loyal and faithful to clients (*fidelity*), honest and forthright with information (*veracity*), and respectful of a person's right to *privacy* and *confidentiality*.

 • • •Thinking Trigger

Which ethical principles appear to be competing for priority in Tanya's predicament? • • •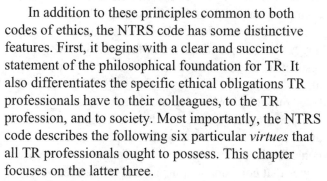

In addition to these principles common to both codes of ethics, the NTRS code has some distinctive features. First, it begins with a clear and succinct statement of the philosophical foundation for TR. It also differentiates the specific ethical obligations TR professionals have to their colleagues, to the TR profession, and to society. Most importantly, the NTRS code describes the following six particular *virtues* that all TR professionals ought to possess. This chapter focuses on the latter three.

1. *Honesty* (being truthful in representing yourself and your profession; being clear about TR practice)

2. *Fairness* (treating people justly and distributing TR services equitably)

3. *Diligence* (being thoughtful and conscientious in the use of time, energy, and resources)

4. *Awareness* (knowing how your personal values, needs, and interests may influence your professional actions)

5. *Integrity* (consistency of character, uncompromising principles, and a steadfast commitment to service)

6. *Competence* (striving to be informed and current in your knowledge and skills, as well as aware of your limitations)

Guidelines for Interpreting Ethics

A code of ethics is not like a rulebook that tells you exactly what to do in all situations. Rather, it contains guiding principles that you interpret and apply to particular circumstances. Both professional organizations have published documents that can help you understand the meaning and application of each ethical principle and rule of conduct. The ATRA publication, *Finding the Path: Ethics in Action* (McFarlane, Keogh-Hoss, Jacobson & James, 1998) contains definitions of each principle, and an explanation of the relationship between the principle and ATRA's standards of practice. Each principle is illustrated through sample dilemmas encountered in practice. The NTRS has also published *Interpretive Guidelines*, which is immensely helpful in understanding why each principle in the NTRS code leads to morally sound and defensible action.

Exhibit 14.2: How far do we go to be helpful?

Tanya knows that she is ethically bound to respect clients' autonomy and their right to refuse to participate in TR programs at the nursing home, but this conflicts with her moral duty to help these clients benefit from her programs. She believes they will benefit more from participating in her sing-along exercise program than sitting in their rooms. She wonders just how firm she ought to be about participation. The Director of Nursing who insists on high program attendance figures to show families and surveyors compounds her dilemma.

Meanwhile, her colleague, Kim, is remarkably successful in getting her clients on the dementia unit to leave their rooms and attend her exercise program. Her strategy is to tell the clients a "little white lie" to get them to attend (e.g., saying that refreshments, a big motivator, will be served). Of course, once they are in the room she gets them exercising to distract them from whatever originally motivated them to come. Kim's rationale: "the fun and physical stimulation the clients experience justifies being a little deceitful. Besides, they'll just forget I mentioned anything about refreshments anyway." Tanya thinks there's something "not right" about Kim's behavior. In both cases, she does not know what she ought to do. She searches for an ethically acceptable response.

Ethical Decision Making

Any attempt to resolve ethical problems depends on your familiarity with a code of ethics, which helps in sorting out competing values and principles. In the earlier example, Tanya was experiencing a conflict between autonomy and beneficence. Her obligation to benefit her clients through activities conflicted with her duty to respect their right to refuse participation. Finding the morally preferred response in such situations requires some orderly thinking. Patricia Shank (1996) provided a thorough explanation of three primary approaches used in ethical decision making. Each approach reflects a particular ethical theory. The *deontological view* holds that there are universal or absolute rules that determine right and wrong behavior, regardless of the consequences. Honoring a client's right to be "free" and self-determining in matters of leisure is considered by many in our profession to be an absolute rule. This ethical principle would be advanced regardless of the consequences to the individual or anyone else. In contrast, the *teleological* or *utilitarian theory* holds that ethical decisions pivot on their consequences. Human action is ethical to the extent that it produces the greatest good or best overall consequences.

The third method, which Shank considers to be the most complex yet the most promising, is the *consequentialist-contextual* method. This approach considers the consequences of each alternative action along with the overall context or circumstances of the situation, including the feelings of the care provider. "The final ethical choice is not based entirely on principles or on rules, but rather on the entirety of the situation" (Shank, 1996, p. 50). While the reasoning process is rational, it is unique in that it includes love, empathy, care, and compassion.

> It is based on interconnectivity that reflects the essence of what it means to be human: that is, as I acknowledge another's uniqueness, there is a paradoxical awareness of sameness. When I make ethical decisions concerning this person, I am simultaneously making ethical decisions about myself; what I do to one, I do to all including myself. (p. 50)

As Shank (1996) stated, "We do ethics every day" (p. 52). She indicated that doing ethics involves an ongoing process of moral reflection, which requires self-awareness, discipline, and practice. Such moral reflection and ethical reasoning depends on three things: an ability to be specific about moral principles or rules, a balanced view of the merits of opposing courses of action, and an appreciation of the situational factors that more fully describe the problem (Sylvester, Voelkl & Ellis, 2001).

Framework for Ethical Reasoning

Table 14.1 contains a six-step process that can be used for ethical reasoning, whether this involves systemic or clinical ethical issues. This framework for ethical reasoning is derived from the models described by Shank (1996), the model contained in *Finding the Path: Ethics in Action*, and a conference presentation by Shank and Lahey (1992). Note that there are many difficult aspects of practice that are not necessarily ethical problems. Likewise, you may experience conflicts between your own self-interests or personal inclination and an ethical principle. In such instances, there is really no conflict; your ethical obligation to act in the interests of your clients *always* outweighs your own personal needs and self-interests. This captures the essence of *virtue ethics*, which focuses on one's character. A virtuous practitioner displays consistently honest, respectful, and compassionate behavior (Sylvester et al., 2001).

Thinking about ethics should not occur only when difficult situations arise and there is a need for immediate action. It is important to find opportunities to consider the ethical dimensions of many contemporary issues that confront health care and human services. This can occur through reading and conversations with other professionals about ethical matters. It also means raising discussions in staff meetings about the moral and ethical bases for decisions about resource allocations and client service priorities. Such behaviors are an important part of being a reflective practitioner and an indication of your commitment to being ethically competent.

Clinical Supervision

The pursuit of professional and ethical competence can be enhanced through clinical supervision. It is described here with a full awareness that it may be seriously lacking for many practitioners, given the large number of recreation therapists who function independently. Yet, it is a support essential to reflective and ethical practice. It is presented with the hope that you will seek it out from others, even in those instances where you are the only recreation therapist in the facility, and that you will give it to others when you time comes.

Clinical supervision primarily concerns a practitioner's professional development and the well-being of clients served by the practitioner (Murray & Shank, 1995). As such, it is essential for developing and maintaining therapeutic competence. It is a process whereby beginning recreation therapists are accountable to a more senior therapist, and in turn they expect to receive direction, education, and support. From here on we refer to this as a relationship between a *supervisor* and a *supervisee*. However, all supervision is not the same. *Managerial* or *administrative supervision* is concerned with making sure practitioners adhere to the regulations of the agency and contribute to organizational efficiency and effectiveness. Managerial supervision is often used for performance evaluation, which is tied to quality improvement within the agency and to a practitioner's adherence to professional standards of practice. While managerial supervision assures that

Table 14.1: Framework for ethical reasoning

Step One: Gather the Facts
What is the issue or the actual events and related behaviors? Who is involved? What is the context of the transaction? What legal or economic aspects pertain to the issue or situation? What is the relationship between the stakeholders (i.e., parties invested in the outcome, such as client, family member, recreation therapist, administrator)?

Step Two: Determine an Ethical Problem Exists
What principles, rights, duties or obligations are in conflict? What are the feelings, needs, and values of each stakeholder in this matter, and how might they be influencing any decision making?

Step Three: Determine Alternatives for Action
Does a real choice exist? What are the possible actions and the ethical principles or rules that pertain to each alternative?

Step Four: Determine the Consequences of Each Alternative Action
What are the consequences for each stakeholder? How are ethical principles enhanced or negated by each course of action?

Step Five: Make a Choice
Choose a course of action with clear ethical justification.

Step Six: Evaluate the Choice
Was the action taken as expected? What were the consequences? What new questions emerged? How does this situation compare to past cases?

tasks are done and services are provided to clients, clinical supervision focuses on a therapist's growth as a reflective practitioner, which ultimately impacts client outcomes.

Defining Clinical Supervision

Bernard and Goodyear (1992) describe clinical supervision as

> an evaluative relationship between senior and junior members of a profession that has the simultaneous purposes of enhancing the professional functioning of the junior member(s), monitoring the quality of professional services offered to the clients she, he, or they see(s), and serving as a gatekeeper for those who enter the particular profession. (p. 4)

Clinical supervision depends on a relationship that is safe, supportive, and nonjudgmental. A supervisee must feel supported enough to reveal limitations without fearing repercussions. Clinical supervision focuses on the TR process as both clients and therapists experience it. It examines the range of thoughts and feelings practitioners have about their work. Clinical supervision is also collaborative—supervisor and supervisee collaborate on ways to increase skills, abilities, and insights pertaining to effective clinical practice. For these reasons, clinical supervision is more likely to support a therapist's abilities and inclination to think critically, reflect, and problem solve.

The need for clinical supervision is not limited to the early years of one's practice. Even with years of practical experience, a TR professional may need clinical supervision until he or she develops *practice wisdom* (Krill, 1990). Practice wisdom is the accumulation of lessons learned and insights gained from years of experience, and the capacity to use these insights in making well-informed, thoughtful decisions about TR practice. Thus, clinical supervision is a critical factor in your development as a competent professional.

Developmental Approaches to Clinical Supervision

Just as all supervision is not the same, the supervisory needs of recreation therapists vary as well. Stoltenberg and Delworth (1987) suggested that supervisees move along three levels of a developmental continuum. Their revised model, the *Integrated Developmental Model* (IDM) of supervision (Stoltenberg, McNeill & Delworth, 1998), has been used widely among many health-related disciplines. The developmental levels reflect how supervisory needs and abilities change over time. Therefore, as the model suggests, supervision ought to be adjusted accordingly. The following sections briefly describe the three developmental levels.

Level 1. Practitioners at this level have some academic training but limited direct experience. This is typical of TR student interns and beginning practitioners entering the field. Practitioners at this level are generally preoccupied with their lack of technical skills and feel uncertain about job tasks and clients' situations, worrying whether their work is correct and acceptable. These preoccupations limit their capacity to consider their clients' perspective or the impact their anxiety and uncertainty has on their clients. Level 1 supervisees depend heavily on supervisors for information, technical direction, and support. Therefore, instructive and emotionally attentive supervision sessions are helpful. At this level, supervisors are like teachers. Supervision should focus on reducing confusion through skill instruction and relieving anxiety through reassurance and positive reinforcement. Over time, confidence grows and the supervisee's desire for autonomy emerges.

Level 2. A resolution of earlier anxiety and an increased comfort and confidence in performing clinical work allows therapists at this level to understand and empathize more with clients. Increased confidence leads to more independent practice and an expectation for taking on more responsibility. However, more independence and responsibility also exposes them to challenges. Increased awareness and understanding reveals the complexity of clinical practice and a realization that there are no "cookbook" approaches that work with all clients all the time. Additionally, recreation therapists at this level may begin to doubt TR practice and realize others may even devalue it. This can shake a practitioner's belief in themselves and their profession. Thus, Level 2 supervisees tend to vacillate between confidence and disillusionment, and this affects their motivation to use clinical supervision. In addition, a conflict between feeling autonomous and feeling dependent on a supervisor for guidance develops. This ambivalence can strain the supervisory relationship.

In keeping with a developmental approach to supervision, supervisors must be flexible and vary their supervisory styles to accommodate the increased independence as well as the ambivalence of Level 2 supervisees. The highly structured and instructive supervision used earlier gives way to offering more choice and collaboration on addressing supervisory issues. A major task for supervision now is to learn how

one's personal characteristics interact with clinical practice. Within a supportive, empathic, and nonjudgmental environment, supervisees explore the impact of their feelings and beliefs on clients. An important approach of the supervisor is to "normalize" the supervisee's struggles as part of normal professional development. This is often accomplished when the supervisor discloses his or her own similar experiences.

Supervision at this developmental stage can be uncomfortable for both supervisor and supervisee. Both may avoid meeting together. The supervisee prefers to remain in a comfort zone and avoid challenges to his or her feelings of autonomy and competence. Very often, confrontation and feedback is met with a defensive attitude. Meanwhile, the supervisor often feels uncomfortable confronting the narrowness or biases in the supervisee's practice, perhaps expecting higher motivation and keener insight. This is especially the case when supervisors are inexperienced themselves, and supervisees have years of experience and resent or reject the assumption that clinical supervision is necessary. However, advancement to higher levels of professional competence is unlikely without being challenged. Ultimately, when a supervisee is open to self-exploration, accepts fluctuations in motivation as normal, and accepts personal responsibility for addressing underdeveloped areas of clinical competence, he or she is ready to transition to Level 3.

Level 3. Therapists at this level have a greater understanding of the complexities of clinical practice and can integrate this with self-awareness and an understanding of the client's context and experience. Therapists at this level possess practice wisdom. Consequently, these therapists rarely have formal supervision. Instead, Level 3 therapists act autonomously and assume responsibility for their professional development. When supervisory feedback is sought, typically through periodic consultation with a colleague, it is received with little if any defensiveness. There is an accurate perception of strengths and weaknesses, and the motivation to move forward with learning and growth is quite stable.

Core Issues and Domains of Practice for Clinical Supervision

Across all developmental levels are three overarching issues that therapists bring to clinical supervision. These may have been evident when reading about each developmental level.

Self-awareness and other-awareness involve cognitive and affective components related to a preoccupation with oneself, awareness of the client's experience, and an enlightened understanding of oneself in relation to others.

Motivation reflects the supervisee's degree of interest, investment, and effort in clinical training and practice. Motivation can be high initially, but can also depend on types of clients and work settings. Motivation is typically stable for practitioners at the most advanced level of development.

Autonomy involves a resolution of the dependence-autonomy conflict. While emerging practitioners are initially dependent on supervisors, effective clinical supervision enables more experienced practitioners to become increasingly autonomous, to the point where the most evolved professionals are well aware of their strengths and weaknesses and can, therefore, assess their need for supervision.

Regardless of developmental level, these are core issues to which clinical supervisors respond. They are reflected in seven specific *domains of practice* that vary across developmental levels (Stoltenberg et al., 1998). Self-awareness, other-awareness, motivation, and autonomy affect each domain of clinical practice. Updating previous work of Murray and Shank (1995), **Table 14.2** (p. 260) describes these domains of clinical practice with an example of how each could be addressed in clinical supervision with a recreation therapist.

Higher levels of clinical competence are not usually achieved on all of the practice domains displayed on Table 14.2. In some cases, particular emphasis is placed on certain issues and not others. For instance, you may have greater self-awareness about your intervention skills and more motivation to increase these competencies. Consequently, you may be more autonomous about learning new techniques without relying on your supervisor. Overall, these domains and the three overarching issues provide a template for making clinical supervision stimulating and worthwhile. These domains are also relevant to self-evaluation and subsequent needs for learning and support.

The chance for a practitioner to advance developmentally depends on the value placed on clinical supervision and, most importantly, the quality of supervision. Because the clinical supervision of TR practice has been found to be alarmingly limited, it will be up to a new generation of TR practitioners to improve this aspect of professional development. The best evidence of this happening is the increased attention to internship supervision and related efforts to help emerging professionals develop their competencies through thoughtful and instructive supervision (Murray, 2000).

Clinical Supervisory Roles

It should be apparent in the previous descriptions that clinical supervisors have three distinct roles: teacher, counselor, and consultant. The most appropriate role for a supervisor to take depends on the issues being addressed and the developmental level of the supervisee. No one will develop at the same pace and in the same ways across all major issues related to professional competence. Consequently, supervisory needs will require that supervisors use a mix of all three roles, which are summarized here.

As a *teacher*, supervisors instruct in methods used in clinical practice through concrete explanations, demonstration, and modeling. They also provide explicit interpretations of the clinical process and help therapists make connections between academic training and real-world applications. This role is prominent with interns and those just entering TR practice. It continues for those who, despite experience, are learning new techniques or ways to work with new client populations.

As a *counselor*, supervisors help supervisees to explore thoughts and feelings that are aroused in the process of working with clients. Supervisees need assistance in recognizing and confronting the impact of wide-ranging feelings—from confidence to demoralization. When needed, supervisors assist in acknowledging any personal issues that hinder effective helping skills, and guiding the supervisee toward resources that can help address such matters. Although this role uses common counseling skills such as empathy and active listening, supervisors *do not* engage supervisees in a therapy relationship.

Finally, the *consultant* role is used with colleagues that have more developed levels of clinical skills yet seek periodic advice and feedback about issues or impending decisions. In these instances the supervisor supports the autonomy of the colleague to ultimately decide on the best use of shared information and other supervisory or consultative feedback.

The Structure and Methods of Clinical Supervision

Supervision should be responsive to practitioners' commitment to pursue competence. This means recognizing the range of pertinent issues and utilizing appropriate supervisory formats and methods. The actual structure and process of clinical supervision depends on several factors, including the value and support the agency gives for its provision. The philosophy, education, and experiences that supervisors and supervisees bring to their relationship also shape clinical supervision. Above all, it is shaped by a shared commitment to competent TR practice in a context of constantly changing service delivery situations.

Structuring Clinical Supervision

An important starting point in any supervisory relationship is a preliminary discussion about expectations of supervision, including supervisor availability and what each hopes to accomplish through supervision. This helps to clarify possibilities and limitations within the relationship and to avoid disappointment or misunderstandings later on. Some tools can be useful for focusing clinical supervision. These include ATRA's *Revised Standards of Practice and Self-Assessment Guide* and *Guidelines for Competency Assessment* self-evaluation tool. In addition to guiding content for supervision, these tools can be used to create performance improvement plans. One's developmental level and corresponding supervisory needs, as described earlier, can be

Table 14.2: Domains of practice addressed in clinical supervision

Domain	Supervision Concerns	Example
Intervention Skills Competence	Therapist's familiarity with and confidence in using a variety of therapeutic modalities.	Supervision focused on learning about group initiative activities and then progressed to learning about processing these activities with various client groups.
Assessment Techniques	Supervisee's confidence in and ability to use assessment methods and techniques with various clients.	Supervision addressed the recreation therapist's adjustment to clients who were nonverbal and required alternative ways to express their preferences and needs.
Interpersonal Assessment	Being aware of and integrating a client's interpersonal dynamics throughout the client–therapist relationship.	After observing several intervention sessions, the supervisor was able to help the recreation therapist make connections between his tendency to take charge and his clients' tendency to be passive and uninvolved.
Client Conceptualization	Therapist's ability to understand her client's total context, not just the functional domains.	Supervision was used to instruct the recreation therapist on ways to obtain pertinent family history and related information about the client's home and community environment.
Individual Differences	Understanding gender, race and cultural differences and their influence on thinking and behavior.	Supervisor assigned specific reading about the meaning of health to people of Asian and Hispanic descent.
Intervention Plans and Goals	Organizing and implementing interventions that aid in goal attainment.	Case presentations were used during group supervision to discuss more creative approaches to helping clients achieve their goals.
Professional Ethics	Exploring how professional ethics and standards of practice intertwine with personal ethics.	Supervision was used to explore the recreation therapist's discomfort with homosexuality in light of the agency's need to make a policy about clients' rights to self-determination, privacy, and sexual expression.

determined by the *Supervisee Levels Questionnaire Revised* (Stoltenberg et al., 1998). Murray's *A Daily Log for the TR Intern* (2000) contains a *Learning Style Inventory*. She also designed a companion *Coaching Style Inventory* for intern supervisors. These two parallel forms (see **Exhibit 14.3**, p. 262) allow student and supervisor to be aware of each others preferred styles of learning and teaching, including sources of motivation, and type and frequency of feedback. It is also important that both partners have a clear understanding of specific performance expectations and the criteria for evaluating performance. Based on this information exchange, a comfortable supervisory structure and process can be negotiated. Three primary formats are used to provide clinical supervision: individual sessions, group sessions and peer supervision.

Individual sessions are the most common format for clinical supervision. These sessions ought to be guided by clearly established expectations between supervisor and supervisee. These expectations include the frequency of sessions, acceptable content, and the methods that will be used. For instance, Level 1 supervisees need the most structure and regularity and are provided with a variety of instructional methods. More advanced practitioners may have arrangements where they are expected to initiate reviews and discussions of their cases without always waiting for the supervisor to determine the content of supervisory sessions. While such arrangements appear to respect the autonomy and clinical competence of these more experienced practitioners, this also runs the risk of avoiding or bypassing clinical reflection. This is especially the case with supervisees who may be reluctant to disclose or discuss their ambivalent feelings about TR practice. Individual supervisory sessions are most helpful when they occur with predictable regularity and in an accepting, open, honest, validating, and supportive environment.

The primary value of *group supervision* is that it exposes individual TR practitioners to the perspectives and insights of others, which can be reassuring, validating, and informative. A supervisor structures discussions about intervention approaches, problems experienced with clients (or with other staff), or any other thoughts and feelings supervisees have about their work. Frequently, group supervision is structured around case presentations. These discussions provide supervisees with ideas, perspectives, or direct feedback that can help with clinical problem solving and can heighten feelings of support. Because it is unlikely that group supervision will involve practitioners who are all at the same level of experience and professional development, it is important that the supervisor in charge keeps the interaction positive and constructive. Less-developed supervisees can learn by listening to and observing more advanced therapists, and more advanced therapists can benefit from instructing their less developed colleagues. When the situation permits, supervisory support groups for student interns appear to help reduce stress and insecurities (Stoltenberg, McNeill & Delworth, 1998).

> ☆• • •Thinking Trigger
>
> What would you tell your internship supervisor about yourself and the ways you would best learn to practice TR?
>
> • • •☆

Peer supervision is another format used occasionally among professionals. This format is best used with individuals who have a commitment to reflective practice and want opportunities to talk with others that can identify with their clinical experiences. Some are motivated to seek peer supervision because they lack adequate supervision in their work setting, and they recognize the importance of professional support. This format appeals to many advanced practitioners because it involves a nonhierarchical relationship of support and consultation. Along with discussing cases and receiving feedback about one's work, peer supervision allows practitioners to discuss larger issues affecting their profession (e.g., reimbursement for services) or career advancement. It also represents a chance to be self-directed and to develop confidence in providing consultation to others. While the idea can be attractive, peer supervision requires a strong commitment to adhering to arrangements made with other professionals and the discipline required to follow through with recommendations made for improving practice.

Methods and Techniques Used in Clinical Supervision

If a clinical supervisor is a mix of educator, counselor and consultant, then various methods and techniques must be used to meet diverse supervisory needs and developmental levels. Any combination of the following methods can be used.

Face-to-face dialogue. This is the primary method for exchanging information, sharing resources, suggesting intervention strategies, and offering encouragement and positive reinforcement. Sessions ought to be flexible enough for either person to bring up topics or any unanticipated issues pertaining to client care. These conversations must occur in a climate of acceptance and support. Supervisory sessions that occur randomly and that have no particular focus run the risk of being unproductive. Either person can feel frustrated and unmotivated to continue. As mentioned earlier, students and those entering practice prefer the most structure and instruction but must also be comfortable enough to admit to making mistakes and feeling unsure about their work.

Exhibit 14.3: Excerpts from the Learning Style and Coaching Style Inventories

The following excerpts are from the *Learning Style* and *Coaching Style Inventories* developed by Murray (2000) for use by TR interns and their supervisors. Students and supervisors are asked to check the responses that best describe their learning and coaching styles and use these parallel inventories to help prepare for clinical supervision. The *Learning Style Inventory* is available in *A Daily Log for the TR Intern* at http://www.nrpa.org. The *Coaching Style Inventory* is available from Boon Murray.

Learning Style Excerpts

PREFERRED SOURCE OF MOTIVATION
Do you prefer to have internship goals and motivation supplied by:
___ Your supervisor's expectations and teaching style?
___ Your university's expectations or requirements or the designated academic liaison's stipulations?
___ Personal expectations, ideas, and interests?
Comments/Suggestions:

RECEIVING SUPERVISION
What type of supervision do you prefer?
___ Direct supervision during a job task or interaction followed by discussion?
___ Distant supervision (supervisor is nearby but not observing) followed by discussion?
___ Discussion before, during, and after a job task or interaction with participants?
Comments/Suggestions:

PREFERRED METHODS OF LEARNING
Rate how much each of the following methods contributes to your ability to learn, where 1=least helpful and 5=most helpful

___ Reading pertinent material from textbooks, articles, or manuals (e.g., a case report)?
___ Seeing live demonstrations?
___ Engaging in classroom lecture or self-paced video instruction?
___ Active participation with hands-on learning?
___ Opportunity for question and answer sessions?
Comments/Suggestions:

Coaching Style Excerpts

PREFERRED SOURCE OF MOTIVATION
Do you prefer to have internship goals set and the intern's motivation supplied by:
___ Your intern's self-described expectations and level of motivation?
___ Your university's expectations or requirements or the designated academic liaison's stipulations?
___ Your professional expectations, work ethic, ideas about practicing TR, and interests?
Comments/Suggestions:

GIVING SUPERVISION
What type of supervision do you consistently offer interns?
___ Direct supervision during a job task or interaction followed by discussion?
___ Distant supervision (supervisor is nearby but not observing) followed by discussion?
___ Discussion before, during, and after a job task or interaction with participants?
Comments/Suggestions:

VARYING COACHING METHODS
Rate how much you utilize each of the following methods to enhance intern's ability to learn job competencies, where 1=least helpful and 5=most helpful

___ Reading pertinent material from textbooks, articles, or manuals (e.g., a case report)?
___ Seeing live demonstrations?
___ Engaging in classroom lecture or self-paced video instruction?
___ Active participation with hands-on learning?
___ Providing opportunity for question and answer sessions?
Comments/Suggestions:

Observation. Supervisees can learn a great deal from observing others who are more experienced. For example, learning group leadership skills through observation and coleadership is effective for inexperienced students and practitioners. It can be helpful for supervisees to observe several therapists. This helps by reinforcing certain procedural skills and presenting a chance to compare and contrast intervention styles and techniques used by various therapists. Observations should focus on something specific, like conducting an assessment interview or opening and closing a group session. Afterward, supervisory sessions can include a reflective discussion about how these procedures went from the perspective of both supervisor and supervisee.

Journaling. Keeping a log of your experiences, thoughts, and feelings is a very useful technique, especially with students and young professionals. Murray's (2000) *A Daily Log for the TR Intern* is an excellent tool for self-mediated learning through reflective writing. Recording impressions helps you look back to interpret your experiences with clients or colleagues. Journaling allows you to express yourself freely and privately and then to select issues or incidents to discuss in supervision. Whether you use your journal to jot down unfamiliar terms that came up in a team meeting, or your feelings about working with a child who has been physically or sexually abused, journaling supports your pursuit of competence. Journaling can also contain other creative–expressive techniques, such as drawing, stories, and metaphors (Lahad, 2000). In addition to helping supervisees understand themselves, therapists also learn about using these same techniques with their clients.

Prescribed Learning Exercises. Supervisors can structure learning by assigning articles to be read and then discussing them during supervision sessions. Assigned readings, instructional videos and other web-based learning materials can expose supervisees to new ideas and perspectives as well as approaches or techniques related to client care. These are helpful ways for supervisees (and supervisors) to keep current with professional literature and technical information pertaining to practice. Supervisees can also be responsible for finding reading materials that they find meaningful and then reporting on it in supervision sessions. A similar learning activity is to have supervisees report on sessions they attended at a professional conference. Discussions can center on how the information or insights gained can be incorporated into their work with clients.

Case Presentations. Perhaps the best way to learn about TR and to expand clinical insights is through case presentations. Each case reflects a therapist's decision making, problem solving and clinical judgment. Assembling the case and presenting it allows staff to appreciate the client and therapist's shared experience and the factors that influenced the care provided. Then, through a reflective discussion with a supervisor or peers, biases can be revealed. This can help inexperienced practitioners to appreciate important issues that shape effective service delivery. This includes the presenter's emotional experience as well as technical skills. For example, a newly graduated recreation therapist made a case presentation about an adolescent female in treatment for an eating disorder. This client was very uncooperative and manipulative. The case discussion helped the supervisor make suggestions about alternative assessment approaches. In addition, the therapist was helped to realize her own discomfort with setting limits with this client and others like her. The therapist was able to appreciate how her tendency to "keep things safe" and her need to keep the client from "going off" actually fed into the client's manipulative style.

Reviewing difficult cases is especially helpful in learning about clinical practice. While there may be a natural tendency to discuss cases that will not raise any questions about the presenter's clinical judgment, recreation therapists can progress to more advanced levels of competence when they have the courage to learn from their mistakes or from the more demanding aspects of their work. Supervisors should encourage supervisees, especially those who are at Level 2, to use more complicated and difficult cases for expanding their theoretical and conceptual understanding of practice. **Table 14.3** (p. 264) contains guidelines for case reviews.

Impediments to Clinical Supervision

The nature of clinical supervision is complicated and there can be impediments. As indicated earlier, advancing to higher developmental levels of clinical competence is not an automatic result of one's accumulating experience. Some therapists are blocked in their development due to lack of motivation, effort, or abilities to work collaboratively with a supervisor. Consequently, supervision stagnates and both supervisor and supervisee find reasons to avoid each other. At best, supervision focuses only on administrative matters.

Another impediment to effective clinical supervision is associated with supervisors themselves. Quite often recreation therapists become supervisors simply because of their seniority. They may not have more practice wisdom than those they are assigned to supervise.

Table 14.3: Guidelines for case reviews

The following is an outline for organizing and presenting a case for clinical review and discussion. The case review increases understanding of TR as a clinical process and objectively considers work with clients so that clinical knowledge and insights increase.

When organizing and presenting a case, remember that you are describing a client–therapist relationship based on a combined set of concerns, hopes, and expectations for specific outcomes. The accomplishments and shortcomings have much to do with this relationship and the context in which it takes place as well as the intervention strategies used.

It is perfectly acceptable to present a case that did not go as well as you had hoped. "Unsuccessful" cases are often most effective from a learning perspective. Willingness to use the presentation as a learning device will ultimately contribute to the clinical learning of all. Remember to protect privacy and confidentiality of the client when discussing this case with people not involved. Obtain permission before discussing the case outside of the agency.

Case Review Guidelines

1. *Identifying Data*. Present pertinent background information, including age, gender, race or ethnicity, education, residence, occupational or social roles, reasons for receiving health or human services, and anticipated length of involvement.

2. *Reason for Referral to TR*. Indicate whether the client was formally referred to TR and for what reasons, or whether you took it upon yourself to initiate contact and why.

3. *Initial Encounter*. Describe the nature of your initial encounter with this client and give the essence of the individual's response to you and TR services. Indicate the level of awareness, trust, receptivity, and mutuality present in this initial stage.

4. *Formal Assessment Process*. Briefly describe the full assessment process indicating what information was gathered, when, and where. State how this information was obtained (e.g., interview, use of client chart/records, specific assessment tool, and others who gave input, including family or other professionals). Describe client's involvement in the assessment process. Describe any feelings you had developed at this point in your relationship. For example, were you comfortable? Did you have any particular hopes or concerns related to working with this client?

5. *Major Concerns*. Describe the primary concerns that you (or the client) concluded from the assessment process, and their relevance to any overall needs for intervention. For example, the assessment process may suggest that the client needs to learn about community recreation resources suitable for wheelchair sports or that the client needs assistance with meeting other residents/clients to decrease social isolation.

6. *The Plan*. Indicate the parameters of the intervention plan, including specific client outcomes, intervention strategies, and the type and frequency of contact.

7. *Progress to Date/Outcomes Achieved*. Describe how the client is progressing toward the intended outcomes and highlight any key developmental, psychosocial, environmental, or functional issues influencing this case. How has your relationship with this client and your use of particular interventions influenced progress toward goals? If this case has been completed, include information on the discharge or termination process. What discharge plans were made?

8. *Discussion*. Keeping in mind steps 1–7, reflect on your involvement with this client. Was there a therapeutic alliance? How did your thoughts and feelings influence your work? What did the client find most meaningful in his or her TR experience? Consider these questions:

- What went well? What did not?
- What did you have most difficulty with?
- What would you have done differently?
- Were any of your expectations or your client's expectations unfulfilled?
- What do you and this client anticipate for the future?
- What did you learn about yourself or about TR practice from this case?
- What questions do you have for those who listen to or read this case review?

Consequently, these supervisors have difficulty nurturing their supervisees, and the inadequacy they feel combined with the frustration supervisees feel leads to resentment and avoidance. Additionally, gender and cultural diversity, as well as differences in lifestyle issues can interfere with establishing an effective supervisory relationship.

Clinical supervision is impeded by the dual relationship that typifies many supervisory arrangements in TR practice. That is, supervisors have responsibility for guiding the reflective process fundamental to clinical supervision as well as evaluating supervisee's performance. Many supervisees are reluctant to honestly share their thoughts and feelings with supervisors who have both responsibilities. For example, suppose you really disliked some clients, or you secretly avoided certain clients because you did not know what to do with them. You might be very reluctant to reveal such feelings for fear that your supervisor might report this on your permanent personnel record, or might not give you a strong recommendation for a promotion or new job. Yet, helpful clinical supervision depends on complete and honest examination of all feelings and how they might influence client interactions.

Supervisors also have a difficult time with dual responsibilities. It is not easy finding a comfortable balance between supporting a supervisee's ambivalent feelings toward clients and work, and being able to objectively evaluate performance. Many supervisors are not comfortable giving evaluative feedback and so they give vague feedback or avoid criticism altogether. Such behavior impedes supervisees' professional development. These difficulties often occur with young TR professionals who are directors of programs despite having recently graduated and having little practical experience themselves.

Perhaps the greatest impediment to clinical supervision is an assumption that competent practice is self-evident and clinical supervision is unnecessary for those with years of experience. Sylvester et al. (2001) remind us that knowledge is both relative and dynamic. Therefore, TR professionals must construct and reconstruct knowledge to promote the well-being of the people they serve. Reflecting on practice through clinical supervision can help with this.

Of course, the chance for clinical supervision may be remote for those who are the lone recreation therapist in their agency. While they are likely to receive some form of managerial supervision, opportunities to reflect on clinical issues specific to TR practice are rare. All of these impediments to effective clinical supervision are real, but they can be circumvented. If you want to make a commitment to pursuing competence through clinical supervision, then you must join together with other TR professionals and advocate for yourselves. For example, you can ask an administrator for support in arranging group supervision, perhaps coordinated by a social worker or psychologist. Peer supervision with TR professionals from your local area is another alternative. Regardless of the mechanism, clinical supervision is essential to developing competence, and the investment in you and your fellow TR professionals pays dividends for clients. It is well worth the extra effort that will be required in arranging and using it.

Summary

Learning to be an effective recreation therapist takes time. It is a journey that extends over your entire career. Given the constant change in health and human services, you will need to continuously reaffirm your personal and professional commitment to pursuing competence and conscientiously examine and refine knowledge and skills. The motivation for excellence must come from within you.

Pursuing competence requires a deliberate process of self-monitoring. Becoming a reflective practitioner captures the essence of this process. Having the courage to examine the moral imperatives of TR practice and the ethical substance of day-to-day work with clients helps ensure professional integrity. Clinical supervision also plays an important role in advancing emotional competence and practice wisdom as well as technical knowledge and skills. These processes involve a core set of skills that contribute to competence and will be needed for career-long learning as well as adjustment to changing conditions within the workplace (Kinney, Witman, Sable & Kinney, 2001). These core skills include maximizing your abilities to deal with uncertainty, communicating effectively with a variety of individuals and groups, managing people and tasks (especially through sound clinical reasoning) and mobilizing innovation and change.

Pursuing competence is difficult to do alone. Reflective practice is a reciprocal process between you and others through discussing ethical matters and engaging in clinical supervision. That is, it has as much to do with what you can offer someone else (even if that person is your supervisor) as it does with what you can get from others. In this sense you are a part of a larger community of professionals who share a commitment to the same principles and ideals, even if practice settings and specific duties differ. All TR professionals share the responsibility of elevating TR practice to the highest, most meaningful level possible for those we serve.

In closing, we offer the following 10 actions that can help you on your journey toward professional competence. The success of your journey will inevitably help the journey of many other TR professionals.

1. Maintain membership in a professional TR organization. Encourage others to do the same and share your resources (e.g., newsletters, professional journal) with them.

2. Periodically review your professional standards of practice and complete a self-assessment at least annually.

3. Know your code of ethics and understand the interpretive guidelines. Ask to have at least one staff meeting devoted to examining an ethical issue relevant to your work setting.

4. Do your part to challenge complacency. Raise questions about TR practice. Engage others in discussions about the moral, theoretical, and practical aspects of practice.

5. Attend local and national professional conferences, but first use the various competency assessments mentioned in this chapter to help you select relevant sessions based on your strengths and need for growth. Share what you learn with others. As you collect your CEUs, ask yourself, *What have I learned and what can I do with this new knowledge?*

6. Join a treatment network sponsored by ATRA or a NTRS Best Practices Committee and use it for sharing, discussion, resources, and support.

7. Read! Share your reading with your supervisor, administrator, and colleagues. Challenge yourself to relate the readings to work with clients.

8. Talk about your work. If you believe in what you do, share this with others either through presentations at local and national professional conferences, or simply through staff in-services.

9. Write about your work. Share your experiences, insights, and opinions by submitting manuscripts to professional journals. Collaborating with others helps to overcome insecurities about writing.

10. Help build the body of knowledge by collaborating on research with others, whether they are in TR or not.

References

Bernard, J. and Goodyear, R. (1992). *Fundamentals of clinical supervision*. Needham Heights, MA: Allyn & Bacon.

Collopy, B. (1996). Bioethics and therapeutic recreation: Expanding the dialogue. In C. Sylvester (Ed.), *Philosophy of therapeutic recreation: Ideas and issues* (Vol. 2, pp. 10–19). Arlington, VA: National Recreation and Park Association.

Dattilo, J. (2000) *Facilitation techniques in therapeutic recreation*. State College, PA: Venture Publishing, Inc.

Fain, G. (1989). Ethics in the therapeutic recreation profession. In D. Compton (Ed.), *Issues in therapeutic recreation: A profession in transition*. Champaign, IL: Sagamore Publishing.

Haas, L. and Malouf, J. (1989). *Keeping up the good work: A practitioner's guide to mental health ethics*. Sarasota, FL: Professional Resources Exchange.

Kinney, T. and Witman, J. (1997). *Guidelines for competency assessment and curriculum planning in therapeutic recreation: A tool for self-evaluation*. Hattiesburg, MS: American Therapeutic Recreation Association.

Kinney, T., Witman, J., Sable, J., and Kinney, J. (2001). Curricular standardization in therapeutic recreation: Professional and university implications. In N. Stumbo (Ed.), *Professional issues in therapeutic recreation: On competence and outcomes* (pp. 87–103). Champaign, IL: Sagamore Publishing.

Krill, D. (1990). *Practice wisdom: A guide for helping professionals*. Newbury Park, CA: Sage Publications.

Lahad, M. (2000). *Creative supervision: The use of expressive arts methods in supervision and self-supervision*. Philadelphia, PA: Kingsley Publishers.

Last, J. and Woolf, S. (1996). Ethical issues in health promotion and disease prevention. In S. Woolf, S. Jonas, and R. Lawrence (Eds.), *Health promotion and disease prevention in clinical practice* (pp. 554–568). Philadelphia, PA: Williams & Wilkins.

McFarlane, N., Keogh-Hoss, M. Jacobson, J., and James, A. (1998). *Finding the path: Ethics in action*. Hattiesburg, MS: American Therapeutic Recreation Association.

Murray B. and Shank, J. (1995). Clinical supervision in therapeutic recreation: Contributing to competent practice. *Annual in Therapeutic Recreation, 5*, 83–93.

Murray, S. B. (2000). *A daily log for the TR intern*. Ashburn, VA: National Therapeutic Recreation Society.

O'Keefe, C. (1994). *Teaching ethics in therapeutic recreation*. Paper presented at the National Recreation and Park Association's NTRS Institute, Minneapolis, MN.

O'Keefe, C. (1999, October). *Ethics in changing times*. Paper presented at the National Recreation and Park Association's NTRS Institute, Salt Lake City, UT.

Riley, B., West, R., and Van Andel, G. (2000). *Revised ATRA standards of practice and self-assessment guide*. Hattiesburg, MS: ATRA.

Salladay, S. (1996, October/November). Rehabilitation, ethics, and managed care. *REHAB Management*, 38–42.

Schon, D. (1983). *The reflective practitioner: How professionals think in action*. New York, NY: Basic Books.

Shank, J. and Lahey, M. (1992, October). *Ethical decisions and the practice of TR*. Paper presented at the NTRS Institute, Cincinnati, OH.

Shank, P. (1996). Doing ethics: Toward the resolution of ethical dilemmas. In C. Sylvester (Ed.), *Philosophy of therapeutic recreation: Ideas and issues* (Vol. 2, pp. 30–56). Arlington, VA: National Recreation and Park Association.

Sneegas, J. (2001). Addressing the need for quality in therapeutic recreation continuing education programs. In N. Stumbo (Ed.), *Professional issues in therapeutic recreation: On competence and outcomes* (pp. 123–137). Champaign, IL: Sagamore Publishing.

Stoltenberg, C., McNeill, B., and Delworth, U. (1998). *IDM Supervision: An integrated developmental model for supervising counselors and therapists*. San Francisco, CA: Jossey-Bass.

Stoltenberg, C. and Delworth, U. (1987). *Supervising counselors and therapists: A developmental approach*. San Francisco, CA: Jossey-Bass.

Sylvester, C. (1986). Wonder, doubt, and thoughtfulness in therapeutic recreation: An invitation to philosophize. *Therapeutic Recreation Journal, 20*(3), 6–10.

Sylvester, C., Voelkl, J., and Ellis, G. (2001). *Therapeutic recreation programming: Theory and practice*. State College, PA: Venture Publishing, Inc.

Author Index

Subject Index

Books by Venture Publishing

Venture Publishing, Inc.
1999 Cato Avenue
State College, PA 16801
Phone: 814-234-4561
Fax: 814-234-1651